Headache

Series Editor

Paolo Martelletti, Roma, Italy

The purpose of this Series, endorsed by the European Headache Federation (EHF), is to describe in detail all aspects of headache disorders that are of importance in primary care and the hospital setting, including pathophysiology, diagnosis, management, comorbidities, and issues in particular patient groups. A key feature of the Series is its multidisciplinary approach, and it will have wide appeal to internists, rheumatologists, neurologists, pain doctors, general practitioners, primary care givers, and pediatricians. Readers will find that the Series assists not only in understanding, recognizing, and treating the primary headache disorders, but also in identifying the potentially dangerous underlying causes of secondary headache disorders and avoiding mismanagement and overuse of medications for acute headache, which are major risk factors for disease aggravation. Each volume is designed to meet the needs of both more experienced professionals and medical students, residents, and trainees.

Igor Petrušić • Yonggang Wang
Editors

Neuroimaging of Headache Disorders

Springer

Editors
Igor Petrušić
Laboratory for Advanced Analysis of Neuroimages
University of Belgrade, Faculty of Physical Chemistry
Belgrade, Serbia

Yonggang Wang
Neurology Centre, Headache Department
Beijing Tiantan Hospital, Capital Medical University
Beijing, China

ISSN 2197-652X ISSN 2197-6538 (electronic)
Headache
ISBN 978-3-031-85401-9 ISBN 978-3-031-85402-6 (eBook)
https://doi.org/10.1007/978-3-031-85402-6

This Springer imprint is published by the registered company Springer Nature Switzerland AG
The registered company address is: Gewerbestrasse 11, 6330 Cham, Switzerland

Foreword

Neuroimaging has played a pivotal role in enhancing our understanding of headache disorders, including migraines, tension-type headaches, and trigeminal autonomic cephalalgias. Key studies have highlighted the contributions of magnetic resonance imaging (MRI), positron emission tomography (PET), and functional imaging techniques in exploring the underlying pathophysiology of these conditions.

MRI and PET have significantly advanced our perception of migraines as a central nervous system disorder. These imaging modalities have helped identify a central migraine generator, clarify the role of cortical spreading depression, and reveal structural abnormalities such as white matter lesions and microstructural brain damage.

In the field of trigeminal autonomic cephalalgias, functional neuroimaging has identified critical brain structures involved in their pathophysiology, particularly the posterior hypothalamus. Resting-state functional MRI has been instrumental in distinguishing brain activation patterns among different subtypes of trigeminal autonomic cephalalgias, providing valuable insights into their mechanisms.

While neuroimaging has greatly improved our knowledge of migraine and cluster headache pathophysiology, its clinical utility remains limited. Nonetheless, in cases where secondary headache is suspected, neuroimaging is essential for confirming the diagnosis. However, for non-acute headaches, its diagnostic value is minimal.

It is undeniable that neuroimaging research has significantly advanced our understanding of migraine by uncovering structural, functional, and biochemical brain changes associated with the disease. These insights continue to refine our comprehension of cortical mechanisms, vascular changes, and potential diagnostic markers. While migraine remains primarily a clinical diagnosis, emerging imaging techniques may enhance our ability to identify and treat this complex neurological disorder.

This is the ultimate objective of this 17th volume of the *Headache Series*—to provide researchers and clinicians with a clear and comprehensive perspective on the contributions of neuroimaging, not only for headache diagnosis but also far beyond.

Unitelma Sapienza University
Rome, Italy

Paolo Martelletti

Preface

This book provides a comprehensive overview of structural and functional neuroimaging findings related to the pathophysiology of primary and secondary headache disorders. It aims to promote best practices in ordering neuroimaging investigations and interpreting findings across various neuroimaging modalities for patients experiencing a wide range of headache types and subtypes.

We hope this book will inspire researchers to leverage cutting-edge neuroimaging technologies and adopt optimized study designs to advance discoveries in headache research. Additionally, this book explores future directions in headache neuroimaging, including the integration of machine learning algorithms for the classification of headache disorders and the prediction of treatment outcomes using diverse neuroimaging approaches.

It has been a privilege to collaborate with internationally recognized experts in headache and neuroimaging, whose contributions have enriched this book with state-of-the-art knowledge from both research and clinical practice. We hope that the comprehensive insights offered in this book will serve as a foundation for future neuroimaging studies, leading to new discoveries and, ultimately, the need for updated editions of this work.

Belgrade, Serbia — Igor Petrušić
Beijing, China — Yonggang Wang

Contents

Chapter 1
Introduction to Neuroimaging Modalities for Headache Experts

Igor Petrušić

1.1 Introduction

All standard images of the head without observable pathology are similar, bearing in mind the corresponding age and sex; every image of the head with pathological findings is unique in its own way, corresponding to its pathological substrate. Understanding imaging modalities is paramount for headache specialists and clinical neuroscientists striving for excellence in diagnosing complex clinical cases of headache and revealing new underlying pathophysiological mechanisms in both primary and secondary types of headache.

The history of imaging modalities reflects an ongoing quest to visualize the human brain and its physiological and pathophysiological processes in ever greater detail, combining physics, engineering, and clinical insights. This journey takes us through a fascinating evolution of technology and scientific understanding. Each modality has its strengths and limitations, forming a comprehensive toolkit for diagnosing and following up on diseases. The first and most accessible imaging modality, that is, X-ray imaging, was discovered by Wilhelm Conrad Roentgen in 1895. Roentgen found that X-rays could penetrate solid objects, producing images of internal structures on photographic plates [1]. X-ray imaging technology evolved over time, leading to advances such as fluoroscopy, which allowed real-time imaging and opened a new field of interventional radiology, and digital subtraction angiography, which is widely used for diagnosing and treating secondary headache disorders [2]. The next imaging modality that emerged in medical practice was ultrasound, which allows visualization of the human body without exposing patients to ionizing radiation and also enables measurement of blood flow utilizing the Doppler effect [3, 4]. Advancements in transcranial Doppler ultrasound have led to

I. Petrušić (✉)
Laboratory for Advanced Analysis of Neuroimages, Faculty of Physical Chemistry, University of Belgrade, Belgrade, Serbia

I. Petrušić, Y. Wang (eds.), *Neuroimaging of Headache Disorders*, Headache,
https://doi.org/10.1007/978-3-031-85402-6_1

important discoveries in the primary headache field [5–9]. In parallel, during the 1960s and 1970s of the twentieth century, single-photon emission computed tomography (SPECT), followed by computed tomography (CT), magnetic resonance imaging (MRI), and positron emission tomography (PET), emerged in the medical field [1, 10]. While CT was, and still is, particularly important in diagnosing secondary types of acute headache disorders (given that the list of differential diagnoses is one of the longest in medicine [11]), MRI has become an indispensable tool for diagnosing primary headache disorders with "red flags" and for designing neuroimaging studies. Although functional MRI (fMRI) has become the predominant neuroimaging method in headache research, a clear message from numerous articles related to headache research is that there is no omnipotent method. All the neuroimaging methods not only provide highly complementary information but also benefit from the synergy of multimodal integration.

A plethora of different imaging modalities are used or are currently being developed for use in medical practice and research. However, this chapter will be limited to those imaging modalities that can be employed in headache diagnosis and research.

1.2 Computed Tomography and Positron Emission Tomography Imaging

The current widely available spiral multidetector technology has revolutionized CT imaging, allowing the production of volumetric images of the entire head within a few seconds, with submillimeter isotropic spatial resolution and high temporal resolution, while considerably reducing radiation dose [12, 13]. However, a drawback of multislice CT is that the data sets consist of thousands of images, particularly when CT angiography or CT perfusion is involved [14, 15].

Native CT (Fig. 1.1) is used for the initial evaluation of many intracranial lesions in the emergency setting, such as examination for acute traumatic brain injury and stroke, since it is especially suited for detecting ischemia, hemorrhage, and skull fractures [16]. Depending on their density compared with that of normal brain tissue, native CT findings are categorized into hyperdense (e.g., acute intracranial hemorrhages, vascular clots, calcifications, lymphomas), isodense (e.g., subacute intracranial hemorrhages), and hypodense (e.g., chronic intracranial hemorrhages, edema, hydrocephalus) [17]. However, it should be kept in mind that native CT is less sensitive for detecting and describing nonhemorrhagic diffuse axonal injury, contusions, early infarction, encephalitis, and brain tumors [18, 19]. Another important piece of information for headache specialists is that there are no absolute contraindications for CT. However, a risk–benefit analysis, as well as adherence to the ALARA (as low as reasonably achievable) principle, is required in pregnant and pediatric patients to prevent or minimize radiation exposure.

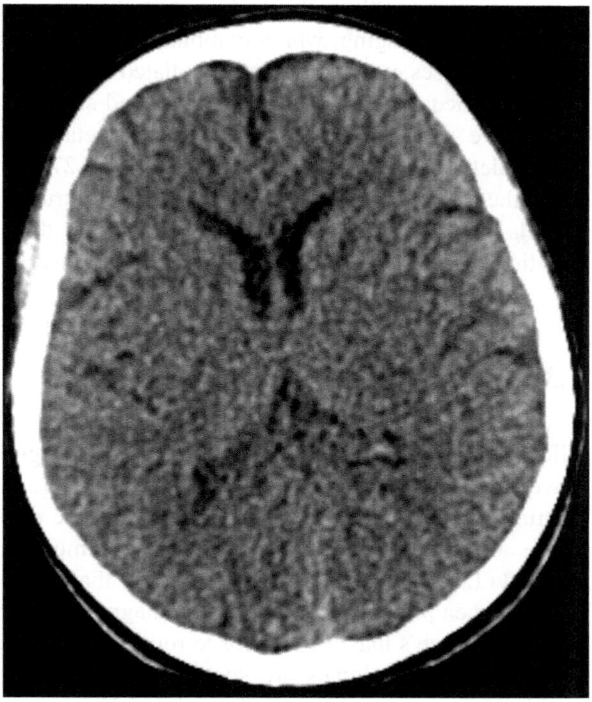

Fig. 1.1 Showcase of normal axial native CT image of the head. (All images presented in the chapter are from the image database of the Laboratory for Advanced Analysis of Neuroimages, Faculty of Physical Chemistry, University of Belgrade)

After the acquisition of the CT data, the images are reconstructed using either a soft tissue algorithm, a bone algorithm, or both [20]. The attenuation value of an individual voxel depends on its contents and can be quantitatively scored in Hounsfield units obtained from a linear transformation of the measured attenuation coefficients (ranging from −1000 Hu [air] to +1000 Hu [cortical bone], with water in the middle [Hu = 0], fat [−100 Hu], cerebrospinal fluid [+5 Hu], soft tissue [+30 to +45 Hu], normal brain tissue [+40 Hu], and hemorrhage [+60 to +90 Hu]) [21]. The bone algorithm provides very sharp images but at the cost of increased image noise, which, in turn, decreases the contrast between soft tissues. In contrast, the soft tissue algorithm focuses on non-osseous structures, displaying them with smoother borders, lower noise, and higher contrast differentiation. Hence, radiologists need to be aware of the drawbacks of these algorithms and should request additional post-processing images if needed. Such post-processing capabilities of the CT images are more demanding for radiologists, but at the same time, they allow individualization of the reconstructions based on the patient's unique anatomy or pathology. Moreover, CT angiography is highly sensitive and specific for identifying underlying vascular lesions, while CT perfusion is sensitive and specific for assessing cerebral blood supply. It records the wash-in and wash-out of the iodine contrast bolus through the cerebral vasculature, enabling the estimation of cerebral blood flow (CBF), cerebral blood volume (CBV), mean transit time (MTT), and time to peak (TTP) parameters [22, 23].

CT imaging hardly finds its place in studying primary headache disorders; however, PET-CT imaging, which combines the sensitivity of nuclear medicine technique that traces radionuclides accumulated in the body and space resolution of CT, allows the acquisition of both functional and anatomical images, providing a comprehensive view of the brain's structure and metabolic processes. This could help in further defining migraine pathophysiology [24–27]. In addition, CT has advantages when the detailed evaluation of small anatomic structures and visualization of small vessels in headache studies are needed. However, this puts demands on thinner collimation, smaller detector sizes, and special reconstruction algorithms [28].

1.3 Magnetic Resonance Imaging

MRI is a noninvasive technique that uses strong magnetic fields and radiofrequency waves to obtain images of body organs and structures by leveraging the complex relationship between the detected signals and the physical–chemical properties of tissue, allowing the generation of images with multiple contrasts [29].

MRI (Table 1.1) is based on the principle that all biological tissues become magnetized when placed in a strong, static magnetic field. Short radiofrequency pulses cause the tissue's magnetic vector to rotate, inducing electric currents in a receiver coil. The electric signals are spatially encoded using magnetic field gradients, enabling image reconstruction through fast Fourier transformation [30]. The signal intensities depend on several tissue parameters, allowing for multiple unique image contrast possibilities [31].

The superiority of MRI over CT lies in its ability to provide excellent contrast between soft tissues, which is reflected in different intensities on grayscale images. The most important parameters that determine image contrast are proton density and characteristic relaxation times: spin–lattice (or longitudinal) relaxation time (T1), which quantifies the rate of energy transfer from the nuclear spin system to neighboring molecules, and spin–spin (or transverse) relaxation time (T2), which quantifies the rate of decay of transversal magnetization toward its equilibrium value [29]. Liquids have a T1 of 1500–2000 ms; tissues predominantly composed of water have intermediate T1 values (400–1200 ms), while fatty tissues exhibit the lowest values (100–150 ms). The spin–spin relaxation time is always shorter than the spin–lattice relaxation time for the observed tissue. Fat has shorter T1 and T2 values compared to water, for which these values are relatively high. T2*, which accounts for inhomogeneities in the magnetic field at both the macroscopic level (due to imperfections in the magnetic field) and the microscopic level (due to variations in tissue susceptibility), is short for both fat and water.

Brain MRI is the most important imaging modality for detecting structural changes in the brain. Numerous MRI neuroimaging techniques exist, including structural (Fig. 1.2), microstructural, functional, spectroscopic, and other advanced MRI methods.

Table 1.1 Structural MRI techniques and the types of images they produce

Type of image	Description	Typical appearance
T1-weighted imaging	Produces high-resolution images with good anatomical detail. These images are produced based on the longitudinal relaxation time (T1) of tissues, which reflects how quickly protons realign with the magnetic field after being disturbed by a radiofrequency pulse	Fat appears as high signal intensity, while CSF and edema appear as low signal intensity. Gadolinium is the most commonly used contrast agent in T1-weighted imaging. It shortens the T1 relaxation time of tissues where it accumulates, leading to a high signal intensity in the resulting images
T2-weighted imaging	Highlights differences in water content, making it useful for detecting edema, inflammation, and other pathological changes. T2-weighted images are based on the T2 relaxation time, which reflects how quickly protons lose phase coherence after being disturbed by a radiofrequency pulse	CSF and edema appear as high signal intensity, while fat appears as low signal intensity
Fluid-attenuated inversion recovery	A T2-weighted sequence with suppressed CSF signal, making it ideal for detecting lesions near the ventricles, such as multiple sclerosis plaques	Pathological lesions appear as high signal intensity, while CSF has low signal intensity
Susceptibility-weighted imaging	Sensitive to magnetic susceptibility differences and useful for detecting blood products, iron deposition, and microhemorrhages	Veins and hemorrhages appear as low signal intensity
Gradient-echo imaging	Sensitive to magnetic field inhomogeneities and used to detect small hemorrhages, calcifications, and other paramagnetic substances. Gradient-echo sequences are often faster than spin-echo sequence	Similar to T2*, with blood products appearing as low signal intensity

CSF cerebrospinal fluid

Moreover, structural MRI is a state-of-the-art technique for studying the brain's morphological features in patients with headache when advanced post-processing neuroimaging methods are applied. The most widely used post-processing methods are voxel-based morphometry and surface-based morphometry [32]. Voxel-based morphometry typically utilizes T1-weighted volumetric MRI scans that undergo several preprocessing steps, including spatial normalization, registration to a standard template (such as the MNI152 template), segmentation, and smoothing. The output of these morphological techniques is then subjected to statistical tests across all brain voxels to identify significant differences between groups of subjects [33]. Although findings from voxel-based morphometry studies are difficult to validate, several studies have shown relatively good correspondence between voxel-based morphometry and manual measurements of specific structural features [34, 35]. In contrast, surface-based morphometry refers to a group of techniques that reconstruct and analyze the cortical surface of the brain, taking into account its highly

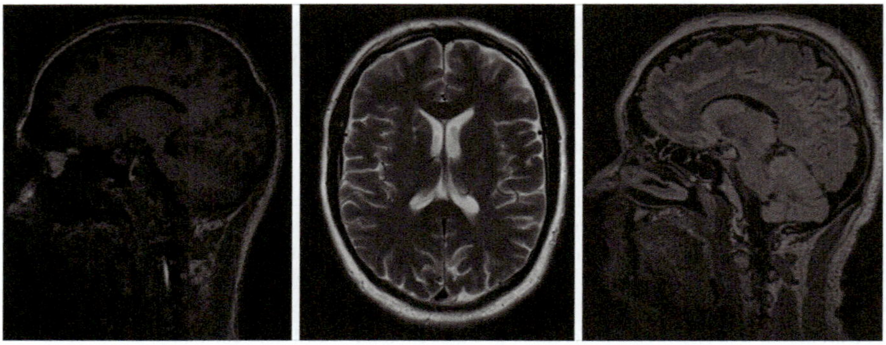

Fig. 1.2 Showcases of normal 3D T1-weighted, axial T2-weighted and 3D FLAIR images of the head

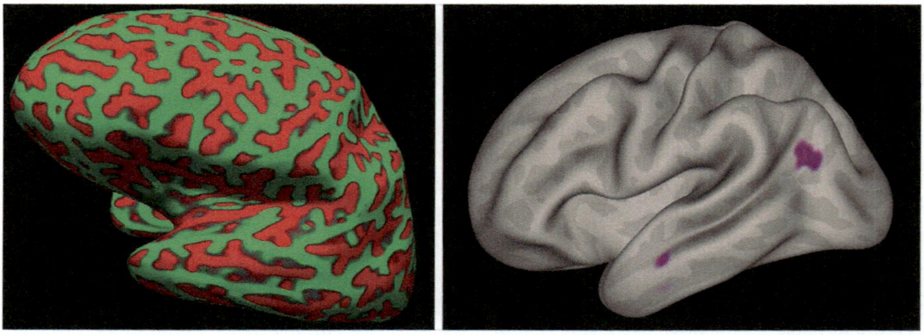

Fig. 1.3 Showcase of inflated representation of the brain as a step of post-processing structural MRI

folded geometry [32]. These techniques allow for the detection of spatially restricted lesions hidden within the brain's gyrification patterns. In surface-based morphometry, the surface of the cortex and the gray/white matter junction are tessellated by polygons, with vertices characterized by coordinates in the x, y, and z planes. These coordinates enable further image processing, such as unfolding and flattening of the surface (Fig. 1.3). After all post-processing steps are performed [36, 37], valuable parameters such as cortical thickness, volume, surface area, and the rate of curvature or gyrification index can be quantified and extracted [38]. Additionally, various post-processing techniques can be used to evaluate the volumes of subcortical structures, such as thalamic nuclei, basal ganglia, amygdala, and brainstem substructures [39–42]. Altogether, advanced structural MRI represents a powerful tool for studying headache disorders, particularly for investigating specific subtypes, such as migraine with aura [43].

Diffusion-weighted imaging measures the self-diffusion of water molecules in tissue. The characteristics of water molecule diffusion can be quantitatively assessed using the apparent diffusion coefficient (ADC) by eliminating the T2-weighting effect. Diffusion-weighted imaging is particularly sensitive to acute ischemic stroke, lymphoma, and high-grade brain tumors, where areas of restricted diffusion appear as regions of high signal intensity. Diffusion tensor imaging (DTI) is a variant of diffusion-weighted imaging that uses the anisotropy of water diffusion to map the distribution of white matter tracts (Fig. 1.4), enabling the assessment of structural connectivity in the brain and quantifying white matter microstructural alterations in subjects [44]. In brief, the DTI technique describes the diffusion process using three eigenvectors and their corresponding eigenvalues (λ1, λ2, λ3) to quantify diffusion in three orthogonal directions [45]. Due to barriers to water diffusion imposed by myelin, cell membranes, and the cytoskeleton, diffusion is greater longitudinally than perpendicularly to axonal fibers, causing diffusion in white matter to be anisotropic. Anisotropy is commonly expressed relative to the magnitude of the diffusion tensor as fractional anisotropy [46]. This index (ranging from 0 to 1) is found to be higher in intact white matter consisting of highly parallel fibers. Further dimensions, such as tensor orientation or mean, axial, and radial diffusivity, are less commonly applied, although they may provide important information in neuroimaging studies. Voxel-wise comparison of DTI post-processed maps between investigated groups is the most commonly used design in DTI studies. However, the tract-based spatial statistics method is also a popular technique due to its reduction of the multiple comparison problem and improved statistical power [47]. In addition, more advanced DTI techniques have been developed, such as neurite orientation dispersion and density imaging (NODDI), which provide additional estimates of tissue microstructure in both gray and white matter by assessing neurite density and fiber orientation dispersion [48]. Moreover, high angular resolution diffusion imaging (HARDI) probabilistic tractography is capable of discriminating multiple fiber populations crossing within the same voxel [49]. Diffusion kurtosis imaging (DKI), based on the non-Gaussian diffusion of water, is considered to reflect diffusion in biological tissues more effectively than DTI [50]. These modalities seem to provide

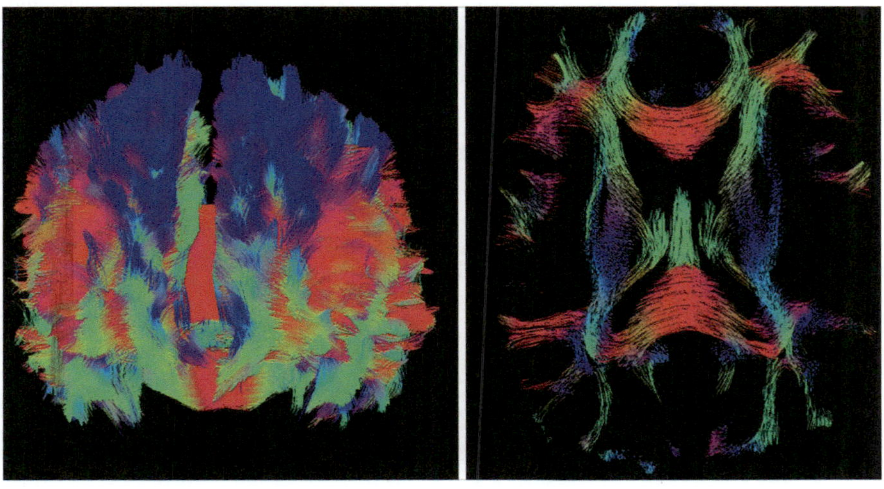

Fig. 1.4 Showcase of tractography representation after post-processed diffusion tensor images

more information for complex structural brain areas; however, they have the disadvantage of longer scan times and require high-quality MRI equipment.

Since fMRI was introduced to the medical community in the early 1990s, it has been considered a revolutionary tool for exploring both healthy and diseased brains [51]. fMRI measures changes in blood-oxygen-level-dependent (BOLD) signals, allowing brain activity to be indirectly assessed with good spatial resolution; some MRI scanners are now capable of imaging voxels as small as 2 mm [52]. fMRI is also used to identify regions of the brain that are active during specific tasks or stimuli [53]. This enables researchers to obtain activation maps superimposed on anatomical images, highlighting areas of increased neural activity and offering insights into how different brain regions are connected and work together. Furthermore, by using fMRI to study brain activity during specific cognitive or motor tasks, researchers can gain insights into how the brain processes information related to perception, memory, language, attention, and decision-making, as well as map motor areas (Fig. 1.5) [54]. Another application of fMRI in neuroimaging studies is the resting-state fMRI technique, which measures brain activity while a person is at rest and not performing any specific task [55]. Advances in resting-state fMRI connectivity analysis have facilitated the characterization of functional connectivity between different brain regions or networks, such as the default mode network, which is active when an individual is awake and at rest. Several post-processing techniques can be used to investigate resting-state fMRI connectivity [54]. Seed-based functional connectivity involves selecting a region of interest (seed) and calculating correlations between the seed region's time series and all other brain voxels. This method enables researchers to examine the functional connectivity between the seed region and the rest of the brain, uncovering networks and connectivity patterns linked to specific brain functions or disorders [54]. Furthermore, independent component analysis (ICA) is a data-driven approach that decomposes fMRI data into spatially independent components, each representing distinct functional networks. This method is useful for identifying resting-state networks and analyzing their alterations in various diseases. Another approach is analysis by graph theory, which provides a framework for describing and quantifying the

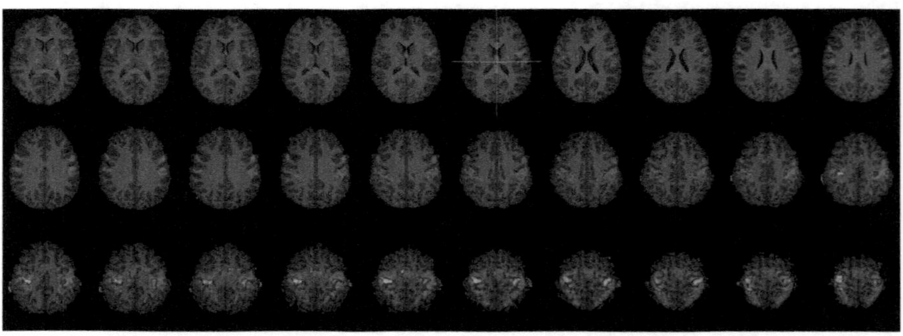

Fig. 1.5 Example of mapping motor areas in hemiplegic migraine patient (blue color) masked with a motor map from healthy controls (green color) using finger-tapping motor task fMRI

topological properties of brain networks derived from fMRI data. Metrics such as node degree, clustering coefficient, and node centrality can be employed to evaluate network organization and detect network-level changes associated with brain disorders [54].

Overall, fMRI is a powerful tool that provides insights into the functioning of the human brain and has a wide range of applications in both primary and secondary headache research. Moreover, by using fMRI to identify brain regions associated with specific headache disorders, researchers can develop new therapies that target these areas. In addition, several other MRI modalities can be utilized in neuroimaging studies of headache disorders (Table 1.2). While MRI is a highly versatile imaging modality, it requires specific knowledge of physical principles to fully exploit its capabilities.

1.4 Ultrasound

Ultrasound imaging is based on the transmission and reflection of high-frequency sound waves. A transducer emits sound waves that penetrate the body and, when reflected by different tissues, create an image based on the varying levels of echo [56]. Since ultrasound does not use ionizing radiation, it is considered safe. In the field of headache research, the most commonly used modality of ultrasound imaging is transcranial Doppler (TCD). TCD is a specialized form of ultrasound that measures the velocity of blood flow through the brain's major arteries. It is particularly useful for assessing cerebral hemodynamics, including cerebral autoregulation and cerebral vasoreactivity, as well as for detecting conditions that affect blood flow to the brain [57]. TCD uses the Doppler effect to measure blood flow velocity. The Doppler effect refers to the change in frequency of sound waves as they reflect off moving objects, such as red blood cells in blood vessels [58]. The transducer is placed on the scalp, allowing sound waves to penetrate the skull and reach the cerebral arteries. The difference in frequency between the emitted and reflected waves, referred to as the "Doppler shift frequency," is directly proportional to the blood flow velocity. Spectral analysis of this signal can produce specific parameters, such as peak systolic velocity, end-diastolic velocity, pulsatility index, and time-averaged mean maximum velocity [59]. These specific parameters can be used to examine cerebrovascular profiles in primary headache disorders [7].

TCD is also used to detect and monitor cerebral vasospasm, which is especially important in conditions such as subarachnoid hemorrhage, a potentially life-threatening situation in which blood vessels constrict, thus reducing blood flow to the brain [60]. Additionally, TCD with a bubble study (contrast-enhanced TCD) can help detect a patent foramen ovale by identifying microembolic signals during the injection of contrast material [61]. Furthermore, TCD can be used to detect spontaneous microembolic signals—high-intensity and short-duration signals representing circulating gaseous or solid particles [62]—which can be utilized in headache research [8].

Table 1.2 Less common MRI modalities used in neuroimaging studies of headache disorders

MRI modality	Key features of modality	Type of image
Perfusion-weighted imaging (PWI)	It assesses blood flow within tissues, used to evaluate stroke, tumors, and other conditions affecting perfusion. There are several techniques, and they are as follows: (1) Dynamic susceptibility contrast (DSC) PWI involves the rapid injection of a gadolinium-based contrast agent and the continuous acquisition of images as the contrast passes through the brain's vasculature. (2) Dynamic contrast-enhanced (DCE) PWI also uses gadolinium contrast but focuses on the rate at which the contrast agent leaks out of the blood vessels and into the extracellular space (useful for evaluating blood–brain barrier integrity). (3) Arterial spin labeling (ASL) is a non-contrast technique that uses magnetically labeled blood water by an inversion pulse proximal to the imaging region as a tracer to measure blood flow	Maps show cerebral blood volume (the total volume of blood within a given amount of brain tissue, measured in mL/100 g), cerebral blood flow (the volume of blood passing through a given amount of brain tissue per unit time, usually measured in mL/100 g/min), mean transit time (the average time it takes for blood to pass through a given volume of brain tissue), and time to peak (the time it takes for the contrast agent to reach its maximum concentration within the tissue after injection)
Magnetic resonance spectroscopy	It provides a biochemical tissue profile by measuring the concentration of various metabolites that differ in their resonance frequency profiles by a few parts per million	Spectra showing peaks or ratios corresponding to different metabolites (e.g., N-acetyl aspartate, choline, glutamate, gamma-aminobutyric acid, creatine, etc.)

(continued)

Table 1.2 (continued)

MRI modality	Key features of modality	Type of image
Chemical exchange saturation transfer (CEST)	It enhances contrast based on the exchange of protons between water and other molecules, used for imaging pH, peptides, glucose, and other metabolites	Contrast-enhanced images indicating specific molecular and biochemical environments of tissues
Magnetic resonance angiography (MRA) and magnetic resonance venography (MRV)	There are several techniques, and they are as follows: (1) Time-of-flight relies on the flow of blood to create contrast between the vessels and surrounding tissue (most commonly used for imaging blood vessels in the head and neck). (2) Phase contrast derives contrast between stationary tissues and flowing blood by manipulating the phase of magnetization, which allows measuring the velocity of blood flow, making it useful for both visualizing vessels and quantifying blood flow. (3) Contrast-enhanced involves the injection of gadolinium contrast to improve the visibility of blood vessels	MRA and MRV can be performed with or without the use of a contrast agent. It is mostly used to detect aneurysms, arteriovenous malformations, and suspected cerebral venous sinus thrombosis or evaluate stroke patients. It can be employed for both 2D and 3D imaging of vessels

Although TCD has numerous benefits in terms of safety, cost-effectiveness, and functional assessment of blood flow that make it indispensable in clinical practice, one should be aware of its limitations, such as low resolution and dependence on the skill and experience of the operator.

1.5 Electroencephalography (EEG) and Magnetoencephalography (MEG)

EEG measures the electrical activity of the brain produced by the synchronous firing of neurons, recording voltage fluctuations resulting from ionic current flows within the neurons [63]. However, one should keep in mind that EEG signals can be contaminated by artifacts from muscle activity, eye movements, and external electrical interference [64].

The EEG signal is typically analyzed in terms of waveforms, which are categorized into frequency bands: delta (0.5–4 Hz), theta (4–8 Hz), alpha (8–13 Hz), beta (13–30 Hz), and gamma (30–100 Hz). The EEG waveforms are described based on their amplitude, location, frequency, symmetry, and reactivity [65]. Recent advances in signal analysis have elevated EEG to a robust brain mapping and imaging method capable of providing detailed spatiotemporal information about brain function and dysfunction. With growing interest in the temporal dynamics of brain networks, and due to its seamless compatibility with other neuroimaging techniques, such as fMRI, EEG is becoming increasingly popular within the neuroimaging community [66]. Moreover, modern EEG systems can be portable, allowing for use in various settings, including at home or work [67].

In addition, visual, somatosensory, and auditory evoked potentials, along with event-related potentials, allow for assessing the brain's electrical response to specific sensory stimuli or cognitive events. These tools are invaluable for evaluating the functional integrity of sensory pathways and studying cognitive processes, making them particularly important in headache research, where they could serve as potential biomarkers [68] or alerts for an early phase of a migraine attack [69].

MEG detects the magnetic fields generated by electrical activity in the brain. These fields are extremely weak (in the femtotesla range) and are detected using highly sensitive devices called superconducting quantum interference devices (SQUIDs) [70]. MEG has a high temporal resolution in milliseconds and provides a more direct measure of brain activity than hemodynamic-based neuroimaging methods, such as fMRI and PET. MEG is widely used in research to study the neural basis of cognitive functions such as perception, memory, and decision-making [71].

1.6 Conclusion

The evolving landscape of neuroimaging has equipped headache specialists with an array of advanced tools to investigate both the structural and functional aspects of the brain. While CT excels in acute settings and provides critical insights into assessing secondary headache, MRI remains central to both clinical diagnosis and research, especially for primary headache disorders. The integration of multiple modalities—ranging from diffusion tensor imaging to fMRI—highlights the importance of complementary approaches to capture the complexity of headache pathophysiology. In parallel, techniques such as ultrasound, EEG, and MEG provide noninvasive and dynamic views of cerebral hemodynamics and electrical activity. This multimodal strategy enables a more comprehensive understanding of headache disorders, paving the way for tailored diagnostic strategies and novel therapeutic interventions. However, given the rapid advancements in neuroimaging technologies, continuous education and interdisciplinary collaboration are essential for headache experts to effectively leverage these tools in both research and clinical practice.

References

1. Scatliff JH, Morris PJ. From Roentgen to magnetic resonance imaging: the history of medical imaging. N C Med J. 2014;75:111–3.

2. Lopez PD. Fluoroscopy history, evolution, and technological advancements: a narrative review. J Med Imaging Radiat Sci. 2024;55:347–53.
3. Reneman RS, Hoeks A, Spencer MP. Doppler ultrasound in the evaluation of the peripheral arterial circulation. Angiology. 1979;30:526–38.
4. Newman PG, Rozycki GS. The history of ultrasound. Surg Clin N Am. 1998;78:179–95.
5. Totaro R, De Matteis G, Marini C, et al. Cerebral blood flow in migraine with aura: a transcranial Doppler sonography study. Headache. 1992;32:446–51.
6. Thomsen LL, Iversen HK, Olesen J. Increased cerebrovascular pCO2 reactivity in migraine with aura – a transcranial Doppler study during hyperventilation. Cephalalgia. 1995;15:211–5.
7. Podgorac A, Petrusic I, Radojicic A, et al. Breath holding index in episodic primary headaches. Vojnosanit Pregl. 2018;75:347–35.
8. Petrusic I, Podgorac A, Zidverc-Trajkovic J, et al. Do interictal microembolic signals play a role in higher cortical dysfunction during migraine aura? Cephalalgia. 2016;36:561–7.
9. Ornello R, Frattale I, Caponnetto V, et al. Cerebral vascular reactivity and the migraine-stroke relationship: a narrative review. J Neurol Sci. 2020;414:116887.
10. Booij R, Budde RPJ, Dijkshoorn ML, et al. Technological developments of X-ray computed tomography over half a century: user's influence on protocol optimization. Eur J Radiol. 2020;131:109261.
11. Evans RW. Diagnostic testing for the evaluation of headaches. Neurol Clin. 1996;14:1–26.
12. Berris T, Gupta R, Rehani MM. Radiation dose from cone-beam CT in neuroradiology applications. AJR Am J Roentgenol. 2013;200:755–61.
13. Booij R, Dijkshoorn ML, Straten van M. Efficacy of a dynamic collimator for overranging dose reduction in a second- and third-generation dual source CT scanner. Eur Radiol. 2017;27:3618–24.
14. Prokop M. Multislice CT angiography. Eur J Radiol. 2000;36:86–96.
15. Enterline DS. CT angiography of the neck and brain. In: Saini S, Rubin GD, Kalra MK, editors. MDCT: a practical approach. Milano: Springer; 2006. p. 151–66.
16. Lolli V, Pezzullo M, Delpierre I, et al. MDCT imaging of traumatic brain injury. Br J Radiol. 2016;89:20150849.
17. Hou Q, Tong E, Gao C, et al. Computed tomography. In: Filippi M, editor. Oxford textbook of neuroimaging. Oxford: Oxford University Press; 2015. p. 3–12.
18. Rath TJ, Hughes M, Arabi M, et al. Imaging of cerebritis, encephalitis, and brain abscess. Neuroimaging Clin N Am. 2012;22:585–607.
19. Bruggeman GF, Haitsma IK, Dirven CMF, et al. Traumatic axonal injury (TAI): definitions, pathophysiology and imaging-a narrative review. Acta Neurochir. 2021;163:31–44.
20. Dzierżak R, Omiotek Z, Tkacz E, et al. Comparison of the classification results accuracy for CT soft tissue and bone reconstructions in detecting the porosity of a spongy tissue. J Clin Med. 2022;11:4526.
21. Kamalian S, Lev MH, Gupta R. Computed tomography imaging and angiography – principles. In: Masdeu JC, González RG, editors. Handbook of clinical neurology. 3rd ed. Amsterdam: Elsevier; 2016. p. 3–20.
22. Huisa BN, Neil WP, Schrader R, et al. Clinical use of CT perfusion for diagnosis and prediction of lesion growth in acute ischemic. Stroke. 2012;23:P114–22.
23. Sabarudin A, Subramaniam C, Sun Z. Cerebral CT angiography and CT perfusion in acute stroke detection: a systematic review of diagnostic value. Quant Imaging Med Surg. 2014;4:282–90.
24. Jassar H, Nascimento TD, Kaciroti N, et al. Impact of chronic migraine attacks and their severity on the endogenous μ-opioid neurotransmission in the limbic system. NeuroImage Clin. 2019;23:101905.
25. Deen M, Hougaard A, Hansen HD, et al. Migraine is associated with high brain 5-HT levels as indexed by 5-HT 4 receptor binding. Cephalalgia. 2019;39:526–32.

26. Torres-Ferrus M, Pareto D, Gallardo VJ, et al. Cortical metabolic and structural differences in patients with chronic migraine. An exploratory 18FDG-PET and MRI study. J Headache Pain. 2021;22:75.
27. Marino S, Jassar H, Kim DJ, et al. Classifying migraine using PET compressive big data analytics of brain's μ-opioid and D2/D3 dopamine neurotransmission. Front Pharmacol. 2023;14:1173596.
28. Lell M, Kachelrieß M. Computed tomography 2.0. Investig Radiol. 2023;58:587–601.
29. Alzola-Aldamizetxebarria S, Fernández-Méndez L, Padro D, et al. A comprehensive introduction to magnetic resonance imaging relaxometry and contrast agents. ACS Omega. 2022;7:36905–17.
30. Hansen MS, Kellman P. Image reconstruction: an overview for clinicians. J Magn Reson Imaging. 2015;41:573–85.
31. Smith HJ, Gjesdal KI. Magnetic resonance – historical and theoretical basis. Tidsskr Nor Laegeforen. 2000;120:931–5.
32. Martin P, Bender B, Focke NK. Post-processing of structural MRI for individualized diagnostics. Quant Imaging Med Surg. 2015;5:188–203.
33. Ashburner J, Friston KJ. Voxel-based morphometry-the methods. NeuroImage. 2000;11:805–21.
34. Good CD, Scahill RI, Fox NC, et al. Automatic differentiation of anatomical patterns in the human brain: validation with studies of degenerative dementias. NeuroImage. 2002;17:29–46.
35. Giuliani NR, Calhoun VD, Pearlson GD, et al. Voxel-based morphometry versus region of interest: a comparison of two methods for analyzing gray matter differences in schizophrenia. Schizophr Res. 2005;74:135–47.
36. Dale AM, Fischl B, Sereno MI. Cortical surface-based analysis. I. Segmentation and surface reconstruction. NeuroImage. 1999;9:179–94.
37. Fischl B, Sereno MI, Dale AM. Cortical surface-based analysis. II: Inflation, flattening, and a surface-based coordinate system. NeuroImage. 1999;9:195–207.
38. Fischl B, Dale AM. Measuring the thickness of the human cerebral cortex from magnetic resonance images. Proc Natl Acad Sci USA. 2000;97:11050–5.
39. Amann M, Andělová M, Pfister A, et al. Subcortical brain segmentation of two dimensional T1-weighted data sets with FMRIB's Integrated Registration and Segmentation Tool (FIRST). Neuroimage Clin. 2014;7:43–52.
40. Iglesias JE, Insausti R, Lerma-Usabiaga G, et al. A probabilistic atlas of the human thalamic nuclei combining ex vivo MRI and histology. NeuroImage. 2018;183:314–26.
41. Iglesias JE, Van Leemput K, Bhatt P, et al. Bayesian segmentation of brainstem structures in MRI. NeuroImage. 2015;113:184–95.
42. Saygin ZM, Kliemann D, Iglesias JE, et al. High-resolution magnetic resonance imaging reveals nuclei of the human amygdala: manual segmentation to automatic atlas. NeuroImage. 2017;155:370–82.
43. Mitrović K, Petrušić I, Radojičić A, et al. Migraine with aura detection and subtype classification using machine learning algorithms and morphometric magnetic resonance imaging data. Front Neurol. 2023;14:1106612.
44. Le Bihan D, Mangin JF, Poupon C, et al. Diffusion tensor imaging: concepts and applications. J Magn Reson Imaging. 2001;13:534–46.
45. Basser PJ, Mattiello J, Le Bihan D. MR diffusion tensor spectroscopy and imaging. Biophys J. 1994;66:259–67.
46. Pierpaoli C, Basser PJ. Toward a quantitative assessment of diffusion anisotropy. Magn Reson Med. 1996;36:893–906.
47. Focke NK, Yogarajah M, Bonelli SB, et al. Voxel-based diffusion tensor imaging in patients with mesial temporal lobe epilepsy and hippocampal sclerosis. NeuroImage. 2008;40:728–37.
48. Zhang H, Schneider T, Wheeler-Kingshott CA, et al. NODDI: practical in vivo neurite orientation dispersion and density imaging of the human brain. NeuroImage. 2012;61:1000–16.

49. Berman JI, Lanza MR, Blaskey L, et al. High angular resolution diffusion imaging probabilistic tractography of the auditory radiation. AJNR Am J Neuroradiol. 2013;34:1573–8.
50. Huang S, Huang C, Li M, et al. White matter abnormalities and cognitive deficit after mild traumatic brain injury: comparing DTI, DKI, and NODDI. Front Neurol. 2022;13:803066.
51. Bandettini PA. Twenty years of functional MRI: the science and the stories. NeuroImage. 2012;62:575–88.
52. Bollmann S, Barth M. New acquisition techniques and their prospects for the achievable resolution of fMRI. Prog Neurobiol. 2021;207:101936.
53. Ebrahimzadeh E, Saharkhiz S, Rajabion L, et al. Simultaneous electroencephalography-functional magnetic resonance imaging for assessment of human brain function. Front Syst Neurosci. 2022;16:934266.
54. Yen C, Lin C-L, Chiang M-C. Exploring the frontiers of neuroimaging: a review of recent advances in understanding brain functioning and disorders. Life (Basel). 2023;13:1472.
55. Lv H, Wang Z, Tong E, et al. Resting-state functional MRI: everything that nonexperts have always wanted to know. AJNR Am J Neuroradiol. 2018;39:1390–9.
56. Carlsen EN. Ultrasound physics for the physician. A brief review. J Clin Ultrasound. 1975;3:69–75.
57. Purkayastha S, Sorond F. Transcranial Doppler ultrasound: technique and application. Semin Neurol. 2012;32:411–20.
58. DeWitt LD, Wechsler LR. Transcranial Doppler. Stroke. 1988;19:915–21.
59. Nicoletto HA, Burkman MH. Transcranial Doppler series part III: interpretation. Am J Electroneurodiagnostic Technol. 2009;49:244–59.
60. Sharma S, Lubrica RJ, Song M, et al. The role of transcranial Doppler in cerebral vasospasm: a literature review. Acta Neurochir Suppl. 2020;127:201–5.
61. Alexandrov AV, Sloan MA, Tegeler CH, et al. Practice standards for transcranial Doppler (TCD) ultrasound. Part II. Clinical indications and expected outcomes. J Neuroimaging. 2012;22:215–24.
62. Dittrich R, Ritter MA, Droste DW. Microembolus detection by transcranial doppler sonography. Eur J Ultrasound. 2002;16:21–30.
63. Biasiucci A, Franceschiello B, Murray MM. Electroencephalography. Curr Biol. 2019;29:R80–5.
64. Jiang X, Bian G-B, Tian Z. Removal of artifacts from EEG signals: a review. Sensors (Basel). 2019;19:987.
65. Parvizi J, Kastner S. Human intracranial EEG: promises and limitations. Nat Neurosci. 2018;21:474–83.
66. Michel CM, Murray MM. Towards the utilization of EEG as a brain imaging tool. NeuroImage. 2012;61:371–85.
67. Vos MD, Debener S. Mobile EEG: towards brain activity monitoring during natural action and cognition. Int J Psychophysiol. 2014;91:1–2.
68. Petrusic I, Jovanovic V, Kovic V, et al. P3 latency as a biomarker for the complexity of migraine with aura: event-related potential study. Cephalalgia. 2022;42:1022–30.
69. Cao Z, Lai K-L, Lin C-T, et al. Exploring resting-state EEG complexity before migraine attacks. Cephalalgia. 2018;38:1296–306.
70. Gross J. Magnetoencephalography in cognitive neuroscience: a primer. Neuron. 2019;104:189–204.
71. Kim JA, Davis KD. Magnetoencephalography: physics, techniques, and applications in the basic and clinical neurosciences. J Neurophysiol. 2021;125:938–56.

Chapter 2
Neuroimaging of Headache Disorders in the Emergency Department

Thien Phu Do, Anders Hougaard, and Christoph J. Schankin

Abbreviations

CNS	central nervous system
CT	computed tomography
ICHD	International Classification of Headache Disorders
MRI	magnetic resonance imaging

2.1 Introduction

Headaches are one of the most common complaints leading to emergency department visits, presenting a significant challenge for healthcare providers [1, 2]. While the majority of headaches encountered in the emergency department are benign and

T. P. Do (✉)
Department of Neurology, Danish Headache Center, Copenhagen University Hospital – Rigshospitalet, Copenhagen, Denmark

Department of Neurology, Copenhagen University Hospital – Herlev and Gentofte, Herlev, Denmark

Danish Knowledge Center on Headache Disorders, Glostrup, Denmark

Department of Clinical Medicine, Faculty of Health and Medical Sciences, University of Copenhagen, Copenhagen, Denmark

A. Hougaard
Department of Neurology, Danish Headache Center, Copenhagen University Hospital – Rigshospitalet, Copenhagen, Denmark

Department of Neurology, Copenhagen University Hospital – Herlev and Gentofte, Herlev, Denmark

Department of Clinical Medicine, Faculty of Health and Medical Sciences, University of Copenhagen, Copenhagen, Denmark

C. J. Schankin
Department of Neurology, Inselspital, Bern University Hospital, University of Bern, Bern, Switzerland

I. Petrušić, Y. Wang (eds.), *Neuroimaging of Headache Disorders*, Headache,
https://doi.org/10.1007/978-3-031-85402-6_2

self-limiting, a small but crucial subset may be indicative of serious underlying conditions, such as intracranial hemorrhage, ischemic stroke, or central nervous system (CNS) infections [3]. Given the relevance of early diagnosis of these conditions for the treatment and often outcome of both the underlying disorder and the headache, the appropriate and timely use of neuroimaging is critical in the emergency department setting.

Neuroimaging serves as a great tool for diagnosing and differentiating between primary headache disorders—such as migraine, tension-type headache, and cluster headache—and secondary headaches caused by structural or vascular abnormalities. The choice of imaging modality, whether computed tomography (CT), magnetic resonance imaging (MRI), or other advanced techniques, depends on a variety of factors including the clinical presentation, patient history, and the need for rapid decision-making in acute scenarios. Logistical considerations, such as accessibility and cost, also play a significant role in determining the appropriate imaging approach.

This chapter explores the current approaches and best practices in the neuroimaging of headaches within the emergency department, emphasizing the importance of balancing the need for accurate diagnosis with considerations of cost, radiation exposure, and the potential for incidental findings. By understanding the role of neuroimaging in the context of headache evaluation, emergency physicians can better navigate the complex decision-making process to improve patient outcomes and ensure appropriate use of resources.

2.2 Epidemiology

Headaches account for approximately 2–4% of all emergency department visits [1, 2], translating to millions of consultations annually and making them one of the most frequent neurological complaints in emergency settings. The burden of headache presentations is substantial, as it spans a wide spectrum of disorders, from benign primary headaches to potentially life-threatening conditions requiring immediate intervention. The high volume of headache-related consultation visits places a considerable demand on healthcare resources, including the use of imaging technologies and specialist consultations.

While headaches can affect individuals of all ages, the highest prevalence of emergency department visits for headaches is observed in those aged 20–50 years [2]. Pediatric and older populations also present with headaches, though the underlying causes and concerns often differ significantly between these age groups—and although fewer older adults seek emergency care for headaches, the incidence and prevalence of secondary headache disorders increase with age, heightening the need for further investigations in this population. The incidence of headaches leading to emergency department visits is higher among women, with a female-to-male ratio of about 3:1 [2]. This gender disparity is particularly evident in migraine cases, which are more common in women. The majority of headache presentations in the emergency department—up to 90%—are primary headache disorders, which include conditions such as migraine, tension-type headaches, and cluster headache [2, 4]. Among these, migraine is the most commonly diagnosed, particularly in younger adults and women. Although less common, secondary headache disorders represent a crucial subset of cases due to their association with serious underlying conditions. These include intracranial hemorrhage, ischemic stroke, meningitis, subarachnoid hemorrhage, and brain tumors. Secondary headaches account for a minority of headache-related emergency department visits [2, 3, 5], but they carry a higher risk of morbidity and mortality; often, successful treatment of headache also depends on the identification and successful treatment of the underlying cause.

A significant proportion of patients presenting with headaches in the emergency department undergo neuroimaging to rule out serious underlying conditions. Approximately 10–30% of patients with headache complaints receive a CT scan [2], while MRI is used less frequently and is typically reserved for cases requiring more detailed imaging. Among those who undergo neuroimaging, the vast majority of scans yield normal results [6], reflecting the predominance of benign headache disorders. Further, in the case of CT, the likelihood of correctly identifying the underlying cause of a headache can be low in some secondary headaches, such as arterial dissections, subacute subarachnoid hemorrhage, spontaneous intracranial hypotension, reversible cerebral vasoconstriction syndrome, and others. Only a small fraction—around 0.5%—exhibit clinically significant findings related to their headache [6]. While the radiation exposure from non-contrast CT scans of the head is relatively low, excessive use of these scans can lead to increased unnecessary exposure. This is particularly concerning for children and young adults, as accumulated radiation may elevate the risk of developing malignancies later in life [7, 8]. These findings highlight the challenge of appropriately selecting patients for neuroimaging to avoid unnecessary testing while ensuring serious conditions are not missed.

2.2.1 Special Populations

2.2.1.1 Children and Adolescents

Headaches account for approximately 1–2% of all pediatric emergency department visits [9–11]. This prevalence is lower than in adults but still represents a significant number of cases annually. In children and adolescents presenting with headaches in the emergency department, neuroimaging is less frequently employed compared to adults, reflecting the lower incidence of secondary headaches in this population. Studies suggest that neuroimaging is performed in about 10–20% of pediatric cases [10, 11], usually when red flags are present or when secondary causes are strongly suspected. Most neuroimaging studies in this group return normal results, consistent with the predominance of primary headache disorders.

2.2.1.2 Pregnancy

Headache is a common acute neurological complaint during pregnancy, accounting for about half of neurological complaints in one US-based cohort [12]. This prevalence reflects the impact of both primary and secondary headache disorders in this population. Headache frequency tends to be higher in the first trimester. Migraine, which is common in the general population, may worsen during this period. The frequency of headaches, particularly migraine attacks, often decreases in the second trimester. Headaches that occur in the third trimester are more concerning for secondary causes, such as preeclampsia, which requires urgent evaluation. Neuroimaging is used selectively in pregnant women due to concerns about fetal exposure to radiation. When imaging is necessary, MRI without contrast is preferred over CT to minimize radiation risks. However, imaging is typically reserved for cases where there is a strong suspicion of a serious underlying condition, such as preeclampsia, cerebral venous thrombosis, or intracranial hemorrhage.

2.2.1.3 Older Adults

Headache accounts for approximately 2–3% of all emergency department visits among older adults [5]. This reflects a lower prevalence compared to younger age groups but underscores the importance of addressing headache complaints in this demographic. The prevalence of primary headache disorders, such as tension-type headache and migraine, tends to decrease with age. However, secondary headaches due to conditions like stroke, tumors, or other intracranial pathologies become more common. Due to the higher likelihood of secondary headaches and the potential for serious underlying conditions, neuroimaging is frequently utilized in older adults presenting with headaches. For the same reason, older age is considered an independent risk factor for secondary headaches with >50 years old considered as the threshold [13, 14].

2.3 Rational Screening and Stratification

Given the wide range of potential causes, from benign primary headaches to serious secondary conditions, employing a rational approach that incorporates both red and green flags is crucial for effective diagnosis and treatment. Red flags are indicators that suggest the presence of secondary headache disorders or potentially serious conditions. If any red flag symptoms are present, further evaluation and neuroimaging are often warranted. Green flags suggest a lower likelihood of secondary pathology and often indicate primary headache disorders. The presence of green flags is reassuring in the absence of red flags.

2.3.1 Red Flags in Headache

A special interest group from the International Headache Society developed the SNNOOP10 list of red flags for headaches (Table 2.1) [3]. While the list does not cover all potential red flags, it highlights the 15 most commonly used indicators and their associated secondary causes. Unfortunately, many of these red flags are based on case series of patients with known secondary headaches (e.g., prevalence of headache among a cohort of patients with an existing cancer diagnosis). As a result, these studies provide data on sensitivity, but specificity and predictive values remain unknown. The sensitivity of the SNNOOP10 list was validated in a single-center cohort study from Spain, where it demonstrated 100% sensitivity for detecting high-risk headaches [16]. However, further prospective studies are needed to validate these findings and assess the list's broader applicability.

2.3.2 Green Flags in Headache

Since red flags are not pathognomonic for their associated conditions, their absence does not rule out a secondary cause. Furthermore, no reliable biomarkers for primary headache disorders have been identified in humans. To address this, "green flags" were introduced in 2021 as indicators suggestive of primary headache disorders (Table 2.2) [17]. Screening for both green and red flags is therefore crucial for a more comprehensive assessment. The presence of a green flag with high specificity increases the likelihood of a primary headache disorder. However, more data are needed to support this concept, as the list was based on expert opinion and has not yet been validated in any clinical cohort.

2.3.3 Diagnostic Approach

Red and green flags serve distinct purposes in headache evaluation. The goal of red flags is to achieve high sensitivity for detecting secondary headaches: the higher the sensitivity, the fewer cases of secondary headache missed. In contrast, the aim of green flags is to achieve high specificity, ensuring that primary headache disorders are accurately identified without overlooking a potential secondary cause.

In the absence of red flags and the presence of green flags, the likelihood of a primary headache disorder is higher than that of a secondary etiology. In such cases, patients can be treated symptomatically during the acute phase and referred for further diagnostic evaluation later. If both red and green flags are absent and the International Classification of Headache Disorders (ICHD) criteria for a primary headache disorder are not met, clinicians should consider a headache specialist (Fig. 2.1). This systematic approach can also guide primary care providers in

Table 2.1 The SNNOOP10 list of red flags for secondary headache disorders

	Sign or symptom	Related secondary etiology	Key points
1	Systemic symptoms including fever	Headache attributed to infection or nonvascular intracranial disorders, carcinoid, or pheochromocytoma	Headache with fever is primarily alarming when accompanied by relevant symptoms (e.g., neck stiffness, decreased consciousness, and neurologic deficit)
2	Neoplasm in history	Neoplasms of the brain; metastasis	A newly developed headache in a patient with neoplasm is highly suspect for an intracranial metastasis
3	Neurological deficit or dysfunction (including decreased consciousness)	Headaches attributed to vascular, and nonvascular intracranial disorders; brain abscess and other infections	Headache occurs in one-fourth of episodes of acute stroke. The severity of headache is not related to the size of the lesion
4	Onset of headache is sudden or abrupt (thunderclap headache)	Subarachnoid hemorrhage and other headaches attributed to cranial or cervical vascular disorders	Thunderclap headache can be the only initial symptom of subarachnoid hemorrhage
5	Older age (after 50 years)	Giant cell arteritis and other headache attributed to cranial or cervical vascular disorders; neoplasms and other nonvascular intracranial disorders	Older individuals with headache have a higher frequency of secondary etiology. The incidence of primary headache disorders is also lower in this age group
6	Pattern change or recent onset of headache	Neoplasms, headaches attributed to vascular, nonvascular intracranial disorders	A recent change of pattern or a newly developed headache can be the only signs of a secondary etiology. Diagnosis is often delayed in these cases
7	Positional headache	Intracranial hypertension or hypotension	Positional headache is the trademark of intracranial hypotension, and the most common cause is a cerebrospinal fluid leak at the spinal level
8	Precipitated by sneezing, coughing, or exercise	Posterior fossa lesions, Chiari malformation	Cough headache is highly predictive of Chiari malformations and posterior fossa lesions
9	Papilledema	Neoplasms and other nonvascular intracranial disorders; intracranial hypertension	A high prevalence of patients with papilledema has a serious underlying pathology

(continued)

Table 2.1 (continued)

	Sign or symptom	Related secondary etiology	Key points
10	Progressive headache and atypical presentations	Neoplasms and other nonvascular intracranial disorders	Progressive headache and atypical headache presentation can be the only signs of serious underlying pathology
11	Pregnancy or puerperium	Headaches attributed to cranial or cervical vascular disorders; post-dural puncture headache; hypertension-related disorders (e.g., preeclampsia); cerebral venous thrombosis; hypothyroidism; anemia; diabetes	Headache during pregnancy and puerperium has a higher risk of severe pathology. More than one-third of individuals presenting to acute care with headache during pregnancy will have a secondary etiology. Most common causes are hypertensive disorders followed by pituitary adenoma or stroke. Other risk factors are no prior headache history, occurring during third trimester, seizures, hypertension, and fever
12	Painful eye with autonomic features	Pathology in posterior fossa, pituitary region, or cavernous sinus. Tolosa–Hunt syndrome. Ophthalmic causes	Patients with presentations of painful eye with autonomic features should undergo neuroimaging as it can be due to a structural lesion. Even typical presentations of cluster headache (or other trigeminal autonomic cephalalgias) can derive from a structural lesion
13	Posttraumatic onset of headache	Acute and chronic posttraumatic headache; subdural hematoma and other headache attributed to vascular disorders	Headache related to trauma should always be explored
14	Pathology of the immune system such as AIDS (acquired immunodeficiency syndrome) or medical immunosuppression	Opportunistic infections	Risk of severe pathology is dependent on the degree of immunosuppression
15	Painkiller overuse or new drug at onset of headache	Medication overuse headache; drug incompatibility	Medication overuse is the most common cause of secondary headache. Onset of headache due to a new drug can be a sign of incompatibility with the given drug

The SNNOOP10 list is a diagnostic tool comprising 15 red flags used to identify potentially serious underlying causes of headaches that require further investigation or immediate intervention [3, 15]

Table 2.2 List of green flags for secondary headaches

	Sign or symptom	Key points
1	The current headache has already been present during childhood	Viral infections are the most common cause of secondary headache in children. In children with chronic headache, the pain is rarely secondary. A life-threatening headache is very unlikely in adults in whom that headache type has already been present during childhood
2	The patient has headache-free days	Most primary headache disorders are paroxysmal. Although recurring secondary headache also occur, they are often caused by trigger factors, such as injury to the head, cerebral ischemia, intracranial hemorrhage, arteritis, arterial dissection, or exposure to a substance, e.g., phosphodiesterase inhibitors or nitric oxide donors. An important exception is intracranial tumors that can also present with recurring headache
3	The headache occurs in temporal relationship with the menstrual cycle	The relationship between pain and menstrual cycle has been validated with a headache diary. Migraine attacks associated with fluctuations in the menstrual cycle are common
4	Close family members have the same headache phenotype	There is a genetic disposition to migraine, cluster headache, and medication overuse headache. The prevalence of genetic vasculopathies is lower than the beforementioned headache disorders
5	Headache occurred or stopped more than 1 week ago	Life-threatening secondary headache generally presents within a few days. Consequently, the more time passed since the headache, the smaller the probability of a life-threatening cause. However, the time passed since onset is unlikely to influence the likelihood of other non-life-threatening secondary causes, e.g., temporomandibular disorder, and persistent posttraumatic headache

Green flags are indicators suggestive of primary headache disorders [15, 17]

determining whether to refer patients for specialized care. Moreover, when patients fulfil the ICHD criteria for a primary headache disorder including the previous occurrence of similar headaches (criterion A of the ICHD), the risk of a secondary etiology is very low also in the emergency department. Still, the presence of red flags should prompt appropriate investigations.

Interestingly, a Spanish working group recently proposed a protocol for optimizing headache management specifically in the emergency department that incorporates several of these red flags [18]. However, further validation in a clinical cohort is needed before this protocol can be widely adopted.

2.4 Conclusions

The appropriate use of neuroimaging is vital for identifying secondary causes of headaches, enabling timely interventions for serious underlying conditions. A systematic assessment of red and green flags, along with a thorough clinical evaluation, is crucial. This dual approach enhances diagnostic accuracy, reduces unnecessary imaging, and optimizes patient outcomes. However, further validation of these flags

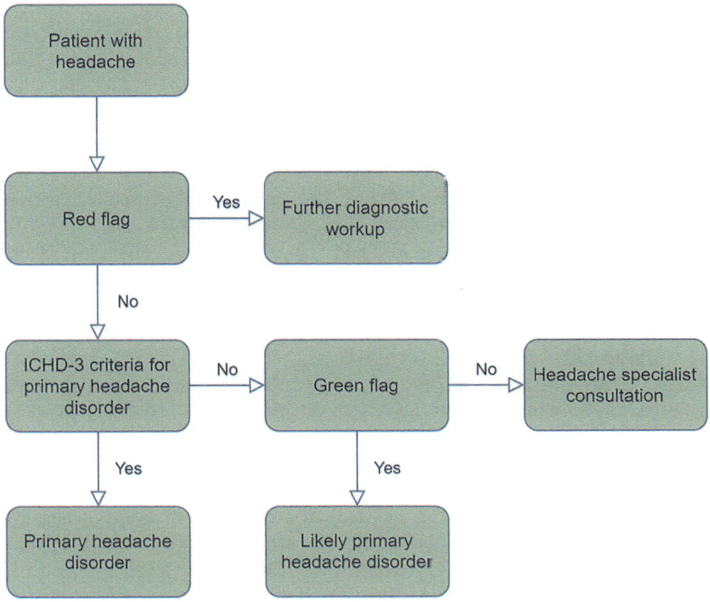

Fig. 2.1 An algorithmic approach to headache disorders. An algorithmic approach to evaluating individuals presenting with headaches involves using the SNNOOP10 list of red flags alongside green flags. If neither red nor green flags are present and the criteria for a primary headache disorder according to the International Classification of Headache Disorders (ICHD) are not met, consultation with a specialist should be considered [15]

in clinical practice is necessary through prospective studies to confirm their specificity and predictive values. Recent initiatives show progress in refining assessment strategies for headache diagnosis, and the continued development of protocols for the rational use of neuroimaging will ultimately improve patient care and enhance resource allocation in emergency medicine.

Key Points

- Headaches are a substantial concern in the emergency department, accounting for 2–4% of all consultations.
- The peak incidence of emergency department visits for headaches occurs in individuals aged 20–50 years, with most neuroimaging in this group yielding nonsignificant findings, as primary headache disorders are the predominant cause.
- Implementing a systematic approach that assesses both red and green flags through a comprehensive clinical evaluation can identify cases where neuroimaging is strictly needed, reduce unnecessary tests, ensure timely treatment, and ultimately improve patient outcomes.

References

1. Burch R, Rizzoli P, Loder E. The prevalence and impact of migraine and severe headache in the United States: updated age, sex, and socioeconomic-specific estimates from government health surveys. Headache J Head Face Pain. 2021;61:60–8. https://doi.org/10.1111/head.14024.
2. Goldstein J, Camargo C, Pelletier A, Edlow J. Headache in United States emergency departments. Cephalalgia. 2006;26:684–90. https://doi.org/10.1111/j.1468-2982.2006.01093.x.
3. Do TP, Remmers A, Schytz HW, et al. Red and orange flags for secondary headaches in clinical practice. Neurology. 2019;92:134–44. https://doi.org/10.1212/WNL.0000000000006697.
4. Minen MT, Boubour A, Wahnich A, et al. A retrospective nested cohort study of emergency department revisits for migraine in New York City. Headache. 2018;58:399–406. https://doi.org/10.1111/head.13216.
5. Munoz-Ceron J, Marin-Careaga V, Peña L, et al. Headache at the emergency room: etiologies, diagnostic usefulness of the ICHD 3 criteria, red and green flags. PLoS One. 2019;14:e0208728. https://doi.org/10.1371/journal.pone.0208728.
6. Jordan JE, Ramirez GF, Bradley WG, et al. Economic and outcomes assessment of magnetic resonance imaging in the evaluation of headache. J Natl Med Assoc. 2000;92:573–8.
7. Pearce MS, Salotti JA, Little MP, et al. Radiation exposure from CT scans in childhood and subsequent risk of leukaemia and brain tumours: a retrospective cohort study. Lancet. 2012;380:499–505. https://doi.org/10.1016/S0140-6736(12)60815-0.
8. Meulepas JM, Ronckers CM, Smets AMJB, et al. Radiation exposure from pediatric CT scans and subsequent cancer risk in The Netherlands. JNCI J Natl Cancer Inst. 2019;111:256–63. https://doi.org/10.1093/jnci/djy104.
9. Burton LJ, Quinn B, Pratt-Cheney JL, Pourani M. Headache etiology in a pediatric emergency department. Pediatr Emerg Care. 1997;13:1–4. https://doi.org/10.1097/00006565-199702000-00001.
10. Rossi R, Versace A, Lauria B, et al. Headache in the pediatric emergency department: a 5-year retrospective study. Cephalalgia. 2018;38:1765–72. https://doi.org/10.1177/0333102417748907.
11. Perry MC, Yaeger SK, Toto RL, et al. A modern epidemic: increasing pediatric emergency department visits and admissions for headache. Pediatr Neurol. 2018;89:19–25. https://doi.org/10.1016/j.pediatrneurol.2018.07.015.
12. Bilello LA, Greige T, Singleton JM, et al. Retrospective review of pregnant patients presenting for evaluation of acute neurologic complaints. Ann Emerg Med. 2021;77:210–20. https://doi.org/10.1016/j.annemergmed.2020.02.014.
13. Cortelli P, Cevoli S, Nonino F, et al. Evidence-based diagnosis of nontraumatic headache in the emergency department: a consensus statement on four clinical scenarios. Headache. 2004;44:587–95. https://doi.org/10.1111/j.1526-4610.2004.446007.x.
14. Locker TE, Thompson C, Rylance J, Mason SM. The utility of clinical features in patients presenting with nontraumatic headache: an investigation of adult patients attending an emergency department. Headache. 2006;46:954–61. https://doi.org/10.1111/j.1526-4610.2006.00448.x.
15. Do TP, la Cour Karottki NF, Ashina M. Updates in the diagnostic approach of headache. Curr Pain Headache Rep. 2021;25:80. https://doi.org/10.1007/s11916-021-00995-8.
16. García-Azorín D, Abelaira-Freire J, González-García N, et al. Sensitivity of the SNNOOP10 list in the high-risk secondary headache detection. Cephalalgia. 2022;42:1521–31. https://doi.org/10.1177/03331024221120249.
17. Pohl H, Do TP, García-Azorín D, et al. Green flags and headache: a concept study using the Delphi method. Headache J Head Face Pain. 2021;61:300–9. https://doi.org/10.1111/head.14054.
18. Membrilla JA, Alpuente A, Gómez-Dabo L, et al. "Code headache": development of a protocol for optimizing headache management in the emergency room. Eur J Neurol. 2024;31:e16484. https://doi.org/10.1111/ene.16484.

Chapter 3
Incidental Neuroimaging Abnormalities in Patients with Headache Disorders

Edina Szabo, Rune H. Christensen, and Robert Semnic

3.1 Introduction

Incidental findings, also known as incidental abnormalities or incidentalomas, are unexpected, previously unknown findings discovered in healthy people or in patients undergoing imaging for an unrelated reason. They are common both in clinical and research settings and occur both in the general population and in people with headache disorders. They can vary from normal anatomical differences to findings that need immediate medical attention. Incidental findings can also be associated with the headache disorders or sometimes even be the underlying cause (i.e., a secondary

The Authors Edina Szabo and Rune H. Christensen contributed equally to this chapter.

E. Szabo (✉)
Department of Anesthesia, Critical Care and Pain Medicine, Beth Israel Deaconess Medical Center, Boston, MA, USA

Department of Anaesthesiology, Harvard Medical School, Boston, MA, USA
e-mail: eszabo@bidmc.harvard.edu

R. H. Christensen
Department of Neurology, Danish Headache Center, Copenhagen University Hospital – Rigshospitalet, Copenhagen, Denmark

Department of Clinical Medicine, Faculty of Health and Medical Sciences, University of Copenhagen, Copenhagen, Denmark

Translational Research Center, Copenhagen University Hospital – Rigshospitalet, Copenhagen, Denmark

R. Semnic
Center for Imaging and Functional Medicine, Uppsala University Hospital, Uppsala, Sweden

Department of Diagnostic and Interventional Radiology, Dubrava University Hospital, Zagreb, Croatia

I. Petrušić, Y. Wang (eds.), *Neuroimaging of Headache Disorders*, Headache,
https://doi.org/10.1007/978-3-031-85402-6_3

headache, see Chap. 4). In individuals with headache disorders, the relative frequency of incidental findings ranges from 13% to 39% [1]. However, these estimates vary depending on the specific abnormality, sociodemographic composition of cohorts, headache disorder, imaging modality and sequence, and clinical setting of the study.

In the present chapter, we outline current knowledge on the prevalence of incidental abnormalities in individuals with headache disorders in comparison to the general population. We also discuss incidental findings commonly reported in headache populations and their possible pathophysiological relevance. Finally, we set out general rules for the management of incidental abnormalities of varying clinical significance in individuals with headache disorders.

3.1.1 Detecting Incidental Findings

Incidental abnormalities in headache disorders are usually identified upon imaging of the brain and head. They are most commonly discovered by magnetic resonance imaging (MRI) or computed tomography (CT). Incidental findings are overall more frequent with MRI, since this modality is more sensitive to the most common incidental findings, such as white matter abnormalities. For MRI, the rate of unexpected findings will also depend on the specific sequence used, since some sequences are more sensitive to certain abnormalities (this being the reason they were developed). For instance, white matter abnormalities are more common on T2-weighted sequences, especially with fluid-attenuated inversion recovery (FLAIR), whereas susceptibility-weighted imaging (SWI) is more sensitive for cavernous malformations and microbleeds (for more on neuroimaging modalities and sequences, see Chap. 1).

3.1.2 Clinical Implications of Incidental Findings

Incidental abnormalities can broadly be categorized as clinically significant or clinically nonsignificant. Clinically significant abnormalities are commonly defined as findings that require further investigation and/or intervention. The latter require appropriate neurological work-up and often referral to subspecialized neurological or neurosurgical departments. Examples of clinically significant incidental findings might include pituitary tumors, multiple sclerosis suspect white matter hyperintensities, and cerebral tumors [2]. Clinically nonsignificant findings can include non-suspect white matter hyperintensities, cerebral microbleeds, and isolated enlarged perivascular space [2]. It should be emphasized that the majority of incidental findings never become symptomatic. This is the case even for many findings that may require further investigations or follow-up visits to monitor.

In some instances, an incidental finding may be the cause of the patient's headache. When there is reasonable evidence to assume this, the patient's headache diagnosis should be reclassified to the appropriate secondary headache disorder, in accordance with the International Classification of Headache Disorders (ICHD) [3]. For some incidental findings, there is sufficient evidence that the finding is causally related to a certain presentation of headache. However, for other incidental abnormalities, the association between the finding and development of headache is less clear. In some scenarios, the incidental finding might also have a scientifically theorized, often partly unelucidated, relationship to the pathophysiology of the disorder; these do not require any clinical intervention or further investigation but can be of research-wise interest. Finally, it is important to note that when imaging is conducted to detect or rule out a suspected lesion that may establish the diagnosis, the finding is by definition not incidental. The utility of imaging in diagnosing secondary headache disorders is discussed in Chap. 4.

3.2 Common Types of Incidental Findings in Headache Disorders

Incidental findings that have been investigated in relation to headache disorders include white matter hyperintensities, infarcts, pineal gland cysts, vascular abnormalities, enlarged perivascular spaces, cerebral microbleeds, and pituitary tumors (for a summary, see Table 3.1).

3.2.1 White Matter Hyperintensities

White matter hyperintensities, also known as white matter lesions, are named after their hyperintense appearance (bright spots) on T2-weighted MRI sequences (Fig. 3.1). They are optimally visualized using a FLAIR sequence, which suppresses signal noise coming from the cerebrospinal fluid.

White matter hyperintensities represent focal areas of increased water, gliosis, and sometimes demyelination. Their origins are multifarious and include vascular insufficiency and inflammatory activity [4]. They are also associated with vascular risk factors such as hypertension, smoking, diabetes, obesity, and age [5–7]. White matter hyperintensities are very common occurrences in otherwise healthy individuals, and most are not associated with any focal or global neurological symptoms [8]. Nevertheless, they can also be the first presentation of serious neurological conditions, most notably multiple sclerosis. This depends on their character as well as their location, where periventricular (surrounding the lateral ventricles), juxtacortical (next to the cortex and/or in the cortex), cerebellar, brainstem, and spinal locations can be a cause for clinical concern [9]. The clinical significance of white

Table 3.1 Common types of incidental findings on neuroimaging of individuals with headache disorders

Incidental finding	Optimal imaging approach	Imaging features	Clinical significance
White matter hyperintensities	FLAIR (MRI)	Hyperintensity on FLAIR and other T2-weighted sequences. Positioned within white matter in the brain, brainstem, or spinal cord. May conflate	Not clinically significant if limited and located in benign areas. Can be suspect if locations fulfill McDonald criteria for multiple sclerosis, or due to extensive distribution and confluence. Both require appropriate neurological work-up
Infarcts	T1-weighted and T2-weighted MRI sequences	Appears hypointense on T1-weighted sequences and hyperintense on T2-weighted sequences If incidental, most often present as minor infarcts in deep brain tissue (lacunar infarcts) or between the perfusion territories of major arteries (watershed infarcts)	In the chronic setting, can warrant the initiation of platelet inhibitor and anti-thrombotic treatment Generally contraindicates triptan treatment. In case of subtle, age-related infarcts (e.g., lacunar), continuation of an existing triptan treatment might be considered under close neurological consultancy
Vascular abnormalities			
Aneurysms	MR angiography, CT angiography	MR and CT angiographies detect unruptured aneurysms Non-contrast CT is preferred in the acute case of raptured aneurysm leading to bleeding in the brain (hemorrhagic stroke) and subarachnoid space (subarachnoid hemorrhage)	Usually asymptomatic until they become large or rupture. Symptoms vary based on the affected blood vessel Rupture causes a hyperacute medical emergency and results in a sudden, intense headache ("thunderclap headache") Headache can occur a few days or weeks before rupture possibly due to a "warning leak"
Arteriovenous malformations	Digital subtraction angiography	Tightly packed feeding arteries supply a central nidus. This is drained by one or more dilated veins. Due to shunting of blood, veins can appear opaque in the arterial phase Rapid blood flow can cause flow voids, a type of MRI artifact, easily visible on T2-weighted MRI images	Requires neurological/ neurosurgical consultation. For asymptomatic malformations, the decision between follow-up or treatment is based on the risk for complications, which depends on characteristics of the arteriovenous malformation The main risk is hemorrhage, often from an associated aneurysm. Seizures represent another risk. The presence of multiple arteriovenous malformations can be part of a syndrome

(continued)

Table 3.1 (continued)

Incidental finding	Optimal imaging approach	Imaging features	Clinical significance
Cavernous malformations	T2-weighted or GRE sequences (MRI)	Groups of small, tightly packed blood vessels, typically shaped like small mulberries or popcorns Challenging to detect on cerebral angiography (due to their low-flow nature) A pattern of mixed hyper- and hypointensities on T1- and T2-weighted images, with a hypointense rim best observed on T2-weighted or GRE sequences. SWI sequence is recommended	Size depends on the number of blood vessels affected. Some people develop multiple lesions Can stay stable without symptoms or can bleed, causing headaches, seizures, stroke, or neurological deficits
Pineal gland cysts	T2-weighted sequences (MRI)	T2 hypointense, cystic appearance, with homogenous internal structure. Most commonly unilocular but can be multilocular Signal intensity similar to that of cerebrospinal fluid on T1- and T2-weighted images. Sometimes with higher T1 signal. On FLAIR images brighter than the cerebrospinal fluid	Benign in the greater majority of cases, with either stable size or slow growth over several years. Should be consulted with neurosurgical units when deciding whether a relevant follow-up plan is indicated In rare cases, large pineal gland cysts may obstruct drainage of cerebrospinal fluid and cause headache, dizziness, and visual disturbances due to hydrocephalus. This requires immediate neurosurgical referral

(continued)

Table 3.1 (continued)

Incidental finding	Optimal imaging approach	Imaging features	Clinical significance
Pituitary tumors	Dedicated pituitary gland protocol with small field of view focused on the gland T1-weighted, T2-weighted sequences, as well as a T1-weighted sequence with dynamic and delayed contrast enhancement (MRI)	Classified based on diameter as microadenomas (<10 mm) or macroadenomas (>10 mm). Enlargement of pituitary gland on T1- and T2-weighted sequences, potentially with deviation of the gland away from the midline. Sometimes slightly hypointense on T2-weighted sequences. Delayed contrast enhancement of adenomas compared to the rest of the gland. Macroadenomas display heterogeneous intensity on T1- and T2-weighted sequences, often with a hypointense rim on T2-weighted sequences Hemorrhage can be visible with SWI sequences	Generally benign. The most common type is an adenoma. Pituitary tumors should be discussed with neurosurgical units for appropriate clinical work-up. Depending on the size, clinical symptoms, and hormone secretion, this may include MRI follow-up, surgical resection, or medical management. Many patients do not require any clinical intervention Symptoms can occur due to mass effects or secretion of hormones. Macroadenomas may compress the optic chiasma, causing loss of peripheral version (tunnel vision). Some adenomas secrete prolactin (prolactinomas), which might be linked to headache Other types include Rathke's pouch tumors and rarely carcinomas
Enlarged perivascular spaces	T2-weighted sequences (MRI)	Brightly hyperintense (on T2-weighted MRI), small, and round structures along the course of the brain's penetrating arteries and veins Can be seen on T1-weighted images as well	Typically, not clinically significant by itself, based on current knowledge. Nevertheless, extensively enlarged perivascular space can be associated with certain diseases, including small vessel diseases such as cerebral amyloid angiopathy. Further neurological follow-up may also be indicated in patients with concomitant neurological symptoms such as cognitive decline
Cerebral microbleeds	SWI sequences (MRI)	Minute hypointense oval lesions of SWI sequences. Can be located in either white matter or the cerebral cortex	Isolated cerebral microbleeds do not warrant clinical action. The presence of numerous cerebral microbleeds can suggest an underlying small vessel disease, such as cerebral amyloid angiopathy. This requires neurological management

Notes: *CT* computed tomography, *FLAIR* fluid-attenuated inversion recovery, *GRE* gradient-echo, *MRI* magnetic resonance imaging, *SWI* susceptibility-weighted imaging

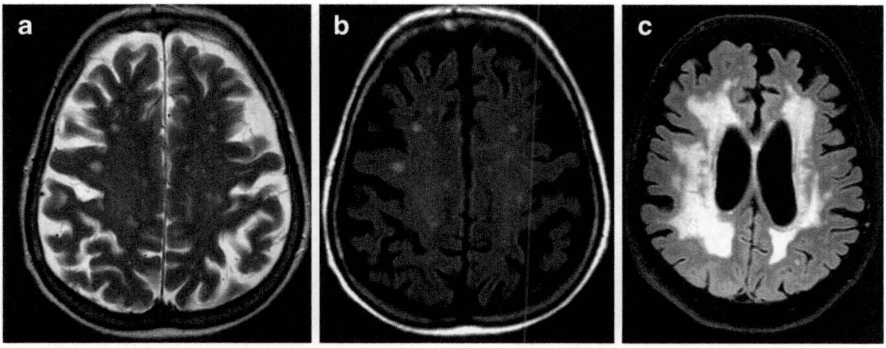

Fig. 3.1 T2-weighted (**a**) and correspondent FLAIR (**b**) transverse image with small subcortical white matter hyperintense lesion. FLAIR (**c**) transverse image—leukoaraiosis in patient with chronic headache with huge, conflating areas of white matter hyperintensities

matter hyperintensities therefore depends entirely on their radiological characteristics, which are systematically assessed using scoring systems such as the Fazekas grade, Scheltens scale, and McDonald criteria. The Fazekas scale rates white matter hyperintensities (periventricular and deep hyperintensities are considered separately) on a 4-point visual scale of increasing severity from 0 (absent) to 3 (irregular periventricular hyperintensities extending into deep white matter/large confluent areas) [10]. Unlike the Fazekas scale, which is more general, the Scheltens scale provides a more detailed assessment by scoring different brain regions separately, typically including the frontal, parietal, occipital, and temporal lobes, as well as subcortical areas [11]. In contrast, the McDonald criteria are a set of guidelines that are specifically developed to diagnose multiple sclerosis including MRI findings related to white matter alterations [9].

In extreme cases, white matter hyperintensities conflate extensively, presenting as leukoaraiosis. Leukoaraiosis can be either without clinical significance or sometimes a manifestation of neurological diseases, such as cerebral autosomal dominant arteriopathy with subcortical infarcts and leukoencephalopathy (CADASIL) [12].

3.2.2 *Infarcts*

Infarcts are areas of necrosis due to ischemia, i.e., reduced blood flow. They are of variable shape, size, and location, with cortical and subcortical involvement. In the chronic setting, infarcts appear as hyperintense on T2-weighted sequences and hypointense on T1-weighted sequences (Fig. 3.2). This is due to the combination of loss of neuronal tissue and its replacement with fluid (encephalomalacia due to liquefactive necrosis) and gliosis [13].

When discovered in patients with headache disorders, the infarct is often due to a

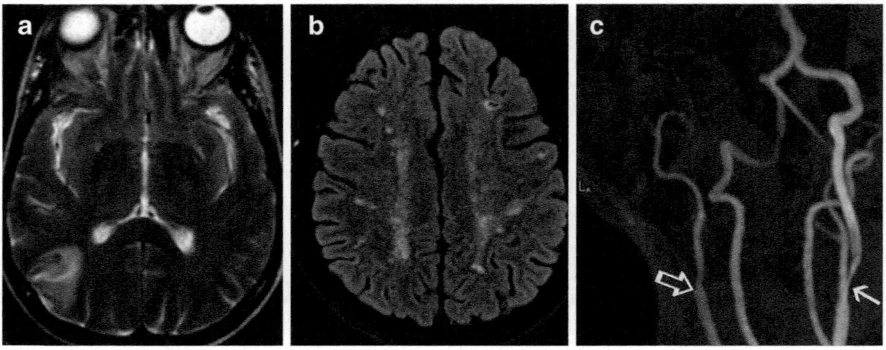

Fig. 3.2 T2-weighted image in transverse plane (**a**). Subacute infarct in the right parietal region as an irregular lesion with high signal intensity. Asymptomatic patient with multiple watershed infarcts in both cerebral hemispheres, between territories of medial and anterior cerebral arteries—T2-weighted transversal image (**b**). 3D time-of-flight (TOF) MR cerebral angiography (**c**) with complete occlusion of the left internal carotid artery (⇨) and severe left carotid stenosis (←)

silent stroke, i.e., asymptomatic. Most commonly, these are so-called lacunar infarcts: small infarcts that occur in deep structures of the brain (most frequently in the basal ganglia, thalamus, pons, and white matter of the internal capsule). Watershed or borderzone infarcts are likewise frequent and occur in the watershed regions between the supply territory of major arteries [14]. Since these regions occur in the brain at the furthest distance from arterial supply, watershed areas are more susceptible to infarction due to hypoperfusion, which can occur with progressed age, carotid artery stenosis, or systemic diseases, such as hypertension and atherosclerosis [15].

In terms of headache, it is important to note that triptans are per se contraindicated in patients with a prior stroke even if the stroke is silent. This is based on conflicting epidemiological data suggesting a possibly higher risk of stroke in individuals using triptans [16, 17]. In a patient with no other vascular risk factors who is perhaps benefitting markedly from triptan use, the decision to discontinue triptans may however require a clinical wagering of pros and cons in the context of silent strokes (e.g., lacunar or watershed infarcts). This is especially true in light of there being no evidence for sumatriptan constricting cerebral arteries based on MR angiography data [18]. Sumatriptan might therefore be a more preferable option in these special scenarios. Nevertheless, a decision to continue treatment should always be made with senior neurological consultancy.

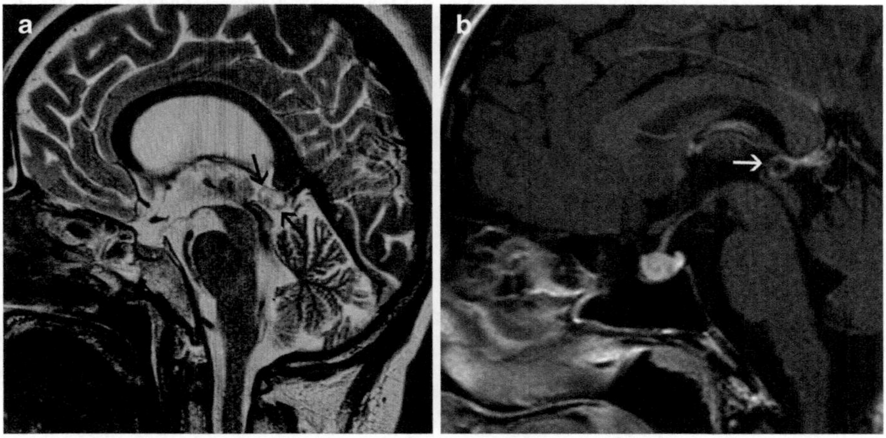

Fig. 3.3 T2-weighted image in sagittal plane (**a**) and contrast-enhanced T1-weighted (**b**). Small pineal gland cyst without compression of midbrain tectum (black →). Regular thin contrast enhancement of the walls (white →)

3.2.3 Pineal Gland Cysts

Pineal gland cysts are fluid-filled spaces within the pineal gland, which is a highly vascularized and secretory neuroendocrine gland in the mid-line of the brain. On MRI scans, pineal cysts can appear round or oval, thin-walled, and well-circumscribed (Fig. 3.3). Pineal cysts typically show signal intensity similar to that of cerebrospinal fluid on T1- and T2-weighted images, but sometimes they have a higher T1 signal. On FLAIR images, they appear brighter than the cerebrospinal fluid [19]. The cysts' contents are homogenous, and they show no restricted diffusion in diffusion-weighted imaging [20].

The majority of pineal gland cysts are asymptomatic and benign, but large pineal cysts may lead to a variety of symptoms, such as headaches, vertigo, visual and oculomotor disturbances, and, in severe cases, seizures and loss of consciousness [21]. However, in many cases, the association between the cyst size and the onset of symptoms has been found to be irrelevant [22, 23]. On rare occasions, pineal cysts can lead to hydrocephalus (increased pressure on the brain due to abnormal buildup of fluid) by blocking the flow of cerebrospinal fluid that may require immediate neurosurgical intervention.

In terms of headache research, it should be noted that most studies investigating pineal cysts include patients suffering from headaches without secondary hydrocephalus who underwent surgical resection. According to a recent meta-analysis among patients (with surgically managed) symptomatic pineal cysts [22], females were more likely to experience headaches than males, while seizures were more frequently observed in males. Additionally, pineal cyst size was negatively associated with headache, visual disturbance, and vertigo.

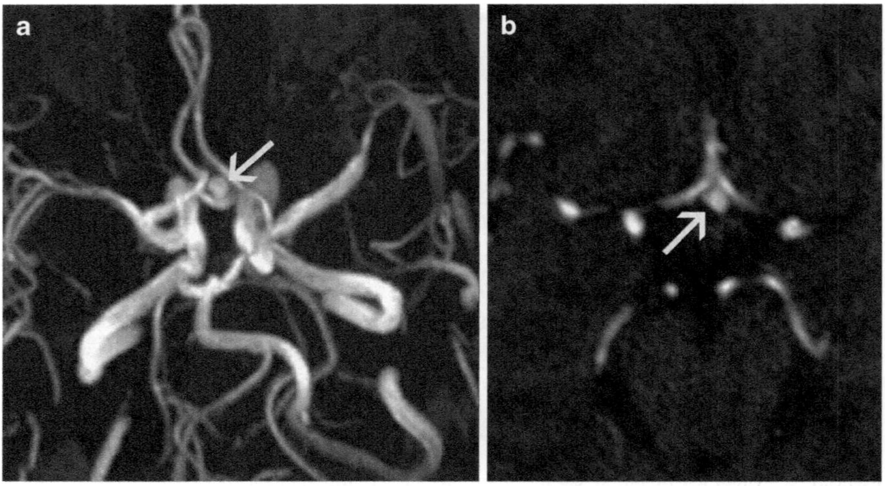

Fig. 3.4 Time-of-flight (TOF) cerebral angiography (**a**) and source MR angiography image (**b**) in patient with anterior communicating saccular aneurysm (A ↙, B ↗)

3.2.4 Vascular Abnormalities

Due to the increasing utilization of MR and CT angiography, which involve either injecting dye or contrast or magnetically labelling blood to outline vessels (for more details, see Chap. 1), incidental vascular findings are frequently discovered [24]. Vascular abnormalities (or anomalies) are also commonly visible on standard neuroimaging sequences, such as T1-weighted imaging [25]. The most common abnormalities are aneurysms, arteriovenous malformations, and cavernous malformations that affect the blood vessels and blood flow in the brain.

Aneurysm is a weak or thin spot in the wall of a brain vessel that balloons or bulges out and fills with blood [26] (Fig. 3.4). An aneurysm is usually asymptomatic until it becomes very large or ruptures, and symptoms vary depending on which blood vessel is affected. Both MR and CT angiographies are capable of detecting aneurysms that have not ruptured, whereas non-contrast CT is the preferred method to acutely identify aneurysms that have ruptured and led to bleeding in the brain (hemorrhagic stroke) and subarachnoid space [27]. The rupture results in the hyperacute and dire medical emergency of subarachnoid hemorrhage, which manifests as an intense, sudden-onset headache ("thunderclap headache"). This requires immediate emergency medical attention. The rupture is sometimes precipitated by a "warning leak" as well, which manifests as a similarly severe, sudden-onset headache days to weeks before the actual rupture.

Arteriovenous malformations in the brain are congenital abnormal connections between arterial and venous vessels, with no capillary structures between them (Fig. 3.5) [28]. On an angiogram, an arteriovenous malformation is seen as a nidus of tightly packed mass of enlarged vessels. Additionally, the fast flow in tangled

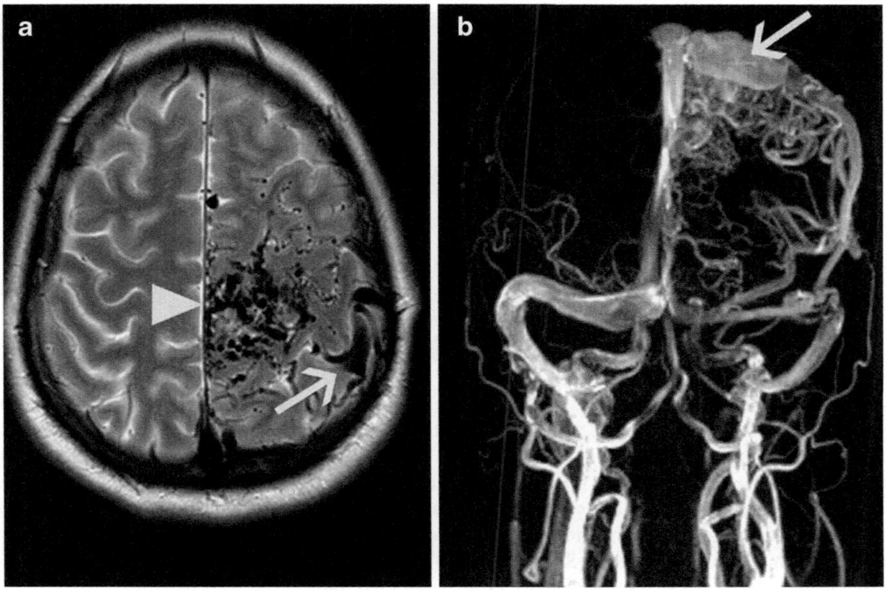

Fig. 3.5 T2-weighted image in transverse plane (**a**) and compressed TOF cerebral angiography (**b**). Huge arteriovenous malformation in the left frontoparietal region (A▷) with prominent drainage vein (A→, B ↙)

blood vessels can generate flow voids (a type of artifact in MRI images when the signal is lost due to the blood flow), easily seen on T2-weighted MRI images as well [29]. Arteriovenous malformations are most commonly detected within the cerebral cortex, brainstem (pons and midbrain), and cerebellum [28, 30]. Complications from these direct arteriovenous communications are dependent on their anatomical location and stage, and they can include stroke, hypoxemia, or local rupture with hemorrhages including subarachnoid [31, 32]. Symptoms of a ruptured arteriovenous malformation include a sudden, severe headache or pain in one area of the head, nausea and vomiting, sensitivity to light, confusion, weakness, fainting, and seizures [33]. This likewise requires immediate neurological attention.

Cavernous malformations or cavernomas are groups of small, tightly packed blood vessels with abnormally thin walls, and they are typically shaped like small mulberries or popcorns [34] (Figs. 3.6 and 3.7). These vessels contain slow-moving or stagnant blood that is usually clotted. Due to their low-flow nature, cavernous malformations can be challenging to detect on cerebral angiography (which is more effective for visualizing high-flow vascular structures) [35]. On MRI, their main characteristics include a reticulated pattern of mixed hyper- and hypointensities (due to the presence of different stages of blood products within the malformation) on T1- and T2-weighted images, with a hypointense rim best observed on T2-weighted or gradient-echo (GRE) sequences [34, 36]. Notably, SWI sequence is highly sensitive for detecting cerebral cavernous malformations. The size of cavernous malformations can vary depending on the number of blood vessels affected, and

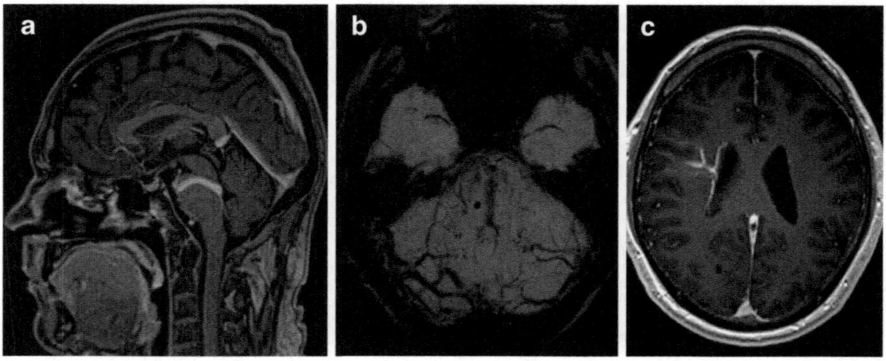

Fig. 3.6 Contrast-enhanced T1-weighted image in sagittal plane (**a**) and transversal image on susceptibility-weighted image (SWI) (**b**). Prominent venous anomaly (developmental venous anomaly; DVA) passes through the midline of the upper pons. One microhemorrhage is present in the pons, on the right side from DVA. Contrast-enhanced T1-weighted image in transverse plane (**c**) in another patient with a classical presentation of DVA with collector branches located in the cortex and subcortical white matter of the right middle frontal gyrus. DVA fusses with periventricular vein network. Transverse SWI image—DVA in the right cerebellar hemisphere with typical appearance of the radiating collector veins "caput medusae"

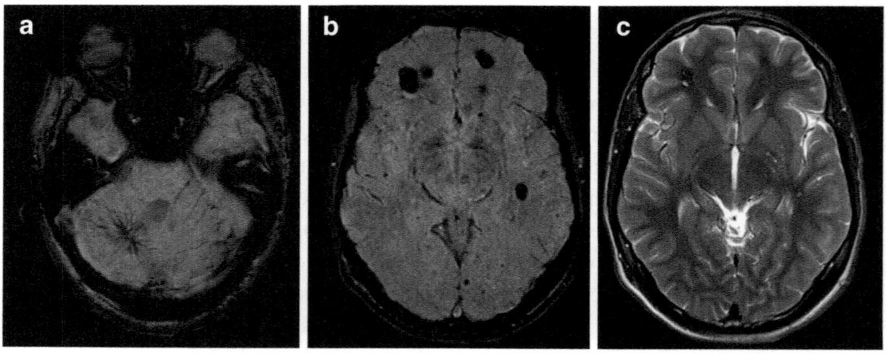

Fig. 3.7 Transverse susceptibility-weighted image (SWI) (**a**)—developmental venous anomaly (DVA) in the right cerebellar hemisphere with the typical appearance of the radiating collector veins "caput medusae". Transverse SWI image (**b**) and correspondent T2-weighted image in another patient—multiple cavernomas in both frontal lobes as rounded low signal intensity changes. One cavernoma can be seen in the left temporal region. Cavernoma in the right frontal region has the appearance of a "popcorn"

some people develop multiple lesions. They may remain stable and never cause symptoms or may bleed one or more times and cause headaches, seizures, stroke, and or neurological deficits [37]. They can also rupture, but they are the least lethal of the three abnormalities.

Taken together, most commonly, the reason for symptoms caused by these vascular abnormalities is the rupture of the vessels leading to intracerebral hemorrhage, and the most frequent symptoms are (secondary) headaches. Despite the absence of evidence for triptans having cerebral vasoconstrictive effects in patients, some authors theorize that triptans could potentially increase the risk of ruptures [38]. Currently, these vascular abnormalities do not contraindicate triptans, though prior cerebral or subarachnoid hemorrhage does [39–41].

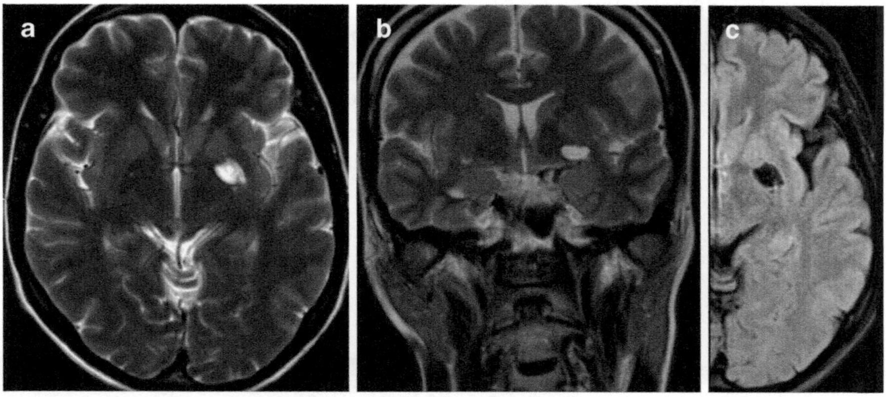

Fig. 3.8 T2-weighted transverse (**a**), coronal image (**b**) and FLAIR coronal image in patient with incidentally discovered singe dilated perivascular spaces at a typical location, under left putamen

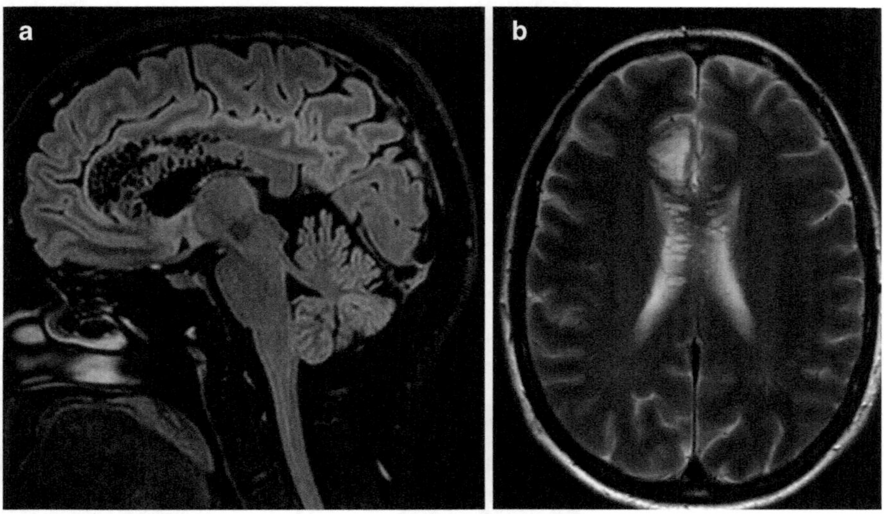

Fig. 3.9 FLAIR image in sagittal plane (**a**) and T2-weighted transversal image (**b**) in patient with incidentally depicted clusters of dilated perivascular spaces with mild mass effect in the region of the right anterior cingulum

3.2.5 Enlarged Perivascular Spaces

Enlarged perivascular space, also known as Virchow–Robin space, can be described by fluid-filled cavities that surround the small blood vessels in the brain (Figs. 3.8 and 3.9). Perivascular spaces are normal anatomical structures, playing a prominent role in the exchange of cerebrospinal and interstitial fluids and in the clearance of waste in the brain [42]. Enlarged perivascular spaces can be detected as hyperintensities on T2-weighted MRI (but they can also be seen on T1-weighted images) [43]. They are mainly distributed in the white matter centrum semiovale, basal ganglia, midbrain, and hippocampus [44–46].

Enlarged perivascular spaces are generally a benign finding, especially in older adults (often considered as part of the normal aging process) [47, 48]. However, when they are extensive or occur at younger age, they could indicate underlying pathological processes, such as cerebral small vessel disease. They are also linked to a heightened risk of headache, dizziness, cognitive decline, dementia, and stroke [48, 49].

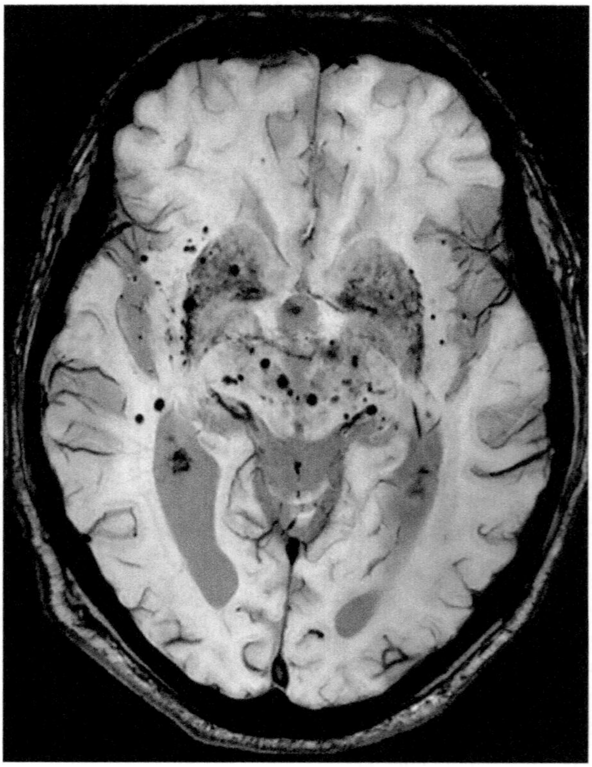

Fig. 3.10 Transverse SWI image. Symmetrical multiple microbleeds in white matter, basal ganglia, and midbrain as a lesion with low signal in patient with hypertensive encephalopathy

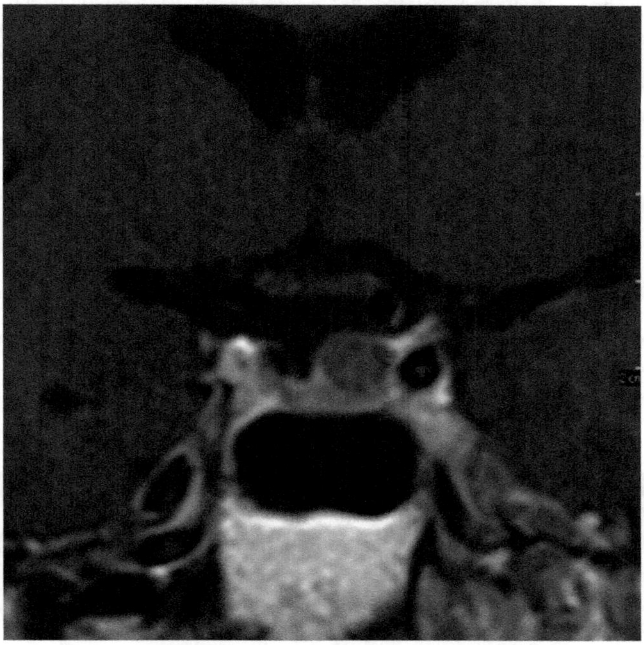

Fig. 3.11 Incidental pituitary microadenoma on contrast-enhanced image of the sella region in coronal plane. Tumor is located in the left side of the pituitary gland

3.2.6 Other Incidental Abnormalities

Cerebral microbleeds, also known as microhemorrhages in the brain, are small, spherical hypointense regions detected with T2*-weighted MRI images, including either GRE or SWI sequences due to their iron content (Fig. 3.10). They likely stem from structural abnormalities or damaged small vessels [50]. Numerous microbleeds can suggest neurological conditions, such as a cerebral amyloid angiopathy, and they might be more common in conditions such as Alzheimer's disease [50]. Nevertheless, isolated microbleeds are not a cause for clinical concern, and they occur with a frequency of approximately 15% in the general population, with the prevalence increasing with age [51].

Pituitary tumors are relatively frequent, occurring in approximately 22.5% of the general population, based on a meta-analysis of imaging studies [52]. Pituitary adenomas are classified based on their size as either the more common microadenomas (diameter $\leq$ 10 mm) or the rarer macroadenomas (diameter > 10 mm) (Fig. 3.11). They are usually benign but can produce symptoms including headache and visual loss (tunnel vision) due to mass effects on the chiasma opticum or surrounding structures. In the context of headache, the prolactin-producing subtype prolactinomas have garnered interest due to a potential involvement of prolactin in headache

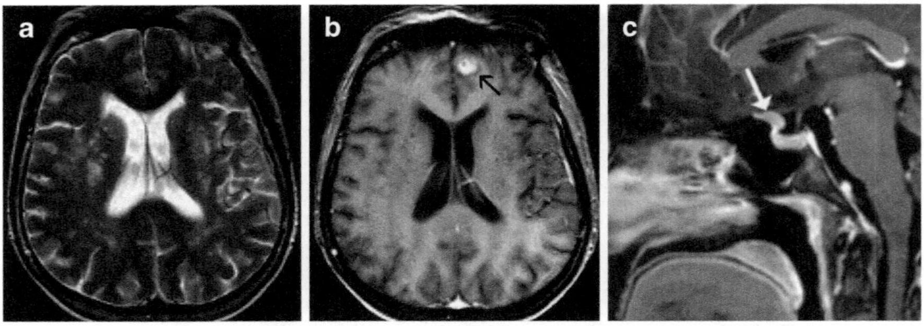

Fig. 3.12 Incidental meningioma, practically non-visible isointense with surrounding brain parenchyma on T2-weighted image (**a**) and clearly visible in the left frontal region after intravenous administration of contrast (**b**). No significant mass effect is seen. Tuberculum sellae meningioma (C)

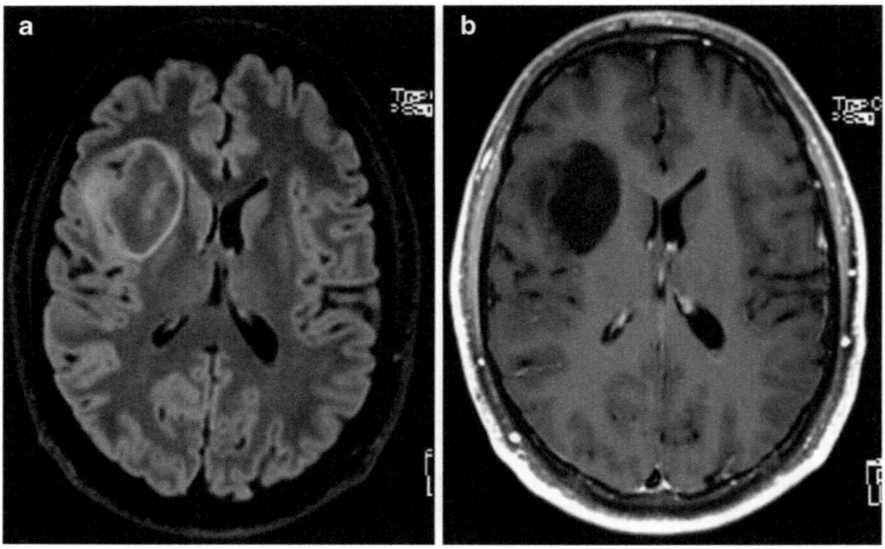

Fig. 3.13 FLAIR transverse (**a**) and contrast-enhanced T1-weighted image (**b**). Expansile tumor in the right middle temporal gyrus with mild mass effect and without contrast enhancement. Pathohistology revealed diffuse astrocytoma

[53, 54]. Furthermore, they have an association with certain rare headache types, including the trigeminal autonomic cephalalgias [55].

Compared to pituitary and pineal gland tumors, other neoplasms are rarer (Figs. 3.12 and 3.13). These may range from benign tumors, such as the more common meningiomas, to aggressive malignancies, such as glioblastomas, and can sometimes produce headache possibly related to mass effects or invasion of pain sensitive tissues, such as bone [56]. They generally require neurosurgical consultation, with some aptly controlled by follow-up visits and others requiring intervention.

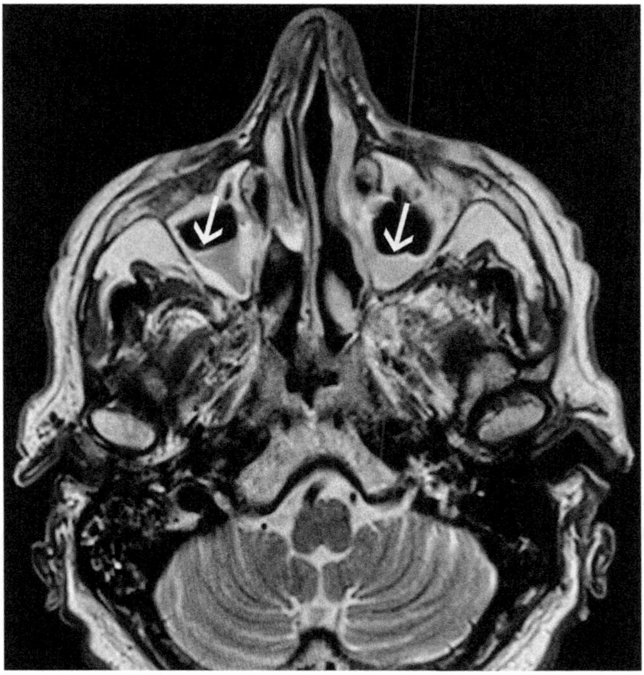

Fig. 3.14 T2-weighted transverse image. Light thickening of the mucosa in both maxillary sinuses with fluid levels (↓)

Sinusitis is a frequent incidental finding, characterized by opacity within the sinus instead of air (Fig. 3.14). It is often not symptomatic [57], but can sometimes warrant clinical examination, especially because it can cause headache symptoms that may mimic exacerbation of headache types, such as migraine or tension-type headache. In turn, sinusitis might be treated symptomatically or with antibiotics, depending on the circumstances.

3.3 Prevalences and Relative Frequencies of Incidental Abnormalities in Individuals with Headache Disorders and the General Population

Estimates of the prevalence of incidental findings in headache disorders vary substantially between studies. A meta-analysis of 41 studies of individuals with a headache disorder and normal neurological examination put the pooled relative frequency of incidental findings at 17.5%, but the estimate was associated with considerable heterogeneity between studies [1]. Estimates in the general population likewise vary considerably from 24.2% to 54.9% even in large, population-based studies [58–61]. It is therefore not clear whether the rate of incidental findings overall differs between individuals with headache disorders as a whole, compared to the general populations.

There might be several reasons for this heterogeneity, since prevalence and relative frequencies of incidental findings depend on a number of factors. These include the pooling of different headache disorders, the combination of patients presenting with an acute headache episode and those with a recurrent headache disorder, as well as the combination of data collected prospectively and retrospectively. Also, the available studies often do not differentiate between headache patients scanned on suspicion of a secondary headache disorder or just incidentally for another reason. They are thereby not generally comparable to truly "incidental findings" that are reported in studies in the general population. Moreover, most studies used a combination of MR or CT, with MR sequences of varying sensitivity to the abnormalities. Other epidemiological challenges include differences in sociodemographic composition of cohorts and that most studies estimated the relative frequency of incidental findings in patients attending tertiary headache centers, which provides only a poor estimate of the prevalence among individuals with headache in the general population. Finally, it should also be noted that in headache populations, some factors increase the likelihood of incidental findings. These include a retrospective study design as well as patient age, given that patients over 40 years old were more likely to have abnormalities [62]. The association between age and incidental findings is similar to what is seen in the general population. Furthermore, up to 8% of patients not responding to migraine and headache treatments had clinically significant MRI findings in one study [62]. On the other hand, this study found no significant results related to sex or the duration of headaches.

3.4 Common Incidental Abnormalities in Different Types of Headaches and Their Possible Pathophysiological Relevance

Studies have suggested distinct rates of specific incidental findings in certain headache disorders, which could potentially be linked to their pathophysiology. In the following, we will cover the most common types of incidental findings in major headache disorders (for a summary, see Table 3.2).

Table 3.2 Current knowledge of incidental findings in major headache disorders

Headache disorder	Type of finding	Potential pathophysiological relevance
Migraine	White matter hyperintensities	White matter hyperintensities might be related to vascular insufficiency. This could be related to, e.g., migraine with aura, but the pathophysiological implication remains uncertain [63] Early studies suggested that migraine was associated with white matter hyperintensities [64] Subsequent studies have continued to yield inconsistent results. Some suggested that white matter hyperintensities are either not or only discretely associated with migraine [66, 67]
	Posterior circulation infarcts	Infarcted tissue might locally irritate the cortex, potentially triggering cortical spreading depression, the neural substrate of aura [73] In a large-scale, population-based sample, infarcts in the posterior circulation were linked to migraine, especially migraine with aura [68, 69] A subsequent population-based sample of individuals with migraine with aura did not find any difference in infarcts in general, compared to healthy controls [66]. However, many patients within this cohort had not experienced aura for years
	Arteriovenous malformations	Arteriovenous malformations might provide local cortical irritation that could trigger cortical spreading depression underlying aura. Arteriovenous malformations have been linked to symptoms resembling migraine with aura [72–74]. However, it is unknown whether occipital arteriovenous malformations are more common in individuals with aura compared to those without or healthy controls
	Enlarged perivascular spaces	Enlarged perivascular spaces may indicate impairment in the brain's glymphatic system [48, 75] Dysfunction or damage to this system could potentially affect migraine development [76] Enlarged perivascular spaces were found to be more prevalent in the centrum semiovale and midbrain in patients with migraine compared to healthy controls [77]. However, there was no significant difference between patients with episodic and patients with chronic migraine. Of note, the study utilized a graded scale instead of directly comparing the number of enlarged perivascular spaces
Tension-type headache	White matter hyperintensities	White matter hyperintensities might arise due to vascular insufficiency in tension-type headache In a large-scale population-based study among middle-aged individuals, the prevalence of abnormal white matter hyperintensities, assessed with Fazekas grade, Scheltens score, and white matter volume, was greater among individuals with frequent or chronic tension-type headache compared to healthy controls, but similar compared to migraine [79, 80]. Nevertheless, it should be noted that their method (based on the Scheltens score and white matter volume) is not validated for this application, warranting cautious interpretation

(continued)

Table 3.2 (continued)

Headache disorder	Type of finding	Potential pathophysiological relevance
New daily persistent headache	White matter hyperintensities	Studies on the link between new daily persistent headache and incidental findings are limited A retrospective analysis of 97 patients found that only 13 had white matter abnormalities, and those patients had a history of migraine or cardiovascular/cerebrovascular risk factors [81]
	Infarcts	None of the 97 patients had infarct-like lesions [81]
Post-traumatic headache	White matter hyperintensities	White matter damage is speculated to play a role in post-traumatic headache genesis, due to disruption of fiber tracts involved in pain and cognitive processing [82] The only study investigating post-traumatic headache (persistent) found no differences in number or frequency of white matter hyperintensities in post-traumatic headache compared to healthy controls [84]. This is despite multiple studies investigating white matter hyperintensities in traumatic brain injury [85–87]
	Cerebral microbleeds	No difference in number or frequency of cerebral microbleeds, in the only study comparing post-traumatic headache to healthy controls [84]
Cluster headache	Pituitary tumors	Pituitary tumors might lead to autonomic imbalance or neuroendocrine disruption that could promote symptoms of cluster headache and (on a casuistic basis) other trigeminal autonomic cephalalgias Early data suggested a possible association between pituitary tumors and cluster headache [91] Subsequent studies were unable to confirm an association, finding tumors in at most 9.3% of cluster headache patients on MRI, comparable to or less than prevalences of 22.5% in a meta-analysis of studies on the general population [52, 93]

3.4.1 Migraine with and without Aura

White matter hyperintensity is the most frequent incidental abnormality in patients with migraine. Several studies using MRI have investigated the association with migraine [63]; however, the clinical significance of these hyperintensities and their relationship with different migraine subtypes and treatment responses are not well understood.

According to one meta-analysis, patients with migraine with aura were at a 1.68-fold higher risk of having white matter hyperintensities than healthy controls [64], whereas there was no significant difference for patients with migraine without aura. A more recent meta-analysis reported greater numbers, with six- and fourfold higher risk in patients with migraine with and without aura, respectively [63]. Besides the presence of aura, older age was found to be another crucial factor for the occurrence of white matter hyperintensities in migraine [63], which is similar to the findings in the general population [65]. However, a female twin study from the Danish Twin Registry found that the ratings of white matter hyperintensities in migraine with aura were not significantly different from that of healthy controls

[66]. This evaluation was based on the Fazekas and Scheltens scores using both FLAIR and T2-weighted images among 172 patients and 139 healthy controls. Volumetric analysis in the whole brain was also performed, but only a weak association was observed between migraine with aura and the total volume of white matter hyperintensities. In line with this finding, a recent study based on data from 1062 participants (45% women) yielded no evidence of higher occurrence of white matter hyperintensities in individuals with migraine (with or without aura) [67]. This study used FLAIR images and Fazekas's sores and involved a follow-up investigation with 393 participants over an average of 3.7 years. No progression of white matter hypersensitivities was detected in migraine; however, the study did find that women with any type of headache, including migraine, had a greater volume of white matter hyperintensities. Overall, these inconsistent results in the literature might be related to the variations in gender distribution among the groups of patients with migraine and the heterogeneous group of healthy controls. Currently, it is therefore not evident that white matter hyperintensities are more prevalent in migraine than in the general population.

Silent brain infarcts are also frequently studied in migraine, especially in migraine with aura. In the population-based CAMERA (Cerebral Abnormalities in Migraine, an Epidemiological Risk Analysis) study, migraine with aura was linked to an increased risk of silent infarcts in the posterior circulation in the cerebellum [68, 69]. The study used both T2-weighted and FLAIR images to detect infarct-like lesions among 161 patients with migraine with aura, 134 patients with migraine without aura, and 140 healthy controls [68]. According to the results, 8.1% of cases with migraine with aura had one or more cerebellar lesions, compared to 2.2% of cases with migraine without aura and 0.7% of healthy controls. However, a subsequent, population-based MRI study with female twins did not confirm this association [66], and according to the most recent meta-analysis on this topic, migraine and silent brain infarction were not related [70].

Notably, headaches that resemble migraines with aura may occur in patients with arteriovenous malformations, carotid aneurysms, or rare ischemic small vessel diseases, such as CADASIL [71, 72]. According to a recent review, in these cases, the migraine attacks with aura are secondary to the cerebrovascular pathology ("symptomatic migraine with aura"), while the evidence confirming the existence of "symptomatic migraine without aura" remains inconclusive [72]. It has been suggested that arteriovenous malformations located in the occipital lobe could be related to cortical spreading depression, which is the neurophysiological correlate of migraine aura [73, 74].

More recently, investigating the severity and distribution of enlarged perivascular spaces has gained attention in migraine research. These spaces are integral to the brain's glymphatic system, which is responsible for clearing metabolic waste and toxic solutes from the brain [48, 75]. Dysfunction or damage to this system could theoretically affect headache development and chronification [76]. In a study involving 231 participants (57 healthy controls, 59 with episodic migraine, and 115 with chronic migraine), the prevalence of high-grade enlarged perivascular spaces was higher (in the centrum semiovale and midbrain) among patients with migraine compared to healthy controls. However, there was no significant difference between patients with episodic and chronic migraine [77]. Nevertheless, it should be noted that the study used a graded scale rather than directly comparing the number of enlarged perivascular spaces, which may limit accuracy. The association of migraine chronification with the glymphatic system remains unclear, and further investigation is needed utilizing automated and unbiased quantitative methods.

3.4.2 Tension-type Headache

Only a relatively low number of studies have investigated incidental findings in tension-type headache (TTH). This is in part because clinical neuroimaging is rarely warranted in this group, especially in the absence of red flags [78]. The majority of the few conducted studies focused on white matter hyperintensities.

Some insights were gained from the HUNT (Trøndelag Health) study, which is a large-scale, population-based MRI investigation among individuals 50–65 years of age [79, 80]. This study enrolled a total of 862 participants, including 94 with frequent or chronic TTH, 91 with migraine, 126 with unclassified headache, and 551 participants who did not have a headache disorder. The participants underwent MRI on the same 1.5 Tesla MRI scanner, using an identical paradigm that comprised a FLAIR sequence. Across two separate reports, the study found that individuals with frequent or chronic TTH were at greater risk of abnormal white matter hyperintensities, compared with healthy controls [79, 80]. This was the case across three different measures, including a Fazekas grade ≥ 2 or being in the upper quartile of the Scheltens score or volume of white matter hyperintensities. The relative frequency of abnormal white matter hyperintensities ranged from 16% to 38%, depending on the measure. However, it should be noted that this usage of the Scheltens score or white matter hyperintensity volume is not validated as a measure of abnormality. In comparison, there were no differences between individuals with migraine and healthy controls. Moreover, TTH was also not at increased risk for any other abnormalities or incidental findings [79].

For both TTH and migraine, one potential explanation for these reports of increased frequency of white matter hyperintensities has been vascular insufficiency. Yet, the small number of studies in TTH, each with their limitations, warrants considerable caution in interpreting the findings. This is especially true considering the surprisingly low proportion of healthy controls which displayed white matter hyperintensities in the studies, compared to what is found in studies of healthy populations [58–61].

3.4.3 New Daily Persistent Headache

Studies investigating the relationship between new daily persistent headache (NDPH) and incidental findings on brain scans are relatively limited. In a retrospective analysis of 97 patients' medical records, only 13 out of 97 patients with NDPH had white matter abnormalities, and those patients had either a history of migraine

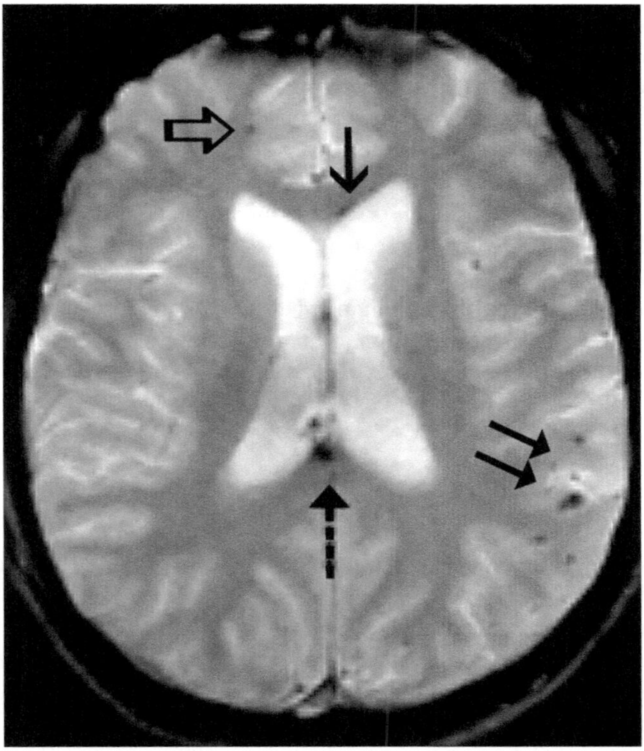

Fig. 3.15 T2 gradient-echo transverse image. Hemorrhagic diffuse axonal lesions in genu (↑) and splenium (↓) of the corpus callosum, frontal on the left side (⇨). Multiple small lesions are seen at the gray–white matter junction of the left parietal lobe (⇉). Transverse SWI image

or comorbid cardiovascular or cerebrovascular risk factors. In addition, none of them had infarct-like lesions [81].

3.4.4 Persistent Post-traumatic Headache

There is considerable interest in incidental findings in post-traumatic headache (PTH), because of the theory that they might represent sequelae of the trauma that could in itself contribute to the development of headache (e.g., by damaging pain processing brain structures or tracts) [82]. Studies on traumatic brain injury (TBI), a common cause of PTH, have suggested the development of white matter hyperintensities or even microbleeds after the brain trauma [83] (Fig. 3.15).

However, only a single study has actually investigated patients with PTH, as defined by the ICHD [3, 84]. The study investigated white matter hyperintensities with FLAIR in a cohort of 96 participants with persistent PTH compared with 96 age- and sex-matched healthy controls. It also investigated chronic microbleeds, minute hemorrhagic lesions, using a sensitive SWI sequence. The study found no difference in relative frequency or number of either white matter hyperintensities or chronic microbleeds in participants with persistent PTH compared to healthy controls [84]. Given that white matter hyperintensities and chronic microbleeds are not considered to resolve with time, this study also argues against a case for these lesions in acute PTH. In this regard, it should be noted that in the case of TBI, white matter abnormalities have been observed and might be associated with TBI severity [85–87]. The reason for the discrepancy between PTH and TBI in general is not perfectly clear but might stem from the studies' focus on mild TBI as opposed to more severe traumas. Yet, this might also be the most representative of persistent PTH, since mild TBI is more common than moderate or severe TBI, and might result in PTH more frequently [88–90].

3.4.5 Cluster Headache

Some lines of evidence have suggested a possible association between pituitary tumors and cluster headache (Fig. 3.11), as well as other trigeminal autonomic cephalalgias [91]. It is speculated that this could be either due to invasion of local structures, such as the cavernous sinus, or secretion of hormones, such as prolactin. These theories are partly based on a series of studies among 84 patients with pituitary tumors, of which 10% reported headache symptoms consistent with a trigeminal autonomic cephalalgia, including 4% with cluster headache [91]. This relative frequency would be considerably greater than the rarity of these diseases in the general population.

However, evidence from individuals with cluster headache have since provided inconsistent results. In a retrospective evaluation of MRI scans from a tertiary headache center, the relative frequency was only 9.3% on dedicated pituitary MRI of 376 cluster headache patients [92]. The majority of these were nonfunctioning pituitary microadenomas (40%; 5 patients). This estimate was comparable or less than the prevalence in the general population, which was as high as 22.5% in a meta-analysis of radiological studies (the majority being microadenomas) [52, 93]. Furthermore, another study only found two symptomatic lesions (a trigeminal schwannoma and a craniopharyngioma) among 130 patients with cluster headache undergoing MRI [94]. Other incidental findings were comparable to the prevalence in the general population. This underlines that the presentation of cluster headache is in the majority of cases a primary headache disorder, in accordance with its current position in the ICHD [3]. It also implies that MRI is not systematically indicated by the presence of cluster headache alone.

3.5 Gaps in the Literature/Future Directions

Several controversies surround the rate of distinct incidental findings in specific headache disorders. These pertain to the presence of white matter hyperintensities and infarcts in migraine, white matter hyperintensities in TTH, and pituitary lesions in cluster headache. Yet, except for migraine, the literature remains very limited. Even among the available studies, only a minority are actually population-based, with most originating from tertiary headache centers. This could potentially bias the estimates, given that such centers usually see the most severely affected cases, which could theoretically be at a greater risk for incidental findings. There is therefore a need for further population-based studies. This becomes a challenge for rare headache disorders, such as NDPH, cluster headache, and other trigeminal autonomic cephalalgias, because of the low occurrence of these disorders in the general population. Since this would necessitate a vast population-based cohort, clinic-based studies might provide the only feasible option for such rare headache disorders. Moreover, it should be noted that much of the extant literature is decades old and used imaging techniques of limited sensitivity by current standards. Future studies using modern approaches such as 3 T field strengths and optimized MRI sequences with dedicated fields of view are therefore warranted. An interesting question is also whether specific clinical features of headache might be associated with a greater risk of incidental findings (e.g., nonresponse to treatment, as suggested in one study [62], and side-locked headache [95]), and thereby expand upon our knowledge of potential "red flags."

3.6 Summary

For people with primary and some secondary headache disorders, there is no robust evidence for incidental findings being more common than in the general population. For migraine, there is conflicting evidence on the role of white matter hyperintensities, with many early studies not having been reproduced. This is likewise the case for reports of posterior circulation infarction in migraine with aura. For many other conditions, such as TTH, PTH, and cluster headache, the data is either very limited, methodologically problematic, or does not support an increased prevalence of incidental findings. Future investigations with modern techniques might impart further knowledge on potential links between incidental findings and headache, especially among the less frequent headache disorders.

References

1. Kamtchum-Tatuene J, Kenteu B, Fogang YF, Zafack JG, Nyaga UF, Noubiap JJ. Neuroimaging findings in headache with normal neurologic examination: systematic review and meta-analysis. J Neurol Sci. 2020;416:116997.
2. Langner S, Buelow R, Fleck S, Angermaier A, Kirsch M. Management of intracranial incidental findings on brain MRI. Rofo. 2016;188:1123–33.
3. Headache Classification Committee of the International Headache Society (IHS). the international classification of headache disorders, 3rd edition. Cephalalgia. 2018;38:1–211.
4. Wardlaw JM, Valdés Hernández MC, Muñoz-Maniega S. What are white matter hyperintensities made of? J Am Heart Assoc. 2015;4:e001140.
5. Breteler MM, van Swieten JC, Bots ML, Grobbee DE, Claus JJ, van den Hout JH, van Harskamp F, Tanghe HL, de Jong PT, van Gijn J. Cerebral white matter lesions, vascular risk factors, and cognitive function in a population-based study: the Rotterdam Study. Neurology. 1994;44:1246–52.
6. Lampe L, Zhang R, Beyer F, Huhn S, Kharabian Masouleh S, Preusser S, Bazin P, Schroeter ML, Villringer A, Witte AV. Visceral obesity relates to deep white matter hyperintensities via inflammation. Ann Neurol. 2019;85:194–203.
7. Wang D-Q, Wang L, Wei M-M, Xia X-S, Tian X-L, Cui X-H, Li X. Relationship between type 2 diabetes and white matter hyperintensity: a systematic review. Front Endocrinol (Lausanne). 2020;11:595962.
8. Habes M, Erus G, Toledo JB, et al. White matter hyperintensities and imaging patterns of brain ageing in the general population. Brain. 2016;139:1164–79.
9. Thompson AJ, Banwell BL, Barkhof F, et al. Diagnosis of multiple sclerosis: 2017 revisions of the McDonald criteria. Lancet Neurol. 2018;17:162–73.
10. Fazekas F, Chawluk JB, Alavi A, Hurtig HI, Zimmerman RA. MR signal abnormalities at 1.5 T in Alzheimer's dementia and normal aging. AJR Am J Roentgenol. 1987;149:351–6.
11. Scheltens P, Barkhof F, Leys D, Pruvo JP, Nauta JJ, Vermersch P, Steinling M, Valk J. A semiquantative rating scale for the assessment of signal hyperintensities on magnetic resonance imaging. J Neurol Sci. 1993;114:7–12.
12. Di Donato I, Bianchi S, De Stefano N, et al. Cerebral autosomal dominant arteriopathy with subcortical infarcts and leukoencephalopathy (CADASIL) as a model of small vessel disease: update on clinical, diagnostic, and management aspects. BMC Med. 2017;15:41.
13. Yilmazer-Hanke D, Mayer T, Müller H-P, et al. Histological correlates of postmortem ultra-high-resolution single-section MRI in cortical cerebral microinfarcts. Acta Neuropathol Commun. 2020;8:33.
14. Gore M, Bansal K, Khan Suheb MZ, Lui F, Asuncion RMD. Lacunar stroke. StatPearls; 2024.
15. Mangla R, Kolar B, Almast J, Ekholm SE. Border zone infarcts: pathophysiologic and imaging characteristics. Radiographics. 2011;31:1201–14.
16. Hall GC, Brown MM, Mo J, MacRae KD. Triptans in migraine: the risks of stroke, cardiovascular disease, and death in practice. Neurology. 2004;62:563–8.
17. Petersen CL, Hougaard A, Gaist D, Hallas J. Risk of stroke and myocardial infarction among initiators of triptans. JAMA Neurol. 2024;81:248–54.
18. Amin FM, Asghar MS, Ravneberg JW, de Koning PJH, Larsson HBW, Olesen J, Ashina M. The effect of sumatriptan on cephalic arteries: A 3T MR-angiography study in healthy volunteers. Cephalalgia. 2013;33:1009–16.
19. Gokce E, Beyhan M. Evaluation of pineal cysts with magnetic resonance imaging. World J Radiol. 2018;10:65–77.
20. Castillo M. Pineal cyst. In: Rossi A, Huang B, Castillo M, Rumboldt Z, editors. Brain imaging with MRI and CT: an image pattern approach. Cambridge: Cambridge University Press; 2012. p. 141–2.

21. Pu Y, Mahankali S, Hou J, Li J, Lancaster JL, Gao J-H, Appelbaum DE, Fox PT. High prevalence of pineal cysts in healthy adults demonstrated by high-resolution, noncontrast brain MR imaging. AJNR Am J Neuroradiol. 2007;28:1706–9.
22. Masina R, Ansaripour A, Beneš V, et al. Surgical treatment of symptomatic pineal cysts without hydrocephalus – meta-analysis of the published literature. Acta Neurochir. 2022;164:61–77.
23. Pitskhelauri DI, Konovalov AN, Abramov IT, Danilov GV, Pronin IN, Alexandrova EV, Serova NK, Sanikidze AZ. Pineal cyst−related aqueductal stenosis as cause of intractable headaches in nonhydrocephalic patients. World Neurosurg. 2019;123:e147–55.
24. Rutman AM, Wangaryattawanich P, Aksakal M, Mossa-Basha M. Incidental vascular findings on brain magnetic resonance angiography. Br J Radiol. 2023;96:20220135.
25. Bashir U, Shah S, Jeph S, O'Keeffe M, Khosa F. Magnetic resonance (MR) imaging of vascular malformations. Pol J Radiol. 2017;82:731–41.
26. Texakalidis P, Sweid A, Mouchtouris N, Peterson EC, Sioka C, Rangel-Castilla L, Reavey-Cantwell J, Jabbour P. Aneurysm formation, growth, and rupture: the biology and physics of cerebral aneurysms. World Neurosurg. 2019;130:277–84.
27. White PM, Teasdale EM, Wardlaw JM, Easton V. Intracranial aneurysms: CT angiography and MR angiography for detection prospective blinded comparison in a large patient cohort. Radiology. 2001;219:739–49.
28. Zyck S, Davidson CL, Sampath R. Arteriovenous malformations of the central nervous system. StatPearls; 2024.
29. Khurana NKR, Raz E, Mohamed AWH, Sotoudeh H, Reddy A, Jones J, Tanwar M. Intracranial cerebrovascular lesions on T2-weighted magnetic resonance imaging. J Clin Imaging Sci. 2024;14:19.
30. Can A, Gross BA, Du R. The natural history of cerebral arteriovenous malformations. Handb Clin Neurol. 2017;143:15–24.
31. Fleetwood IG, Steinberg GK. Arteriovenous malformations. Lancet. 2002;359:863–73.
32. Halim AX, Johnston SC, Singh V, McCulloch CE, Bennett JP, Achrol AS, Sidney S, Young WL. Longitudinal risk of intracranial hemorrhage in patients with arteriovenous malformation of the brain within a defined population. Stroke. 2004;35:1697–702.
33. Al-Shahi R, Warlow C. A systematic review of the frequency and prognosis of arteriovenous malformations of the brain in adults. Brain. 2001;124:1900–26.
34. Zyck S, Gould GC (2024) Cavernous venous malformation. StatPearls.
35. Vollherbst DF, Bendszus M, Möhlenbruch MA. Vascular malformations of the brain and its coverings. J Neuroendovasc Ther. 2020;14:285–94.
36. Wang KY, Idowu OR, Lin DDM. Chapter 24: radiology and imaging for cavernous malformations. In: Spetzler RF, Moon K, Almefty RO, editors. Handbook of clinical neurology. Elsevier; 2017. p. 249–66.
37. Salman RA-S, Hall JM, Horne MA, et al. Untreated clinical course of cerebral cavernous malformations: a prospective, population-based cohort study. Lancet Neurol. 2012;11:150–6.
38. Baron EP. Headache, cerebral aneurysms, and the use of triptans and ergot derivatives. Headache. 2015;55:739–47.
39. Flemming KD, Chiang C-C, Brown RD, Lanzino G. Safety of select headache medications in patients with cerebral and spinal cavernous malformations. Cephalalgia Reports. 2021;4:25158163211062254.
40. Roberto G, Piccinni C, D'Alessandro R, Poluzzi E. Triptans and serious adverse vascular events: Data mining of the FDA Adverse Event Reporting System database. Cephalalgia. 2014;34:5–13.
41. U.S. Food and Drug Administration (2023) *Imitrex (Sumatriptan)*.
42. Lam MA, Hemley SJ, Najafi E, Vella NGF, Bilston LE, Stoodley MA. The ultrastructure of spinal cord perivascular spaces: implications for the circulation of cerebrospinal fluid. Sci Rep. 2017;7:12924.

43. Potter GM, Chappell FM, Morris Z, Wardlaw JM. Cerebral perivascular spaces visible on magnetic resonance imaging: development of a qualitative rating scale and its observer reliability. Cerebrovasc Dis. 2015;39:224–31.
44. Adams HHH, Hilal S, Schwingenschuh P, et al. A priori collaboration in population imaging: the uniform neuro-imaging of Virchow-robin spaces enlargement consortium. Alzheimers Dement. 2015;1:513–20.
45. Barisano G, Lynch KM, Sibilia F, Lan H, Shih N-C, Sepehrband F, Choupan J. Imaging perivascular space structure and function using brain MRI. NeuroImage. 2022;257:119329.
46. Wardlaw JM, Benveniste H, Nedergaard M, et al. Perivascular spaces in the brain: anatomy, physiology and pathology. Nat Rev Neurol. 2020;16:137–53.
47. Yang S, Chang MC. Chronic pain: structural and functional changes in brain structures and associated negative affective states. Int J Mol Sci. 2019;20 https://doi.org/10.3390/ijms20133130.
48. Yang Y, Wang M, Luan M, Song X, Wang Y, Xu L, Zhong M, Zheng X. Enlarged perivascular spaces and age-related clinical diseases. Clin Interv Aging. 2023;18:855–67.
49. Ding J, Sigurðsson S, Jónsson PV, Eiriksdottir G, Charidimou A, Lopez OL, van Buchem MA, Guðnason V, Launer LJ. Large perivascular spaces visible on magnetic resonance imaging, cerebral small vessel disease progression, and risk of dementia: the age, gene/environment susceptibility-Reykjavik study. JAMA Neurol. 2017;74:1105–12.
50. Martinez-Ramirez S, Greenberg SM, Viswanathan A. Cerebral microbleeds: overview and implications in cognitive impairment. Alzheimers Res Ther. 2014;6:33.
51. Poels MMF, Vernooij MW, Ikram MA, Hofman A, Krestin GP, van der Lugt A, Breteler MMB. Prevalence and risk factors of cerebral microbleeds: an update of the Rotterdam scan study. Stroke. 2010;41:S103–6.
52. Ezzat S, Asa SL, Couldwell WT, Barr CE, Dodge WE, Vance ML, McCutcheon IE. The prevalence of pituitary adenomas: a systematic review. Cancer. 2004;101:613–9.
53. Al-Karagholi MA-M, Kalatharan V, Ghanizada H, Dussor G, Ashina M. Prolactin in headache and migraine: a systematic review of preclinical studies. Headache. 2023;63:577–84.
54. Al-Karagholi MA-M, Kalatharan V, Ghanizada H, Gram C, Dussor G, Ashina M. Prolactin in headache and migraine: a systematic review of clinical studies. Cephalalgia. 2023;43:3331024221136286.
55. Cittadini E, Matharu MS. Symptomatic trigeminal autonomic cephalalgias. Neurologist. 2009;15:305–12.
56. Schankin CJ, Krumbholz M, Sostak P, Reinisch VM, Goldbrunner R, Straube A. Headache in patients with a meningioma correlates with a bone-invasive growth pattern but not with cytokine expression. Cephalalgia. 2010;30:413–24.
57. Ali AHA, Serhan OO, Alsharif MHK, et al. Incidental detection of paranasal sinuses abnormalities on CT imaging of the head in Saudi adult population. PLoS One. 2022;17:e0270764.
58. Håberg AK, Hammer TA, Kvistad KA, Rydland J, Müller TB, Eikenes L, Gårseth M, Stovner LJ. Incidental intracranial findings and their clinical impact; the HUNT MRI study in a general population of 1006 participants between 50-66 Years. PLoS One. 2016;11:e0151080.
59. Lohner V, Lu R, Enkirch SJ, Stöcker T, Hattingen E, Breteler MMB. Incidental findings on 3 T neuroimaging: cross-sectional observations from the population-based Rhineland Study. Neuroradiology. 2022;64:503–12.
60. Tobe RH, Tu L, Roberts M, et al. Age, Motion, Medical, and Psychiatric Associations With Incidental Findings in Brain MRI. JAMA Netw Open. 2024;7:e2355901.
61. Vernooij MW, Ikram MA, Tanghe HL, Vincent AJPE, Hofman A, Krestin GP, Niessen WJ, Breteler MMB, van der Lugt A. Incidental findings on brain MRI in the general population. N Engl J Med. 2007;357:1821–8.
62. Alturkustani A, Bock Y, Bajunaid K, Lingawi S, Baeesa S. Significant incidental brain magnetic resonance imaging findings in migraine headache patients: retrospective cross-sectional study. Clin Neurol Neurosurg. 2020;196:106019.

63. Zhang W, Cheng Z, Fu F, Zhan Z. Prevalence and clinical characteristics of white matter hyperintensities in Migraine: a meta-analysis. Neuroimage Clin. 2023;37:103312.
64. Bashir A, Lipton RB, Ashina S, Ashina M. Migraine and structural changes in the brain. Neurology. 2013;81:1260–8.
65. Zhuang F-J, Chen Y, He W-B, Cai Z-Y. Prevalence of white matter hyperintensities increases with age. Neural Regen Res. 2018;13:2141–6.
66. Gaist D, Garde E, Blaabjerg M, et al. Migraine with aura and risk of silent brain infarcts and white matter hyperintensities: an MRI study. Brain. 2016;139:2015–23.
67. Schramm SH, Tenhagen I, Jokisch M, Gronewold J, Moebus S, Caspers S, Katsarava Z, Erbel R, Stang A, Schmidt B. Migraine or any headaches and white matter hyperintensities and their progression in women and men. J Headache Pain. 2024;25:78.
68. Kruit MC, van Buchem MA, Hofman PAM, Bakkers JTN, Terwindt GM, Ferrari MD, Launer LJ. Migraine as a risk factor for subclinical brain lesions. JAMA. 2004;291:427–34.
69. Kruit MC, Launer LJ, Ferrari MD, van Buchem MA. Infarcts in the posterior circulation territory in migraine. The population-based MRI CAMERA study. Brain. 2005;128:2068–77.
70. Espanol A, Lerebours F, Calviere L, Bonneville F, Ducros A, Larrue V, Gollion C. Silent brain infarct in migraine: systematic review and meta-analysis. Rev Neurol. 2024;180:486–93.
71. Guey S, Mawet J, Hervé D, Duering M, Godin O, Jouvent E, Opherk C, Alili N, Dichgans M, Chabriat H. Prevalence and characteristics of migraine in CADASIL. Cephalalgia. 2016;36:1038–47.
72. Thomsen AV, Sørensen MT, Ashina M, Hougaard A. Symptomatic migraine: a systematic review to establish a clinically important diagnostic entity. Headache J Head Face Pain. 2021;61:1180–93.
73. Galletti F, Sarchielli P, Hamam M, Costa C, Cupini LM, Cardaioli G, Belcastro V, Eusebi P, Lunardi P, Calabresi P. Occipital arteriovenous malformations and migraine. Cephalalgia. 2011;31:1320–4.
74. Kupersmith MJ, Vargas ME, Yashar A, Madrid M, Nelson K, Seton A, Berenstein A. Occipital arteriovenous malformations. Neurology. 1996;46:953–7.
75. Mestre H, Kostrikov S, Mehta RI, Nedergaard M. Perivascular spaces, glymphatic dysfunction, and small vessel disease. Clin Sci. 2017;131:2257–74.
76. Vittorini MG, Sahin A, Trojan A, et al. The glymphatic system in migraine and other headaches. J Headache Pain. 2024;25:34.
77. Yuan Z, Li W, Tang H, et al. Enlarged perivascular spaces in patients with migraine: a case–control study based on 3T MRI. Ann Clin Transl Neurol. 2023;10:1160–9.
78. Do TP, Remmers A, Schytz HW, Schankin C, Nelson SE, Obermann M, Hansen JM, Sinclair AJ, Gantenbein AR, Schoonman GG. Red and orange flags for secondary headaches in clinical practice: SNNOOP10 list. Neurology. 2019;92:134–44.
79. Honningsvåg L-M, Hagen K, Håberg A, Stovner LJ, Linde M. Intracranial abnormalities and headache: A population-based imaging study (HUNT MRI). Cephalalgia. 2016;36:113–21.
80. Honningsvåg L-M, Håberg AK, Hagen K, Kvistad KA, Stovner LJ, Linde M. White matter hyperintensities and headache: a population-based imaging study (HUNT MRI). Cephalalgia. 2018;38:1927–39.
81. Rozen TD. New daily persistent headache: a lack of an association with white matter abnormalities on neuroimaging. Cephalalgia. 2016;36:987–92.
82. Defrin R. Chronic post-traumatic headache: clinical findings and possible mechanisms. J Man Manip Ther. 2014;22:36–44.
83. Trifan G, Gattu R, Haacke EM, Kou Z, Benson RR. MR imaging findings in mild traumatic brain injury with persistent neurological impairment. Magn Reson Imaging. 2017;37:243–51.
84. Ashina H, Christensen RH, Al-Khazali HM, Iljazi A, Tolnai D, Eigenbrodt AK, Larsson HBW, Schytz HW, Lindberg U, Amin FM. White matter hyperintensities and cerebral microbleeds in persistent post-traumatic headache attributed to mild traumatic brain injury:

a magnetic resonance imaging study. J Headache Pain. 2023;24:15. https://doi.org/10.1186/s10194-023-01545-w.
85. Berginström N, Nordström P, Nyberg L, Nordström A. White matter hyperintensities increases with traumatic brain injury severity: associations to neuropsychological performance and fatigue. Brain Inj. 2020;34:415–20.
86. Brett BL, Klein AP, Vazirnia P, Omidfar S, Guskiewicz KK, McCrea M, Meier T. White matter hyperintensities and microstructural alterations in contact sport athletes from adolescence to early midlife. J Neurotrauma. 2024;41:2307. https://doi.org/10.1089/neu.2023.0609.
87. Patel JB, Wilson SH, Oakes TR, Santhanam P, Weaver LK. Structural and volumetric brain MRI findings in mild traumatic brain injury. AJNR Am J Neuroradiol. 2020;41:92–9.
88. Ashina H, Porreca F, Anderson T, Amin FM, Ashina M, Schytz HW, Dodick DW. Post-traumatic headache: epidemiology and pathophysiological insights. Nat Rev Neurol. 2019;15:607–17.
89. Management of Concussion/mTBI Working Group. VA/DoD clinical practice guideline for management of concussion/mild traumatic brain injury. J Rehabil Res Dev. 2009;46:CP1-68.
90. Nampiaparampil DE. Prevalence of chronic pain after traumatic brain injury: a systematic review. JAMA. 2008;300:711–9.
91. Levy MJ, Matharu MS, Meeran K, Powell M, Goadsby PJ. The clinical characteristics of headache in patients with pituitary tumours. Brain. 2005;128:1921–30.
92. Grangeon L, O'Connor E, Danno D, Ngoc TMP, Cheema S, Tronvik E, Davagnanam I, Matharu M. Is pituitary MRI screening necessary in cluster headache? Cephalalgia. 2021;41:779–88.
93. Vassiliadi DA, Tsagarakis S. Endocrine incidentalomas – challenges imposed by incidentally discovered lesions. Nat Rev Endocrinol. 2011;7:668–80.
94. Pérez-Pereda S, Madera J, González-Quintanilla V, et al. Is conventional brain MRI useful for the diagnosis of cluster headache in patients who meet ICHD-3 criteria? Experience in three hospitals in Spain. J Neurol Sci. 2022;434:120122.
95. Sjaastad O, Bakketeig LS. The rare, unilateral headaches. Vågå study of headache epidemiology. J Headache Pain. 2007;8:19–27.

Chapter 4
Neuroimaging Studies of Secondary Headaches

Catherine D. Chong, Richa Chirravuri, Dani Smith, Igor Petrušić, and David García-Azorín

4.1 Neuroimaging Studies of Headache Attributed to Trauma or Injury to the Head and/or Neck

Worldwide, approximately 69 million people experience traumatic brain injury each year [1], and post-traumatic headache (PTH) is the most common and debilitating symptom following mild traumatic brain injury (mTBI) [2–4]. According to the most recent version of the International Classification of Headache Disorders (ICHD-3) criteria [5], PTH, which is considered a secondary headache disorder, requires that the headache develops within 7 days of the TBI or within 7 days of regaining consciousness. Although PTH can occur following moderate or severe TBI, it is most common following mTBI. The most common phenotype of PTH is migraine-like or tension-type headache [6]. Although estimates vary between studies, approximately 25–50% of individuals continue to experience headache for 3 months or longer and develop persistent PTH [3].

Results of prior studies using cross-sectional imaging designs suggest that PTH is associated with changes in cortical structure and function. Imaging studies comparing individuals with PTH to healthy controls identified brain alterations

C. D. Chong (✉) · R. Chirravuri · D. Smith
Department of Neurology, Mayo Clinic, Phoenix, AZ, USA
e-mail: chong.catherine@mayo.edu

I. Petrušić
Laboratory for Advanced Analysis of Neuroimages, Faculty of Physical Chemistry, University of Belgrade, Belgrade, Serbia

D. García-Azorín

Department of Neurology, Hospital Universitario Rio Hortega, Valladolid, Spain

Faculty of Medicine, Department of Medicine, Dermatology and Toxicology, University of Valladolid, Valladolid, Spain

I. Petrušić, Y. Wang (eds.), *Neuroimaging of Headache Disorders*, Headache,
https://doi.org/10.1007/978-3-031-85402-6_4

linked to mTBI and PTH [7, 8]. Other studies, which compared individuals with mTBI and PTH to those with mTBI without PTH, have helped to disentangle brain changes related to PTH from those related to mTBI [9]. Additionally, comparisons between individuals with PTH and those with migraine have revealed shared alterations in brain structure and function as well as alterations that are unique to each headache disorder [7, 10, 11].

While these cross-sectional designs are valuable for identifying brain structural and functional differences associated with PTH, they do not provide insights into the temporal dynamics of brain regions and mechanisms involved in headache recovery or persistence.

In this review, we summarize findings from longitudinal imaging studies that examine brain changes in patients at multiple time points following mTBI, focusing on changes associated with headache recovery or headache persistence. We also review cross-sectional studies that have associated brain alterations in individuals with PTH, with measures of headache burden aiming to identify regions associated with headache persistence (see Table 4.1).

Table 4.1 Brain alterations in individuals with post-traumatic headache

Authors	Imaging time points and imaging modality	Comparison groups	Findings
Longitudinal studies			
Burrowes et al. [12]	Post-mTBI: 10 days 1 month 6 months 18 months *Longitudinal* T1-weighted: 3T (regional brain volume)	mTBI + PTH (n = 19) mTBI − PTH (n = 31) HC (n = 21)	*PTH vs. non-PTH*: Decrease in gray matter volume over four time points in two clusters 1. l middle temporal gyrus, l superior temporal gyrus, and l parietal operculum 2. r inferior temporal gyrus, r middle temporal gyrus, r angular gyrus, r supramarginal gyrus, r superior temporal gyrus, r primary somatosensory cortex, and r primary motor cortex *mTBI + PTH and mTBI − PTH vs HC*: Decrease in gray matter volume in 4 clusters (over 10 days and 6 months) including: 1. l parietal and frontal operculum, l superior temporal gyrus, l middle temporal gyrus 2. l angular gyrus and l parietal junction 3. r middle and superior frontal gyrus 4. r superior temporal gyrus, r supramarginal gyrus, r primary sensory and primary motor cortex

(continued)

Table 4.1 (continued)

Authors	Imaging time points and imaging modality	Comparison groups	Findings
Obermann et al. [13]	Post-mTBI: 14 days 3 months 12 months *Longitudinal* T1-weighted:1.5T (regional brain volume)	mTBI + PTH* ($n = 32$) HC ($n = 30$) *12 patients continued to have headache after 3 months post-mTBI	*14 days to 3 months post-mTBI*: Decrease in gray matter volume in bilateral anterior cingulate and bilateral dorsolateral prefrontal cortex, right superior frontal gyrus, and left middle frontal in individuals that had PPTH at 3 months ($n = 12$) There were no changes in gray matter volume for individuals that had headache recovery at 3 months post-mTBI ($n = 20$) Regional gray matter volume changes normalized along with headache resolution at 1 year, except for one patient who had persistent headache and medication overuse
Xu et al. [15]	Post-mTBI: 7 days (acute) 1 month (subacute) *Longitudinal* T1-weighted: 3T (regional cortical thickness and cortical surface area)	mTBI + PTH ($n = 36$) HC ($n = 34$) All individuals with PTH had cognitive improvement and improvement in headache-related disability (HIT-6) at 1-month follow-up	*Acute PTH vs. HC*: Less cortical thickness in left caudal anterior cingulate cortex and left insula and less cortical surface area in superior frontal gyrus in acute PTH *Longitudinal changes: Acute PTH to subacute PTH*: Improved cortical thickness in left caudal anterior cingulate cortex and left insula and improved cortical surface area in superior frontal gyrus Improved cortical thickness in left caudal anterior cingulate and left insula and larger superior frontal surface area was related to improvement in headache related disability (HIT-6) and cognitive function

(continued)

Table 4.1 (continued)

Authors	Imaging time points and imaging modality	Comparison groups	Findings
Xu et al. [14]	Post-mTBI: 7 days (acute) 1 month (subacute) *Longitudinal* T1-weighted: 3T (structural covariance of regional brain volume)	mTBI + PTH ($n = 36$) HC ($n = 34$) All individuals with PTH had cognitive improvement and improvement in headache-related disability (HIT-6) at 1-month follow-up	Comparison of structural covariance patterns between the acute (aPTH) and the subacute phase (sPTH) of individuals with PTH: *aPTH vs. HC*: Abnormal normalized clustering coefficient in aPTH compared to HCs *sPTH vs. HCs*: No significant difference in normalized clustering coefficient between the groups *aPTH vs. HC*: Altered nodal degree in the right frontal pole, abnormal nodal efficiency in the right rostral middle frontal and frontal pole, and altered nodal betweenness centrality in the left lateral orbitofrontal and right frontal pole in aPTH *sPTH vs. HC*: Altered nodal degree in the right caudal middle frontal, abnormal nodal efficiency in the right caudal middle frontal, and altered nodal betweenness centrality in widespread regions, including the right caudal middle frontal, left frontal pole, and right superior parietal lobule in sPTH
Cross-sectional studies			
Chong et al. [26]	Post-mTBI: 0–59 days *Cross-sectional* T1-weighted and T2* imaging: 3T (thalamic sub-volume and iron accumulation)	mTBI + PTH ($n = 52$) HC ($n = 55$)	*mTBI + PTH vs. HC*: Less volume in LGN and more T2* iron deposition (lower T2*) in left LGN in mTBI + PTH **mTBI + PTH: Positive correlation between left LGN T2* iron deposition and SCAT-5 symptom severity (SCAT-5, total score) at baseline (0–59 days post-mTBI) Positive correlation between left LGN T2* iron deposition and maximum headache intensity at 3 months post-mTBI

(continued)

Table 4.1 (continued)

Authors	Imaging time points and imaging modality	Comparison groups	Findings
Lemme et al. [28]	Post-mTBI: 3–4 months *Cross-sectional* T1-weighed and T2-weighted: 3T (regional brain volume and rs-fc)	Resolved PTH ($n = 18$) PPTH ($n = 21$) HC ($n = 20$) Children and young adults ages 12–24	*PPTH vs. HC*: Stronger fc between inf. frontal gyrus and cerebellum in PPTH *Resolved PTH vs. HC*: Weaker fc of cerebellum with temporal lobe in those with resolved PTH *PPTH vs. resolved PTH*: Stronger fc between the l frontal parietal/lateral prefrontal cortex and the r rostral prefrontal cortex in PPTH *Resolved PTH vs PPTH*: There were no group differences in brain structure for the regions explored
Li et al. [20]	Post-mTBI: 0–7 days *Cross-sectional* T2-weighted: 3T (static and dynamic rs-fc of 9 networks; independent component analysis)	50 mTBI + PTH 39 mTBI − PTH	*mTBI + PTH vs. mTBI − PTH* <u>Static fc</u>: mTBI + PTH had weaker network fc between the salience network and the sensorimotor network and the visual network and default mode network and stronger fc between the salience network and the executive control network and stronger connectivity between the sensorimotor network and the default mode network <u>Dynamic fc:</u> mTBI + PTH had increased connectivity alterations in state 2 between the DMN with the cerebellar network, between the DMN with sensorimotor network, and between the auditory network and cerebellar network and weaker fc alterations between the DMN and the visual network (state 4) **There was a positive association between the number of transitions and headache frequency and a negative correlation between state 1 dwell time and cognitive function (MoCA scores)

(continued)

Table 4.1 (continued)

Authors	Imaging time points and imaging modality	Comparison groups	Findings
Li et al. [19]	Post-mTBI: 0–7 days *Cross-sectional* Arterial spin labeling:3T (rs-fc)	mTBI + PTH (*n* = 48) mTBI − PTH (*n* = 46) Perfusion-based functional connectivity maps of six insular subdivisions	*mTBI + PTH vs. mTBI − PTH*: Stronger rs perfusion-based fc between the anterior insula and middle cingulate cortex and between posterior insula and supplementary motor area in individuals with mTBI + PTH mTBI + PTH had weaker perfusion-based fc between the posterior insula and r thalamus **Changes in the perfusion-based fc of the left posterior insula/dorsal anterior insula with the left thalamus/middle cingulate cortex were significant correlated with headache intensity and fc of the left posterior insula with the right thalamus were associated with headache frequency
Lu et al. [22]	Acute PTH *Cross sectional* T2-weighted: 3T (hypothalamus seeded rs-fc)	44 mTBI + PTH 27 mTBI − PTH 43 HC	*mTBI + PTH vs. mTBI − PTH*: Individuals with PTH had weaker fc between l hypothalamus with right middle frontal gyrus (MFG) and r medial superior frontal gyrus (mSFG) and weaker fc between r hypothalamus with r middle frontal gyrus **Higher headache frequency and headache intensity correlated with weaker l hypothalamus to r middle frontal gyrus and right medial superior frontal gyrus connectivity in individuals with mTBI + PTH
Nikolova et al. [27]	Post-mTBI: 0–59 days *Cross-sectional* T2* and T2-weighted: 3T (iron accumulation and rs-fc)	mTBI + PTH (*n* = 60) HC (*n* = 60)	*mTBI + PTH vs. HC:* Higher iron accumulation (lower T2*) in l post cingulate and bilateral cuneus and stronger fc between bilateral cuneus and r cerebellar regions in mTBI + PTH **For individuals with mTBI + PTH, there was a positive association between higher iron accumulation in the left posterior cingulate with mTBI symptom severity (SCAT-5, total score) and higher iron accumulation in the left cuneus with headache frequency

(continued)

Table 4.1 (continued)

Authors	Imaging time points and imaging modality	Comparison groups	Findings
Niu et al. [16]	Post-mTBI: 7 days *Cross-sectional* T2-weighted: 3 T (PAG seeded rs-fc)	mTBI + PTH (*n* = 54) mTBI – PTH (*n* = 16) HC (*n* = 46)	*mTBI + PTH vs. HC*: Weaker fc of PAG with DMN (bilateral precuneus, r. inf. parietal lobule, r. angular gyrus) and stronger PAG fc with temporal gyrus in those with mTBI + PTH *mTBI + PTH*: Negative correlation between HIT-6 and fc of PAG with r. precuneus and the PAG and r inf. parietal lobule *mTBI – PTH*: No significant correlation between HIT-6 and fc **Weaker fc of PAG with and bilateral precuneus and between PAG and r inf parietal lobule predicted headache persistence at 3 months post-mTBI with 89% accuracy

mTBI + PTH mild traumatic brain injury and post-traumatic headache, *mTBI – PTH* mild traumatic brain injury without post-traumatic headache, *r* right, *l* left, *inf* inferior, *HC* healthy controls, *DMN* default mode network, *rs-fc* resting-state functional connectivity, *T* tesla, *PPTH* persistent post-traumatic headache, *PAG* periaqueductal gray, *LGN* lateral geniculate nucleus, *SCAT-5* Sport Concussion Assessment Tool—5th edition.

4.1.1 Mechanisms of Headache Recovery and Persistence in Headache Attributed to Injury

Several studies have utilized T1-weighted imaging to examine longitudinal brain structural changes in individuals with PTH following mTBI.

Burrows and colleagues [12] investigated brain volume changes over four time points (10 days, 1 month, 6 months, and 18 months post-injury) in individuals with mTBI, comparing those with PTH to those without PTH and healthy controls (HC). PTH status was determined via a self-report questionnaire at the final follow-up. The results indicated progressive bilateral volume loss in PTH patients over 18 months in two clusters: the right anterior to parietal region and the left temporal to opercular region, as compared to mTBI patients without PTH.

A study by Obermann et al. examined gray matter volume changes in individuals with PPTH 3 months post-whiplash injury [13]. Reduced gray matter volume was observed in the anterior cingulate cortex, dorsolateral prefrontal cortex (DLPFC), right superior frontal cortex, and left middle frontal cortex at 2 weeks and 3 months post-injury. These structural changes normalized at 1 year in individuals who experienced headache resolution.

Xu et al. [14] conducted a longitudinal imaging study in individuals with acute PTH who recovered within 1-month post-mTBI. At 7 days post-injury, individuals showed reduced cortical thickness in the left caudal anterior cingulate cortex and left insula, as well as reduced cortical surface area in the superior frontal gyrus, compared to HC. At 1-month post-mTBI, cortical thickness and surface area had normalized.

Mediation analyses suggested that normalization in cortical thickness and surface area was associated with cognitive symptom recovery and reduced headache-related disability, as measured by the Headache Impact Test-6 (HIT-6).

In a follow-up study with the same cohort, Xu and colleagues [15] examined cortical thickness structural covariance networks, finding an abnormal normalized clustering coefficient in patients with acute PTH, which then normalized by 1 month. The study also reported widespread nodal network alterations in prefrontal brain regions during the acute and subacute phases compared to HC.

Cross-sectional functional imaging studies have used blood–oxygenation-level-dependent (BOLD) imaging, arterial spin labeling (ASL), and T2* imaging to examine resting-state functional connectivity, cerebral blood flow, and iron deposition in individuals with PTH, respectively, and explored associations between headache burden (headache frequency, headache intensity, and headache-related disability) with brain connectivity patterns.

In one study, Nui et al. investigated resting-state functional connectivity patterns of the periaqueductal gray (PAG) [16], a known brain region involved in pain modulation and the pathogenesis of migraine [17, 18]. Compared to healthy controls, individuals with acute PTH exhibited reduced PAG connectivity with regions of the default mode network, specifically the bilateral precuneus, right inferior parietal lobule, and right angular gyrus, and increased connectivity between the PAG and the temporal gyrus. Notably, reduced PAG connectivity with the bilateral precuneus and right inferior parietal lobule accurately predicted headache persistence at 3 months with 89% accuracy, suggesting that altered PAG connectivity may play a crucial role in the persistence of PTH symptoms and could serve as a potential biomarker for identifying individuals at risk of developing PPTH.

Li et al. [19] found that, compared to individuals with mTBI without PTH, those with PTH had stronger resting-state perfusion-based connectivity between the anterior insula and middle cingulate cortex and between the posterior insula and supplementary motor area, as well as weaker connectivity between the posterior insula and right thalamus. Notably, weaker connectivity between the left posterior insula and right thalamus was associated with increased headache frequency.

In a prior resting-state functional connectivity study, the authors Li et al. [20] also reported alterations in static and dynamic resting-state functional connectivity patterns in those with mTBI with PTH compared to those with mTBI without PTH. Individuals with PTH had weaker functional connectivity between regions of the salience and sensorimotor network and altered dynamic functional connectivity mainly involving the default mode network. The number of dynamic functional connectivity transitions, indicating network instability, related to headache frequency. These results align with a prior study [21] in those with mTBI with severe headache pain compared to those with moderate headache pain (study not included in this review), which demonstrated lower resting-state activity in the right insula, bilateral premotor cortex, and left parietal cortex. Decreased connectivity of the insula, particularly with regions involved in sensory and affective processing, may reflect alterations in pain modulation, potentially contributing to heightened pain sensitivity and persistent headache symptoms.

Lu et al. [22] reported altered resting-state functional connectivity in individuals with PTH following mTBI compared to individuals with mTBI without PTH. Their findings showed weaker connectivity between the left hypothalamus and both the right middle frontal gyrus and right medial superior frontal gyrus in those with PTH. This reduced hypothalamic to frontal connectivity in individuals with PTH correlated with higher headache frequency. The hypothalamus is widely considered as the "regulator" of the migraine attack [23–25] and has also been implicated as being involved in PTH [10]. This potential overlap in hypothalamic involvement in migraine and PTH could suggest some similarities in the neurobiological pathways that may be involved in the maintenance of headaches in both headache disorders.

Two studies, one by Chong et al. [26] and another by Nikolova et al. [27], used T2* imaging to assess iron deposition in individuals with acute PTH compared to HC. Their findings showed more iron accumulation in the lateral geniculate nucleus, posterior cingulate, and bilateral cuneus. Iron deposition in the cuneus was associated with higher headache frequency, while iron accumulation in the lateral geniculate nucleus correlated with greater headache intensity at 3 months post-injury, suggesting that neuroinflammation or oxidative stress as measured by T2* could play a role in headache burden.

Lemme et al. [28] examined structural brain volume and functional connectivity patterns in children and young adults aged 12–24. Their findings indicated stronger connectivity in prefrontal regions but no significant differences in brain volume among those with persistent headaches compared to those whose headaches resolved within 3–4 months following mTBI.

The findings in this review should be interpreted with caution due to the limited availability of research articles. Only one study has assessed brain changes in pediatric populations, resulting in a very limited understanding of the neuromechanisms underlying PTH in children and adolescents. Interpreting functional and structural imaging results in individuals with PTH following mTBI is challenging due to variations in study design and methodology. Differences in patient populations, including those studied at different time points post-injury, contribute to inconsistent findings. Additionally, the use of various imaging modalities and diverse post-processing techniques further complicates data comparability. Criteria for defining headache recovery also vary across studies, making it difficult to correlate imaging findings with clinical outcomes.

Findings from longitudinal studies indicate reductions over time in cortical thickness, surface area, and volume in frontal regions (including the superior frontal gyrus, anterior cingulate, insula, DLPC, and primary motor cortex) as well as in temporal-parietal regions (such as the superior and inferior temporal gyrus, supramarginal gyrus, and primary somatosensory cortex) in individuals with

PTH. Reduced cortical volume, thickness, and area can be detected as early as several weeks after injury and align with cross-sectional studies, which have shown reduced cortical thickness in the frontal and parietal regions in individuals with PPTH compared to HC [29]. Importantly, some data suggest that structural alterations may partially normalize over time in individuals with headache improvement, indicating potential mechanisms of neuroplasticity.

Furthermore, cross-sectional functional imaging studies indicate reduced functional connectivity of frontal regions with the hypothalamus and the PAG. This reduced connectivity was associated with increased headache frequency and was predictive of headache persistence. These findings align with prior data that suggest altered rs-fc between the PAG and frontal regions (including the DMN and sensorimotor networks) are relevant for distinguishing individuals with PPTH with high and low headache disability [30]. Studies have found abnormal functional connectivity between the insula and the thalamus and an association between decreased lateral geniculate nucleus integrity and headache persistence.

In summary, these preliminary data suggest progressive alterations in brain structure and weaker functional connectivity in individuals with PTH persistence following mTBI, particularly in regions associated with pain integration, modulation, and cognitive control.

Abnormalities in network connectivity, and clustering coefficients, in prefrontal regions in adults as well as in children further highlight disruptions in brain networks relevant for pain modulation and cognitive control [28]. These results are consistent with prior studies that have shown diminished pain inhibitory capacity using conditioned pain modulation testing in individuals with PPTH [31, 32]. Furthermore, network instability in the DLPC and reduced connectivity of the salience network (including regions such as the insula and the anterior cingulate) [33] with the PAG and the hypothalamus may compromise the brain's capacity to modulate pain signals and regulate cognitive control. This network dysregulation could contribute to heightened pain sensitivity, impaired pain inhibition, and PPTH.

4.2 Neuroimaging of Headache Attributed to Cranial or Cervical Vascular Disorder

Imaging is necessary to diagnose a headache attributed to cranial or cervical vascular disorder. Headache can be a manifestation of stroke, usually together with other neurological symptoms of hyper-acute onset. Headache has been associated with certain stroke etiologies, such as intracranial hemorrhage or cerebral venous sinus thrombosis. However, headache is common in acute ischemic stroke, where approximately 15% of patients report it during the acute phase [34]. It could be argued that given the high prevalence of primary headache disorders, in many of these cases, headaches could arise from a transient worsening of a pre-existing headache [35, 36]; nevertheless, in more than half of the cases of acute headache attributed to ischemic stroke, prior history of headache disorders was inexistent [34]. Another traditional reasoning is to associate headache to certain acute ischemic stroke etiologies, such as arterial dissection. In this regard, not all patients with cervical artery dissection report headache as presenting symptom [37], and the most frequent causes of acute headache attributed to ischemic stroke were cardioembolic stroke and posterior circulation strokes, regardless of their etiologies [34]. Between 10% and 15% of patients who experience an acute ischemic stroke report persistence of the headache 3 months after the acute phase [38–40]. Prior history of headache seems more associated with the persistence of headache following cervicocephalic arterial dissection [38, 40]. When this occurs during the peri-acute phase, a possible complication must be ruled out. The association between headache and hemorrhagic transformation is controversial [41–43].

In addition, headache may be a symptom of an intracranial hypertension syndrome, which can occur in certain scenarios, such as malignant stroke [44] or cerebral venous sinus thrombosis [45]. In the case of cerebral venous sinus thrombosis, headache can suggest a raised intracranial pressure, but also other complications, including intracranial hemorrhages, dural venous sinus distension, or venous infarcts [46]. The dynamic pathophysiology of venous thrombosis requires close monitoring and frequent evaluation of patients [47], to adapt the treatment to the possible underlying complications [47, 48].

For all these reasons, imaging in patients with headache must be comprehensive. Physicians must be vigilant because, in many patients, it is important not only to detect that the patient has a stroke but also to identify the stroke etiology. The treatment and prognosis of certain etiologies vary; therefore, treatment and work-up must be adapted accordingly [49, 50].

In general, in addition to plain computerized tomography (CT) images, angio-CT should be performed, and when the timing or presence of a stroke is not certain, a perfusion imaging modality should be considered too [51]. If the diagnosis is not certain or clear, additional studies and sequences should be considered, including CT venography, magnetic resonance imaging (MRI), and digital subtraction angiography (DSA) [52]. Table 4.2 summarizes the main imaging findings in acute ischemic stroke [53].

Table 4.2 The main imaging findings in acute ischemic stroke

Imaging modality	Findings
Computerized tomography	Hyperdense vessel sign Loss of gray–white matter differentiation Hypoattenuation of deep nuclei Cortical hypodensity
CT perfusion	Ischemic penumbra and core
CT angiography	Vessel occlusion Atherosclerosis Dissection signs
Magnetic resonance imaging	Increased diffusion weight imaging signal and reduced apparent diffusion coefficient Hyperintensity and cortical contrast enhancement in T2/FLAIR sequences

4.3 Neuroimaging of Headache Attributed to Nonvascular Intracranial Disorder

The group 7 of the International Classification of Headache Disorders includes a wide range of disorders [5]. Table 4.3 lists the disorders included into this group. Headache is often the symptom that led to the diagnosis [54, 55], and imaging is usually key in the diagnosis of most of these cases [54, 55].

In the case of intracranial hypertension, imaging findings that may suggest a raised intracranial pressure include effacement of the ventricles, basal cisterns and other CSF spaces, loss of gray–white matter differentiation, and ultimately brain herniation [56]. Imaging is necessary also in the differential diagnosis between primary and secondary causes of these, including cerebral venous sinus thrombosis, hydrocephalus, drugs, infections, hormonal disorders, or space-occupying lesions [57, 58]. Table 4.4 summarizes the typical imaging findings of idiopathic intracranial hypertension [59].

On the other face of the coin, intracranial hypotension can be suspected based on imaging findings in patients with orthostatic or atypical headache. Indeed, lumbar puncture may worsen the syndrome, and it is currently not recommended as a first-line diagnostic measure; however, up to 19% of patients may have a normal brain magnetic resonance findings [60]. Imaging findings include diffuse enhancement of the pachymeninges in contrast-enhanced sequences, engorgement of the venous sinuses, subdural fluid collections, sagging brain, and pituitary hyperemia and enlargement [60–62].

Sarcoidosis and other granulomatous disorders can manifest in various ways, with headache being one of the possibilities [63, 64]. From the imaging perspective, findings can occur from the skull to the parenchyma, including pachymeningeal and leptomeningeal involvement, with cranial nerve involvement and pituitary and hypothalamic abnormalities within the most typical features. Brain lesions are usually adjacent to gray matter and show a homogeneous enhancement [65–67].

Table 4.3 Disorders included in group 7 of the international classification of headache disorders

Group	Name	Disorders
7.1	Headache attributed to increased cerebrospinal fluid (CSF) pressure	
7.1.1		Headache attributed to idiopathic intracranial hypertension (IIH)
7.1.2		Headache attributed to intracranial hypertension secondary to metabolic, toxic, or hormonal cause
7.1.3		Headache attributed to intracranial hypertension secondary to chromosomal disorder
7.1.4		Headache attributed to intracranial hypertension secondary to hydrocephalus
7.2	Headache attributed to low cerebrospinal fluid (CSF) pressure	
7.2.1		Post-dural puncture headache
7.2.2		Cerebrospinal fluid (CSF) fistula headache
7.2.3		Headache attributed to spontaneous intracranial hypotension
7.3	Headache attributed to noninfectious inflammatory intracranial disease	
7.3.1		Headache attributed to neurosarcoidosis
7.3.2		Headache attributed to aseptic (noninfectious) meningitis
7.3.3		Headache attributed to other noninfectious inflammatory intracranial disease
7.3.4		Headache attributed to lymphocytic hypophysitis
7.3.5		Syndrome of transient headache and neurological deficits with cerebrospinal fluid lymphocytosis (HaNDL)
7.4	Headache attributed to intracranial neoplasia	
7.4.1		Headache attributed to intracranial neoplasm
7.4.1.1		Headache attributed to colloid cyst of the third ventricle
7.4.2		Headache attributed to carcinomatous meningitis
7.4.3		Headache attributed to hypothalamic or pituitary hyper- or hyposecretion
7.5	Headache attributed to intrathecal injection	
7.6	Headache attributed to epileptic seizure	
7.6.1		Ictal epileptic headache
7.6.2		Postictal headache
7.7	Headache attributed to Chiari malformation type I (CM1)	
7.8	Headache attributed to other nonvascular intracranial disorder	

Table 4.4 Imaging findings of idiopathic intracranial hypertension

Region	Findings
Venous system	Transverse sinus stenosis, internal jugular vein stenosis
Ventricles	Slit-like ventricles
Arachnoid space	Empty sella turcica, Meckel cave enlargement, prominent perivascular spaces, arachnoid pits, enlarged oculomotor cistern
Orbits	Optic nerve sheath distention, posterior globe flattening, optic nerve tortuosity, optic nerve head protrusion, optic nerve head enhancement

Headache is the first and isolated manifestation of brain tumors in around 8% of cases [68], but up to 48–60% of patients present it during the course of the disease [69, 70]. Headache was reported as non-specific in most cases [69–72]; however, the presence of a secondary cause can be suspected based on the presence of red flags [71, 72]. In these patients, imaging is crucial in the diagnosis of intracranial neoplasms [73]. In the diagnosis of brain neoplasms, age, past history of the patient, and the imaging pattern can suggest the underlying etiology [74]. The most common primary tumors are neuroepithelial tumors, mostly astrocytoma, followed by ependymoma, medulloblastoma, and oligodendroglioma. Meningiomas, pituitary tumors, vestibular schwannoma, primary central nervous system lymphoma, and pineal tumors are less prevalent [75, 76].

Chiari I malformation is another disorder that can only be diagnosed in vivo by imaging. It is characterized by the caudal descent of the cerebellar tonsils through the foramen magnum [77]. The most frequent clinical presentation is asymptomatic [78]. Whenever symptomatic, occipital headache precipitated by cough or Valsalva maneuver is typical [79]. The degree of tonsillar herniation has been associated with the presence of headache [79]. In patients with headache precipitated by cough, it is more common to find a secondary cause, mostly Chiari I malformation, than a primary cough headache [80].

4.4 Neuroimaging of Headache Attributed to Infection

Headache disorders and meningitis are within the top neurological contributors to Disability-Adjusted Life Years [81]. The International Classification of Headache Disorders (ICHD) differentiates between headache attributed to intracranial or systemic infections [5]. In the first case, headache is one of the commonest symptoms of bacterial meningitis (83–87% of cases, [82, 83]), viral meningitis (91% of cases [84, 85]), and encephalitis (73% of cases [86]). Headache is part of the meningeal irritation syndrome, wherein the case of bacterial, viral, mycobacterial, or fungal meningitis is caused by the activation of meningeal nociceptors either by the action of the pathogen and its virulence factors or as collateral damage of the immune system response [87].

In the diagnosis of the infection, for example, in meningitis, brain imaging may look normal, and unless post-contrast sequences are acquired, the typical imaging symptoms may not be evident. Table 4.5 shows the typical CT imaging findings and MRI findings of bacterial meningitis.

Table 4.5 Imaging findings of uncomplicated bacterial meningitis

Imaging modality	Findings
Computerized tomography	Sulcal effacement Hyperattenuation of gray matter
Magnetic resonance	Increased T2/FLAIR signal in the cortex
Post-contrast imaging	Leptomeningeal enhancement

Table 4.6 Clinical features of meningeal irritation syndrome and intracranial hypertension

Feature	Meningeal irritation syndrome	Raised intracranial pressure syndrome
Worsening factors	Physical activity, head movements	Decubitus, Valsalva
Associated symptoms	Photophobia, phonophobia, nausea, vomiting	Nausea, vomiting, blurred vision, diplopia
Clinical signs	Kernig, Brudzinski, Jolt	Papilledema, increased blind spot, VI nerve palsy

In some cases, it may reflect the presence of certain complications, such as intracranial hypertension, cerebral venous sinus thrombosis, abscesses, or infective angiitis [88, 89]. Imaging is crucial to detect most of these complications. Table 4.6 shows the clinical features of the two most frequent symptoms associated to headache attributed to intracranial infections, meningeal irritation, and intracranial hypertension [90, 91].

In the case of intracranial hypertension, headache is within the most common symptoms [92]. Imaging findings include increased perioptic nerve space within the nerve sheath, posterior globe flattening, optic nerve tortuosity, venous sinus stenosis, empty *sella turcica*, and slit-like ventricles [93]. Its early detection is crucial, to avoid persistent morbidity by a prompt management [94]. However, the integration of clinical symptoms and signs and the specific evaluation of imaging findings may increase the sensitivity and specificity of imaging biomarkers, since the imaging markers are not neither sensitive nor specific when evaluated in isolation [94, 95].

Headache is the most frequent symptom of abscesses, observed in 69% of cases [96]. Imaging is necessary to diagnose this complication and define the phase of the lesion. This is relevant for both selecting the optimal treatment and ensuring the adequate treatment response. Table 4.7 summarizes the imaging findings depending on the stage of the brain abscess [97–101].

As in most secondary causes of headache, some patients may remain with headache after the acute phase. In bacterial meningitis, around 31% of adult patients of a study with community-acquired bacterial meningitis remained with headache 12 months after the acute phase, with pre-existing headache, higher neutrophilic count in the cerebrospinal fluid, and brain abscesses associated with the persistence of the headache [102]. In the case of encephalitis, about 13–21% of patients exhibited persistent headache following resolution of the infection [103–106]. In some of these cases, such as headache in patients with long effects of coronavirus disease (COVID-19), regular protocols for CT and MRI mostly show normal findings [106]. However, advanced post-processing of MRI may show subtle differences, such as lower cortical gray matter volume and cortical thickness in the inferior frontal and the fusiform cortex [107, 108]. Also, resting-state functional connectivity points to weakened functional connections between the cingulate, hippocampal gyri, parietal, temporal, and frontal gyri [109]. In addition, white matter changes have been reported in post-COVID-19 syndrome associated with headache, compared with healthy controls, with higher axial diffusivity in corona radiata, and

Table 4.7 The imaging findings depending on the stage of the brain abscess

Phase	CT findings	MRI findings
Early cerebritis	Normal CT Cortico-subcortical hypodensity with mass effect Little or absence of enhancement	Iso-hypointense in T1; hyperintense in T2/FLAIR; T1 C+ with no enhancement or minimal enhancement; DWI/ADC: restricted diffusion
Late cerebritis	Similar to early cerebritis, but more defined, still irregular Rim-enhancing lesion with a hypodense center	Progressive enhancement, peripheral and not well defined; progressive restricted diffusion
Early encapsulation	Outer hypodense and inner hyperdense rim (double rim sign); ring of iso-/hyperdense tissue, of uniform thickness; central low attenuation (fluid/pus); surrounding low density (vasogenic edema)	T1: Central low isointensity, peripheral hypointensity (vasogenic edema), ring enhancement T2/FLAIR: Central high intensity (does not attenuate on FLAIR). Peripheral high intensity (vasogenic edema), capsule visible as a slightly lower signal than the rim DWI/ADC: High DWI signal centrally, with true restricted diffusion. Peripheral or patchy restricted diffusion SWI: Low-intensity rim
Late encapsulation	Progressive central necrosis; decreased surrounding edema	
Complications	Ventriculitis (ependyma enhancement); obstructive hydrocephalus	

internal and external capsules, as well as lower fractional anisotropy and higher radial diffusivity in the corpus callosum and left hemisphere [108, 110]. However, the specificity of these changes regarding headache associated with post-COVID-19 syndrome is still to be determined. Moreover, patients with new-onset headache, 1 week after vaccination with an adenovirus vector-based vaccine, should undergo neuroimaging to rule out cerebral venous thrombosis and intracranial hemorrhage [111].

4.4.1 Encephalitis

Imaging is also important in the diagnosis of encephalitis; however, this diagnosis can be made with a fully normal imaging study [112]. Imaging is usually nonspecific, and despite some findings that may be linked to a certain cause, microbiological tests remain the gold standard of etiologic diagnosis. Table 4.8 summarizes

Table 4.8 The imaging findings of some of the commonest encephalitis causes

Diagnosis	Typical imaging findings	CT findings	MRI findings
Herpes simplex encephalitis [113–115]	Bilateral asymmetrical involvement of the limbic system, medial temporal lobes, insular cortices, and inferior frontal lobes Basal ganglia sparing	Normal findings Hypodensity within the anterior and medial temporal lobe and insular cortex	T1: General edema in the affected region, hyperintense signal if hemorrhages T1C+: Enhancement later, localized in gyral, leptomeningeal, ring or diffuse T2: Hyperintensity of white matter and cortex DWI/ADC: More sensitive than T2, cytotoxic edema
Cytomegalovirus [115, 116]	Meningoencephalitis ventriculitis with/without ependymitis	Hydrocephalus	T2: Periventricular hyperintensity No mass effect Enhancement of the ependymal surface
Flavivirus [117, 118]			T2: Hyperintensity in the basal ganglia and/or thalamus DWI/ADC: Restricted diffusion in the basal ganglia and/or thalamus
Dengue [119–122]	Typical involvement of thalami, basal ganglia, cortico-subcortical gray matter, and deep white matter	Hyperdense intraparenchymal lesions if hemorrhages	T2/FLAIR: Hyperintense signal in the affected areas DWI/ADC: Restricted diffusion in the affected areas. Double doughnut sign SWI: Microhemorrhages are common
Japanese [121, 123, 124]	Bilateral thalamic involvement Midbrain, pons, cerebellum, basal ganglia lesions	Symmetric or asymmetric bilateral thalamic hypodensities	T2/FLAIR hyperintensity in the affected regions DWI/ADC: Variable restricted diffusion T1: Hypodensity in affected regions SWI: If hemorrhages are present
Rabies [125–127]	Predilection of gray matter structure	Normal Non-specific hypoattenuation of the brainstem, mesial temporal lobes, basal ganglia, or periventricular white matter Hemorrhage, cerebral swelling	T2/FLAIR hyperintensity in the basal ganglia, thalami, hypothalamic, brainstem, limbic system, spinal cord, frontal and parietal lobes Spinal cord involvement

(continued)

Table 4.8 (continued)

Diagnosis	Typical imaging findings	CT findings	MRI findings
Nipah [128–130]	Small, round lesions in white matter, temporal lobe, pons, and peduncles The lesions may be confluent	Normal	T1: Hyperintense lesions. No edema or mass effect T1C+: Normal T2/FLAIR Hyperintensity on the affected lesions DWI/ADC: Restricted diffusion
Tick-borne [131, 132]	Involvement of thalamus, basal ganglia, cerebellum, and anterior horns of the spinal cord	Normal/unspecific	T1: Involvement of meninges in the cerebellar folia and the basal cisterns T2/FLAIR: Focal or diffuse hyperintensities in the affected regions
Human herpesvirus 6 [133]	Mesial temporal lobes involvement Extratemporal involvement is unusual and, whenever present, circumscribed to the surrounding areas of temporal lobes	Normal/unspecific	T2/FLAIR: Hyperintensity on the affected regions DWI/ADC: Restricted diffusion in the affected regions
Epstein–Barr virus [134, 135]		Normal/unspecific	T2/FLAIR: Hyperintensity in multiple regions, mostly within the sub-cortical white matter and deep gray nuclei DWI: High diffusion signal
Malaria [136–138]	Ischemic and hemorrhagic changes in the deep white matter, cortex, basal ganglia, thalami or cerebellum	Cerebral edema Thalamic hypoattenuation Cerebellar white matter hypoattenuation	T2/FLAIR: Non-specific hyperintensities in the bilateral periventricular white matter, corpus callosum, occipital subcortex, basal ganglia, and thalamic regions DWI/ADC: Restricted diffusion if ischemic lesions SWI: Microbleeds within the infarcted tissue

the imaging findings of some of the commonest encephalitis causes. Headache could be present in patients with encephalitis; nevertheless, most patients will exhibit other accompanying neurological and systemic symptoms [113–138].

4.5 Conclusions

This chapter highlights the pivotal role of neuroimaging in advancing our understanding of secondary headache disorders, offering insights into their pathophysiology and diagnosis. Furthermore, this chapter emphasizes the importance of multimodal imaging approaches, which combine structural, functional, and metabolic data, to uncover unique patterns associated with secondary headaches. However, despite significant progress, several challenges remain, particularly in standardizing imaging protocols and integrating advanced imaging modalities into routine clinical practice.

References

1. Dewan M, Rattani A, Gupta S, et al. Estimating the global incidence of traumatic brain injury. J Neurosurg. 2018;130:1080–97.
2. Lucas S, Hoffman JM, Bell KR, et al. Characterization of headache after traumatic brain injury. Cephalalgia. 2012;32:600–6.
3. Lucas S, Hoffman JM, Bell KR, Dikmen S. A prospective study of prevalence and characterization of headache following mild traumatic brain injury. Cephalalgia. 2014;34:93–102.
4. GBD 2015 Disease and Injury Incidence and Prevalence Collaborators. Global, regional, and national incidence, prevalence, and years lived with disability for 310 diseases and injuries, 1990–2015: a systematic analysis for the Global Burden of Disease Study 2015. Lancet. 2016;388:1545–602.
5. Headache Classification Committee of the International Headache Society (IHS). The international classification of headache disorders, 3rd edition. Cephalalgia. 2018;38:1–211.
6. Labastida-Ramírez A, Benemei S, Albanese M, et al. Persistent post-traumatic headache: a migrainous loop or not? The clinical evidence. J Headache Pain. 2020;21:55.
7. Gilkey SJ, Ramadan NM, Aurora TK, Welch KM. Cerebral blood flow in chronic posttraumatic headache. Headache. 1997;37:583–7.
8. Sarmento E, Moreira P, Brito C, et al. Proton spectroscopy in patients with post-traumatic headache attributed to mild head injury. Headache. 2009;49:1345–52.
9. Alhilali LM, Delic J, Fakhran S. Differences in callosal and forniceal diffusion between patients with and without postconcussive migraine. AJNR Am J Neuroradiol. 2017;38:691–5.
10. Dumkrieger G, Chong CD, Ross K, et al. Static and dynamic functional connectivity differences between migraine and persistent post-traumatic headache: a resting-state magnetic resonance imaging study. Cephalalgia. 2019;39:1366–81.
11. Chong CD, Berisha V, Ross K, et al. Distinguishing persistent post-traumatic headache from migraine: classification based on clinical symptoms and brain structural MRI data. Cephalalgia. 2021;41:943–55.

12. Burrowes SAB, Rhodes CS, Meeker TJ, et al. Decreased grey matter volume in mTBI patients with post-traumatic headache compared to headache-free mTBI patients and healthy controls: a longitudinal MRI study. Brain Imaging Behav. 2020;14:1651–9.
13. Obermann M, Nebel K, Schumann C, et al. Gray matter changes related to chronic posttraumatic headache. Neurology. 2009;73:978–83.
14. Xu H, Xu C, Guo Y, et al. Abnormal longitudinal changes of structural covariance networks of cortical thickness in mild traumatic brain injury with posttraumatic headache. Prog Neuro-Psychopharmacol Biol Psychiatry. 2024;133:111012.
15. Xu H, Xu C, Gu P, et al. Neuroanatomical restoration of salience network links reduced headache impact to cognitive function improvement in mild traumatic brain injury with post-traumatic headache. J Headache Pain. 2023;24:43.
16. Niu X, Bai L, Sun Y, et al. Disruption of periaqueductal grey-default mode network functional connectivity predicts persistent post-traumatic headache in mild traumatic brain injury. J Neurol Neurosurg Psychiatry. 2019;90:326–32.
17. Welch KM, Nagesh V, Aurora SK, Gelman N. Periaqueductal gray matter dysfunction in migraine: cause or the burden of illness? Headache. 2001;4:629–37.
18. Dominguez C, Lopez A, Ramos-Cabrer P, et al. Iron deposition in periaqueductal gray matter as a potential biomarker for chronic migraine. Neurology. 2019;92:e1076–85.
19. Li F, Zhang D, Ren J, et al. Connectivity of the insular subdivisions differentiates posttraumatic headache-associated from nonheadache-associated mild traumatic brain injury: an arterial spin labelling study. J Headache Pain. 2024;25:103.
20. Li F, Lu L, Shang S, et al. Altered static and dynamic functional network connectivity in post-traumatic headache. J Headache Pain. 2021;22:137.
21. Flowers M, Leung A, Schiehser DM, et al. Severities in persistent mild traumatic brain injury related headache is associated with changes in supraspinal pain modulatory functions. Mol Pain. 2021;17:17448069211037881.
22. Lu L, Li F, Wang P, et al. Altered hypothalamic functional connectivity in post-traumatic headache after mild traumatic brain injury. J Headache Pain. 2020;21:93.
23. Schulte LH, May A. The migraine generator revisited: continuous scanning of the migraine cycle over 30 days and three spontaneous attacks. Brain. 2016;139:1987–93.
24. Lerebours F, Boulanouar K, Barège M, et al. Functional connectivity of hypothalamus in chronic migraine with medication overuse. Cephalalgia. 2019;39:892–9.
25. Chen Z, Chen X, Liu M, et al. Volume of hypothalamus as a diagnostic biomarker of chronic migraine. Front Neurol. 2019;10:606.
26. Chong CD, Nikolova S, Dumkrieger G, et al. Thalamic subfield iron accumulation after acute mild traumatic brain injury as a marker of future post-traumatic headache intensity. Headache. 2023;63:156–64.
27. Nikolova S, Chong C, Li J, et al. Brain structural and functional abnormalities associated with acute post-traumatic headache: iron deposition and functional connectivity. J Headache Pain. 2024;25:88.
28. Lemme J, Holmes S, Sibai D, et al. Altered brain network connectivity underlies persistent post-traumatic headache following mild traumatic brain injury in youth. J Neurotrauma. 2021;38:1632–41.
29. Chong CD, Berisha V, Chiang CC, et al. Less cortical thickness in patients with persistent post-traumatic headache compared with healthy controls: an MRI study. Headache. 2018;58:53–61.
30. Monroe KS, Schiehser DM, Parr AW et al. Biological markers of brain network connectivity and pain sensitivity distinguish low coping from high coping Veterans with persistent post-traumatic headache. medRxiv [Preprint]; 2024. https://doi.org/10.1101/2024.09.16.24313761
31. Vanier C, Santhanam P, Rochester N, et al. Symptom persistence relates to volume and asymmetry of the limbic system after mild traumatic brain injury. J Clin Med. 2024;13:5154.

32. Defrin R, Riabinin M, Feingold Y, et al. Deficient pain modulatory systems in patients with mild traumatic brain and chronic post-traumatic headache: implications for its mechanism. J Neurotrauma. 2015;32:28–37.
33. Menon V, Uddin LQ. Saliency, switching, attention and control: a network model of insula function. Brain Struct Funct. 2010;214:655–67.
34. Lebedeva ER, Ushenin AV, Gurary NM, et al. Headache at onset of first-ever ischemic stroke: clinical characteristics and predictors. Eur J Neurol. 2021;28:852–60.
35. GBD 2021 Diseases and Injuries Collaborators. Global incidence, prevalence, years lived with disability (YLDs), disability-adjusted life-years (DALYs), and healthy life expectancy (HALE) for 371 diseases and injuries in 204 countries and territories and 811 subnational locations, 1990–2021: a systematic analysis for the Global Burden of Disease Study 2021. Lancet. 2024;403:2133–61.
36. Hussein M, Ali M, Abdelghaffar M, et al. Frequency, characteristics, and predictors of headache attributed to acute ischemic stroke. Rev Neurol (Paris). 2023;179:1000–7.
37. Wang Y, Cheng W, Lian Y. The headache and neck pain in ischemic stroke patients caused by cervicocerebral artery dissection. A case-control study. J Stroke Cerebrovasc Dis. 2019;28:557–61.
38. Martins BP, Mesquita I, Sousa JM, et al. Persistent headache attributed to past cervicocephalic artery dissection: clinical characteristics and contributors to headache persistence. Cephalalgia. 2023;43:3331024221144782.
39. Lebedeva ER, Ushenin AV, Gurary NM, et al. Persistent headache after first-ever ischemic stroke: clinical characteristics and factors associated with its development. J Headache Pain. 2022;23:103.
40. de Oliveira FAA, Dourado-Filho MG, Sampaio Rocha-Filho PA. Persistent headache attributed to past ischemic stroke: a prospective cohort study. Headache. 2024;64:48–54.
41. Kablau M, Kreisel SH, Sauer T, et al. Predictors and early outcome of hemorrhagic transformation after acute ischemic stroke. Cerebrovasc Dis. 2011;32:334–41.
42. Chaudhry SA, Kwon SY, Kneale H, et al. Post-IV thrombolytic headache and hemorrhagic transformation risk in acute ischemic stroke. Neurol Clin Pract. 2016;6:22–8.
43. Ge WQ, Chen J, Pan H, et al. Analysis of risk factors increased hemorrhagic transformation after acute ischemic stroke. J Stroke Cerebrovasc Dis. 2018;27:3587–90.
44. Heiss WD. Malignant MCA infarction: pathophysiology and imaging for early diagnosis and management decisions. Cerebrovasc Dis. 2016;1:1–7.
45. Wang Y, Shen X, Wang P, Fang Q. Clinical characteristics of cerebral venous sinus thrombosis patients with new-onset of headache. BMC Neurol. 2023;23:56.
46. García-Azorín D, Monje MHG, González-García N, et al. Presence of red flags in patients with cerebral venous sinus thrombosis admitted to the emergency department because of headache: a STROBE compliant cohort-study. Medicine (Baltimore). 2020;99:e20900.
47. Mehta A, Danesh J, Kuruvilla D. Cerebral venous thrombosis headache. Curr Pain Headache Rep. 2019;23:47.
48. Ranjan R, Ken-Dror G, Sharma P. Pathophysiology, diagnosis and management of cerebral venous thrombosis: a comprehensive review. Medicine (Baltimore). 2023;102:e36366.
49. Powers WJ, Rabinstein AA, Ackerson T, et al. Guidelines for the early management of patients with acute ischemic stroke: 2019 update to the 2018 guidelines for the early management of acute ischemic stroke: a guideline for healthcare professionals from the American Heart Association/American Stroke Association. Stroke. 2019;50:e344–418.
50. Saposnik G, Bushnell C, Coutinho JM, et al. Diagnosis and management of cerebral venous thrombosis: a scientific statement from the American Heart Association. Stroke. 2024;55:e77–90.
51. Grau García M, Pérez Bea M, Angulo Saiz A, et al. Update on imaging in code stroke. Radiologia (Engl Ed). 2023;65:S3–S10.
52. Kumar M, Hu S, Beyea S, Kamal N. Is improved access to magnetic resonance imaging imperative for optimal ischemic stroke care? J Neurol Sci. 2023;446:120592.

53. Potter CA, Vagal AS, Goyal M, et al. CT for treatment selection in acute ischemic stroke: a code stroke primer. Radiographics. 2019;39:1717–38.
54. Diener HC, Johansson U, Dodick DW. Headache attributed to non-vascular intracranial disorder. Handb Clin Neurol. 2010;97:547–87.
55. Obermann M, Holle D, Naegel S, Diener HC. Headache attributable to nonvascular intracranial disorders. Curr Pain Headache Rep. 2011;15:314–23.
56. Kareemi H, Pratte M, English S, Hendin A. Initial diagnosis and management of acutely elevated intracranial pressure. J Intensive Care Med. 2023;38:643–50.
57. Friedman DI, Jacobson DM. Diagnostic criteria for idiopathic intracranial hypertension. Neurology. 2002;59:1492–5.
58. Kilic K, Korsbæk JJ, Jensen RH, Cvetkovic VV. Diagnosis of idiopathic intracranial hypertension – the importance of excluding secondary causes: a systematic review. Cephalalgia. 2022;42:524–41.
59. Beier D, Korsbæk JJ, Bsteh G, et al. Magnetic resonance imaging signs of idiopathic intracranial hypertension. JAMA Netw Open. 2024;7:e2420138.
60. D'Antona L, Merchan MAJ, Vassiliou A, et al. Clinical presentation, investigation findings, and treatment outcomes of spontaneous intracranial hypotension syndrome: a systematic review and meta-analysis. JAMA Neurol. 2021;78:329–37.
61. Wang SJ. Spontaneous intracranial hypotension. Continuum (Minneap Minn). 2021;27:746–66.
62. Wu JW, Wang SJ. Spontaneous intracranial hypotension: clinical presentation, diagnosis, and treatment strategies. Neurol Clin. 2024;42:473–86.
63. Tana C, Azorin DG, Cinetto F, et al. Common clinical and molecular pathways between migraine and sarcoidosis. Int J Mol Sci. 2023;24:8304.
64. Fritz D, van de Beek D, Brouwer MC. Clinical features, treatment and outcome in neurosarcoidosis: systematic review and meta-analysis. BMC Neurol. 2016;16:220.
65. Smith JK, Matheus MG, Castillo M. Imaging manifestations of neurosarcoidosis. AJR Am J Roentgenol. 2004;182:289–95.
66. Shah R, Roberson GH, Curé JK. Correlation of MR imaging findings and clinical manifestations in neurosarcoidosis. AJNR Am J Neuroradiol. 2009;30:953–61.
67. Lord J, Paz Soldan MM, Galli J, et al. Neurosarcoidosis: longitudinal experience in a single-center, academic healthcare system. Neurol Neuroimmunol Neuroinflamm. 2020;7:e743.
68. Vázquez-Barquero A, Ibáñez FJ, Herrera S, et al. Isolated headache as the presenting clinical manifestation of intracranial tumors: a prospective study. Cephalalgia. 1994;14:270–2.
69. Valentinis L, Tuniz F, Valent F, et al. Headache attributed to intracranial tumours: a prospective cohort study. Cephalalgia. 2010;30:389–98.
70. Schankin CJ, Ferrari U, Reinisch VM, et al. Characteristics of brain tumour-associated headache. Cephalalgia. 2007;27:904–11.
71. Pfund Z, Szapáry L, Jászberényi O, et al. Headache in intracranial tumors. Cephalalgia. 1999;19:787–90.
72. Palmieri A, Valentinis L, Zanchin G. Update on headache and brain tumors. Cephalalgia. 2021;41:431–7.
73. Hadidchi S, Surento W, Lerner A, et al. Headache and brain tumor. Neuroimaging Clin N Am. 2019;29:291–300.
74. Gritsch S, Batchelor TT, Gonzalez Castro LN. Diagnostic, therapeutic, and prognostic implications of the 2021 World Health Organization classification of tumors of the central nervous system. Cancer. 2022;128:47–58.
75. McNeill KA. Epidemiology of brain tumors. Neurol Clin. 2016;34:981–98.
76. Miller KD, Ostrom QT, Kruchko C, et al. Brain and other central nervous system tumor statistics, 2021. CA Cancer J Clin. 2021;71:381–406.
77. Elster AD, Chen MY. Chiari I malformations: clinical and radiologic reappraisal. Radiology. 1992;183:347–53.

78. Meadows J, Kraut M, Guarnieri M, et al. Asymptomatic Chiari type I malformations identified on magnetic resonance imaging. J Neurosurg. 2000;92:920–6.
79. Pascual J, Oterino A, Berciano J. Headache in type I Chiari malformation. Neurology. 1992;42:1519–21.
80. Pascual J, González-Mandly A, Martín R, Oterino A. Headaches precipitated by cough, prolonged exercise or sexual activity: a prospective etiological and clinical study. J Headache Pain. 2008;9:259–66.
81. GBD 2016 Neurology Collaborators. Global, regional, and national burden of neurological disorders, 1990–2016: a systematic analysis for the Global Burden of Disease Study 2016. Lancet Neurol. 2019;18:459–80.
82. van de Beek D, de Gans J, Spanjaard L, et al. Clinical features and prognostic factors in adults with bacterial meningitis. N Engl J Med. 2004;351:1849–59.
83. Bijlsma MW, Brouwer MC, Kasanmoentalib ES, et al. Community-acquired bacterial meningitis in adults in The Netherlands, 2006–14: a prospective cohort study. Lancet Infect Dis. 2016;16:339–47.
84. Petersen PT, Bodilsen J, Jepsen MPG, et al. Clinical features and prognostic factors in adults with viral meningitis. Brain. 2023;146:3816–25.
85. Jakobsen A, Skov MT, Larsen L, et al. Herpes simplex virus 2 meningitis in adults: a prospective, nationwide, population-based cohort study. Clin Infect Dis. 2022;75:753–60.
86. Babaei A, Shatizadeh Malekshahi S, et al. Prevalence and clinical manifestations of herpes simplex virus infection among suspected patients of herpes simplex encephalitis in Shiraz, Iran. Virusdisease. 2021;32:266–71.
87. Lin AL, Safdieh JE. The evaluation and management of bacterial meningitis: current practice and emerging developments. Neurologist. 2010;16:143–51.
88. Kanamalla US, Ibarra RA, Jinkins JR. Imaging of cranial meningitis and ventriculitis. Neuroimaging Clin N Am. 2000;10:309–31.
89. Kojan S, Al-Jumah M. Infection related cerebral venous thrombosis. J Pak Med Assoc. 2006;56:494–7.
90. Rehder D. Idiopathic intracranial hypertension: review of clinical syndrome, imaging findings, and treatment. Curr Probl Diagn Radiol. 2020;49:205–14.
91. Iguchi M, Noguchi Y, Yamamoto S, et al. Diagnostic test accuracy of jolt accentuation for headache in acute meningitis in the emergency setting. Cochrane Database Syst Rev. 2020;6:CD012824.
92. Barkatullah AF, Leishangthem L, Moss HE. MRI findings as markers of idiopathic intracranial hypertension. Curr Opin Neurol. 2021;34:75–83.
93. El-Hajj VG, Pettersson I, Gharios M, et al. Detection and management of elevated intracranial pressure in the treatment of acute community-acquired bacterial meningitis: a systematic review. Neurocrit Care. 2024;41:228–43.
94. Bsteh G, Marik W, Macher S, et al. Impact of rater experience and referral question on detecting magnetic resonance imaging features of idiopathic intracranial hypertension. Eur J Neurol. 2023;30:3314–21.
95. Agid R, Farb RI, Willinsky RA, et al. Idiopathic intracranial hypertension: the validity of cross-sectional neuroimaging signs. Neuroradiology. 2006;48:521–7.
96. Haimes AB, Zimmerman RD, Morgello S, et al. MR imaging of brain abscesses. AJR Am J Roentgenol. 1989;152:1073–85.
97. Hartmann M, Jansen O, Heiland S, et al. Restricted diffusion within ring enhancement is not pathognomonic for brain abscess. AJNR Am J Neuroradiol. 2001;22:1738–42.
98. Cartes-Zumelzu FW, Stavrou I, Castillo M, et al. Diffusion-weighted imaging in the assessment of brain abscesses therapy. AJNR Am J Neuroradiol. 2004;25:1310–7.
99. Toh CH, Wei KC, Chang CN, et al. Differentiation of pyogenic brain abscesses from necrotic glioblastomas with use of susceptibility-weighted imaging. AJNR Am J Neuroradiol. 2012;33:1534–8.
100. Patel K, Clifford DB. Bacterial brain abscess. Neurohospitalist. 2014;4:196–204.

101. Schwitter J, Branca M, Bicvic A, et al. Long-term sequelae after viral meningitis and meningoencephalitis are frequent, even in mildly affected patients, a prospective observational study. Front Neurol. 2024;15:1411860.
102. Van RN, Tubiana S, De Broucker T, et al. Persistent headaches one year after bacterial meningitis: prevalence, determinants and impact on quality of life. Eur J Clin Microbiol Infect Dis. 2023;42:1459–67.
103. Brouwer MC, Coutinho JM, van de Beek D. Clinical characteristics and outcome of brain abscess: systematic review and meta-analysis. Neurology. 2014;82:806–13.
104. Rocha ND, de Moura SK, da Silva GAB, et al. Neurological sequelae after encephalitis associated with herpes simplex virus in children: systematic review and meta-analysis. BMC Infect Dis. 2023;23:55.
105. Ungureanu A, van der Meer J, Bicvic A, et al. Meningitis, meningoencephalitis and encephalitis in Bern: an observational study of 258 patients. BMC Neurol. 2021;21:474.
106. Tana C, Bentivegna E, Cho S-J, et al. Long COVID headache. J Headache Pain. 2022;23:93.
107. Douaud G, Lee S, Alfaro-Almagro F, et al. SARS-CoV-2 is associated with changes in brain structure in UK Biobank. Nature. 2022;604:697–707.
108. Planchuelo-Gómez A, García-Azorín D, Guerrero AL, et al. Structural brain changes in patients with persistent headache after COVID-19 resolution. J Neurol. 2023;270:13–31.
109. Planchuelo-Gómez A, García-Azorín D, Guerrero Peral AL, et al. Gray matter cortical changes in patients with persistent headache after COVID-19 infection: an exploratory study. The international headache congress – IHS and EHF joint congress 2021: Virtual. 8–12 September 2021. J Headache Pain. 2021;22:103.
110. Planchuelo-Gómez A, García-Azorín D, Guerrero Peral AL, et al. White matter microstructural alterations in patients with persistent headache after COVID-19 infection: an exploratory study. The international headache congress – IHS and EHF joint congress 2021: Virtual. 8–12 September 2021. J Headache Pain. 2021;22:103.
111. García-Azorín D, Do TP, Gantenbein AR, et al. Delayed headache after COVID-19 vaccination: a red flag for vaccine induced cerebral venous thrombosis. J Headache Pain. 2021;22:108.
112. Bewersdorf JP, Koedel U, Patzig M, et al. Challenges in HSV encephalitis: normocellular CSF, unremarkable CCT, and atypical MRI findings. Infection. 2019;47:267–73.
113. Solbrig MV, Hasso AN, Jay CA. CNS viruses—diagnostic approach. Neuroimaging Clin N Am. 2008;18:1–18.
114. Bradshaw MJ, Venkatesan A. Herpes simplex virus-1 encephalitis in adults: pathophysiology, diagnosis, and management. Neurotherapeutics. 2016;13:493–508.
115. Smith AB, Smirniotopoulos JG, Rushing EJ. From the archives of the AFIP: central nervous system infections associated with human immunodeficiency virus infection: radiologic-pathologic correlation. Radiographics. 2008;28:2033–58.
116. John KJ, Gunasekaran K, Sultan N, Iyyadurai R. Cytomegalovirus ventriculoencephalitis presenting with hydrocephalus in a patient with advanced HIV infection. Oxf Med Case Rep. 2019;2019:omz104.
117. Solomon T. Flavivirus encephalitis. N Engl J Med. 2004;351:370–8.
118. Turtle L, Griffiths MJ, Solomon T. Encephalitis caused by flaviviruses. QJM. 2012;105:219–23.
119. Mishra A, Pandey S. Generalized dystonia/parkinsonism and double-doughnut sign in dengue encephalitis. Mov Disord Clin Pract. 2020;7:585–6.
120. Chatur C, Balani A, Kumar A, et al. "Double doughnut" sign – could it be a diagnostic marker for dengue encephalitis? Neurol India. 2019;67:1360–2.
121. Pichl T, Wedderburn CJ, Hoskote C, et al. A systematic review of brain imaging findings in neurological infection with Japanese encephalitis virus compared with Dengue virus. Int J Infect Dis. 2022;119:102–10.
122. Vanjare HA, Mannam P, Mishra AK, et al. Brain imaging in cases with positive serology for dengue with neurologic symptoms: a clinicoradiologic correlation. AJNR Am J Neuroradiol. 2018;39:699–703.

123. Kumar S, Misra UK, Kalita J, et al. MRI in Japanese encephalitis. Neuroradiology. 1997;39:180–4.
124. Misra UK, Kalita J, Jain SK, Mathur A. Radiological and neurophysiological changes in Japanese encephalitis. J Neurol Neurosurg Psychiatry. 1994;57:1484–7.
125. Laothamatas J, Hemachudha T, Mitrabhakdi E, et al. MR imaging in human rabies. AJNR Am J Neuroradiol. 2003;24:1102–9.
126. Co SJ, Mackenzie IR, Shewchuk JR. Rabies encephalitis. Radiographics. 2015;35:235–8.
127. Awasthi M, Parmar H, Patankar T, Castillo M. Imaging findings in rabies encephalitis. AJNR Am J Neuroradiol. 2001;22:677–80.
128. Sarji SA, Abdullah BJ, Goh KJ, et al. MR imaging features of Nipah encephalitis. AJR Am J Roentgenol. 2000;175:437–42.
129. Goh KJ, Tan CT, Chew NK, et al. Clinical features of Nipah virus encephalitis among pig farmers in Malaysia. N Engl J Med. 2000;342:1229–35.
130. Lim CC, Lee KE, Lee WL, et al. Nipah virus encephalitis: serial MR study of an emerging disease. Radiology. 2002;222:219–26.
131. Mansfield KL, Johnson N, Phipps LP, et al. Tick-borne encephalitis virus – a review of an emerging zoonosis. J Gen Virol. 2009;90:1781–94.
132. Horger M, Beck R, Fenchel M, et al. Imaging findings in tick-borne encephalitis with differential diagnostic considerations. AJR Am J Roentgenol. 2012;199:420–7.
133. Noguchi T, Yoshiura T, Hiwatashi A, et al. CT and MRI findings of human herpesvirus 6-associated encephalopathy: comparison with findings of herpes simplex virus encephalitis. AJR Am J Roentgenol. 2010;194:754–60.
134. Luzuriaga K, Sullivan JL. Infectious mononucleosis. N Engl J Med. 2010;362:1993–2000.
135. Shian WJ, Chi CS. Epstein-Barr virus encephalitis and encephalomyelitis: MR findings. Pediatr Radiol. 1996;26:690–3.
136. Patankar TF, Karnad DR, Shetty PG, et al. Adult cerebral malaria: prognostic importance of imaging findings and correlation with postmortem findings. Radiology. 2002;224:811–6.
137. Looareesuwan S, Laothamatas J, Brown TR, Brittenham GM. Cerebral malaria: a new way forward with magnetic resonance imaging (MRI). Am J Trop Med Hyg. 2009;81:545–7.
138. Yadav P, Sharma R, Kumar S, Kumar U. Magnetic resonance features of cerebral malaria. Acta Radiol. 2008;49:566–9.

Chapter 5
Neuroimaging Studies of Migraine Without Aura

Gianluca Coppola, Francesco Casillo, Gabriele Sebastianelli, Chiara Abagnale, Federica Genovese, and Roberta Messina

5.1 Introduction

Despite significant advancements in our understanding of the pathophysiology of migraine pain, the molecular foundation for the onset of migraine disease remains unresolved. Compelling evidence indicates that the mechanisms responsible for the initiation of migraine pain engage the nerve terminals of the trigeminovascular system, especially those of its first division, which innervate the tiny meningeal arteries of the dura mater. At such threshold, the secretion of vasoactive polypeptides begins, initiating sterile inflammation, accompanied by the release of proinflammatory chemicals from mast cells [1]. It is widely accepted that prolonged reactions activate second- and third-order neurons of the trigeminovascular system, leading to cortical sensitization and subsequent pain perception. Which brain structure initiates this sterile inflammation? For certain individuals, the dysfunction and its initiation are predominantly peripheral, with indications of brain structure involvement being secondary to a neuromodulation mechanism due to the recurrence of episodes [2]. Conversely, the presence of premonitory symptoms prior to an attack, which may manifest up to 48 h before the onset of pain, along with accompanying symptoms such as photophobia and cutaneous allodynia, even during the variable pain-free interval, indicates the existence of one or more central generators that trigger the migraine reaction [3–5]. For some, a functional anomaly underlies the

G. Coppola (✉) · F. Casillo · G. Sebastianelli · C. Abagnale
Department of Medico-Surgical Sciences and Biotechnologies, Sapienza University of Rome Polo Pontino ICOT, Latina, Italy
e-mail: gianluca.coppola@uniroma1.it

F. Genovese · R. Messina
Neuroimaging Research Unit and Neurology Unit, IRCCS San Raffaele Scientific Institute, Milan, Italy

Vita-Salute San Raffaele University, Milan, Italy

I. Petrušić, Y. Wang (eds.), *Neuroimaging of Headache Disorders*, Headache,
https://doi.org/10.1007/978-3-031-85402-6_5

condition, whereas for others, there exists a micro- and/or macrostructural modification of the central generator(s) [6]. The progress in this research domain has been facilitated by the concurrent enhancement of neuroimaging techniques, enabling the visualization of activation sites as well as the understanding of their microscopic and macroscopic structures, metabolic activities, and hemodynamic functions, both at rest and during tasks, in relation to other brain structures to establish brain networks.

This chapter summarizes the findings of structural and functional imaging investigations in episodic migraine without aura (MO), illustrating how neuroimaging has enhanced our comprehension of their etiology. This book will evaluate and discuss studies including individuals with migraine with aura (MA), chronic migraine, and pediatric migraine cases in other chapters. At the conclusion of this chapter, we will offer insights for prospective research in the field.

5.2 Structural Investigations in Episodic Migraine Without Aura

Structural magnetic resonance imaging (MRI) offers reliable and high-resolution assessments of brain morphology, exhibiting greater test–retest reliability than functional MRI. The two predominant methodologies utilizing structural MRI data are voxel-based morphometry (VBM) and surface-based morphometry (SBM). VBM is a user-friendly and automated method for assessing variations in gray (GM) and white (WM) matter volume throughout the entire brain. In contrast to VBM, which solely evaluates and GM and WM volume, SBM may analyze additional cortical attributes like cortical thickness (CT), sulcal depth, gyrification index, and surface area [7]. Among the various techniques used to acquire MRI data, DTI is the most sensitive to microstructural changes, as it estimates the diffusivity of water molecules along the fiber bundles of WM in the three main orthogonal directions of diffusion [8].

5.2.1 Voxel-Based Morphometry (VBM) Studies

Over the past two decades, neuroimaging research on migraine has broadened also thanks to the advent of morphometric techniques aimed at identifying GM volume alterations related to migraine [9–14]. The first VBM study on a small cohort of participants (11 MA, 17 MO, and 11 healthy controls [HCs]) reported no significant GM volume differences between patients with migraine and controls [15]. While some subsequent studies replicated these findings [12, 16], more recent investigations have demonstrated both increases and decreases in GM volume across various brain regions, including those associated with nociceptive and visual functions, in MO and MA patients [17–22].

Migraine patients showed significant GM alterations in various brain regions that are crucial for pain perception, including areas involved in sensory processing, emotion, cognition, and pain modulation. The regions showing an increase in GM volume were the bilateral amygdala, temporal poles, left hippocampus, left parahippocampus, right superior frontal gyrus, and precentral gyrus. In contrast, regions displaying a reduction in GM volume included the bilateral middle frontal gyrus, left orbitofrontal cortex (OFC), inferior parietal gyrus, left posterior cingulate cortex (PCC), insula, bilateral rolandic operculum, and the superior and inferior colliculi [10, 17, 23–27]. Notably, the reduction in GM volume in the left insula and the increase in the left parahippocampus were the most consistently reported changes across multiple studies, underscoring their potential involvement in the pathophysiology of migraine [23, 25]. Another area frequently reported to show GM volumetric alterations in migraine patients is the cerebellum. However, the findings have been inconsistent, with some studies reporting an increase in GM volume while others showing a decrease [10, 17, 24, 26, 27].

In a study evaluating the long-term outcomes of migraine patients, patients with poor outcomes (defined as a decrease in headache days of less than 50%) exhibited higher GM volume in the bilateral cerebellum and the right precentral gyrus compared to the healthy controls, as well as lower GM volume in the left posterior cingulate gyrus. Furthermore, patients with poor outcomes exhibited increased GM volume in the bilateral cerebellum compared to those with a positive outcome (defined as a decrease in headache days by at least 50%). Additionally, cerebellar GM volume was associated with the frequency of headaches experienced over 2 years [24]. While the exact pattern of these volumetric changes in the cerebellum remains unclear, the available data suggest that the cerebellum may play a role in the underlying mechanisms of migraine. It might serve as a communication hub between the cortex and brainstem. Volumetric changes have also been identified at the brainstem level, including a reduction in the volume of the periaqueductal gray matter (PAG), locus coeruleus, median raphe nuclei, dorsal pons, and spinal trigeminal nucleus [10, 27].

In a recent morphometric study involving a large cohort of 84 patients with migraine (52 migraine with aura, 32 migraine without aura) and 35 healthy controls, results revealed that patients with migraine had decreased GM volume in the V3 and V5 visual areas of the right occipital cortex compared to the controls [28]. Notably, this reduction was observed irrespective of the presence of migraine aura or disease activity, suggesting that these structural changes may be long-standing and shared across migraine subtypes, potentially reflecting common underlying pathophysiological traits.

Only a limited number of studies have integrated data on structural and functional brain alterations in individuals with migraine [13, 20, 29]. The value of combining various imaging techniques in migraine research is highlighted by the fact that distinct imaging metrics reveal complementary information about the underlying biological processes. This enhances our understanding of the complex mechanisms of migraine, which may not be fully grasped by a single imaging modality alone. Mehnert et al. [20] using VBM and functional magnetic resonance imaging (fMRI) during nociceptive trigeminal stimulation showed concurrent functional and structural alterations of the cerebellum. Two later studies [29, 30] combined the data from resting-state (RS) fMRI and VBM. The first revealed altered functional connectivity (FC) in networks associated with pain and visual processing, specifically highlighting reduced connectivity in the default mode network (DMN) and increased connectivity in the salience network (SN), which may underlie the heightened sensory perception in patients with MO [29]. The second studied 21 MO patients and 21 HCs and found that migraine patients had significantly decreased GM volume in the left medial prefrontal cortex, dorsal anterior cingulate cortex (ACC), right occipital lobe, cerebellum, and brainstem. Focusing on the dorsal ACC, whose GM volume negatively correlated with disease duration, the study revealed increased FC with the bilateral middle temporal lobe, OFC, and left dorsolateral prefrontal cortex. These findings suggest that frequent nociceptive input may lead to structural and functional alterations, particularly in areas involved in pain processing and cognitive functions such as dorsal ACC [30]. Collectively, these studies proved that a multimodal imaging approach is essential for a comprehensive understanding of the structural and functional brain changes associated with migraine without aura, providing insights into the underlying biological mechanisms.

The precise biological underpinnings of cortical structural changes in migraine remain elusive. A central question is whether these brain alterations are a consequence of repeated migraine attacks or pre-existing factors contributing to migraine development [31]. Recent morphometric studies have identified volumetric abnormalities in visual and pain-related brain regions in both pediatric and adult migraine patients, suggesting these structural abnormalities may be intrinsic to migraine pathophysiology [32, 33]. Conversely, other studies have found a significant association between brain alterations and patients' clinical characteristics, such as the duration of their disease and the frequency of migraine attacks, suggesting that the migraine brain may undergo adaptive processes in response to the disease burden [11, 18, 29, 34]. This hypothesis is further strengthened by the evidence of longitudinal GM volume changes. Research has demonstrated that migraine patients experienced both increases and decreases in the volume of nociceptive regions over a 4-year period, which were associated with their disease activity (Fig. 5.1) [35]. In line with the dynamic nature of migraine, with its fluctuating ictal and interictal phases, VBM studies have also revealed that structural brain changes in migraine patients are not static but can vary depending on the disease state [22, 34]. Indeed, Coppola et al. [36] found that GM volume in the left temporal pole and bilateral insula increased during the ictal phase of migraine, while GM volume in the right inferior parietal lobule and right inferior temporal gyrus decreased during the interictal phase. These findings suggest distinct GM volume patterns in temporoparietal regions involved in pain processing, which may vary depending on the disease phase. Taken together, these results suggest that the observed brain changes may arise from the interplay between predisposing brain factors and experience-dependent responses.

Another critical question is whether the morphometric brain abnormalities identified through MRI scans are specific to migraine or are shared with other headache and chronic pain conditions. Studies have revealed distinct patterns of brain activity and structure in migraine patients compared to individuals with tension-type

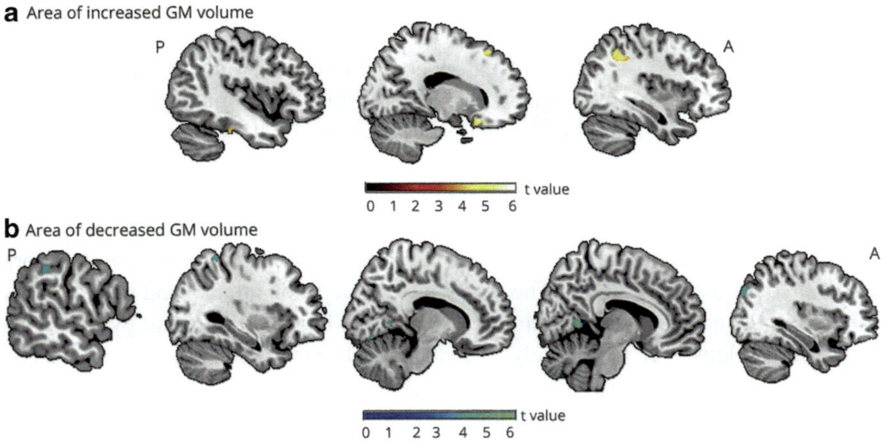

Fig. 5.1 Longitudinal changes in gray matter volume in migraine patients over a 4-year period revealed the following findings: (**a**) In comparison to controls, migraine patients exhibited an increase in gray matter volume in the right inferior parietal gyrus, left inferior temporal gyrus, and the right superior and inferior frontal gyri. (**b**) Conversely, migraine patients showed a reduction in gray matter volume relative to controls in the left supramarginal and superior parietal gyri, as well as in the right lingual and middle occipital gyri. (Used from Messina et al. [22] with permission. Abbreviations: *A* anterior, *P* posterior)

headache (TTH), persistent post-traumatic headaches, and other chronic pain disorders [37, 38]. One study, which involved 56 patients with episodic and chronic migraine and 49 patients with episodic and chronic TTH, focused on volumetric brain differences, highlighting that migraine and TTH were associated with different structural patterns. Specifically, compared to patients with TTH, patients with migraine experienced GM volume reduction in the bilateral putamen, cerebellum, right caudate, precuneus, middle frontal gyrus, and left superior frontal gyrus. These structural differences suggested that while migraine and TTH share some common clinical features, they may have divergent underlying mechanisms [37].

To sum it up, the exact implications of GM volumetric alterations in migraine remain uncertain. Inconsistent findings, including conflicting reports of increased and decreased GM volume, hinder definitive conclusions. Factors such as patient populations, sample sizes, statistical methods, and MRI scanner variations contribute to the variability observed across studies [14]. Moreover, VBM solely measures GM volume, disregarding potential influences of cortical thickness and surface area [7].

5.2.2 *Surface-Based Morphometry (SBM) Studies*

Numerous researchers have examined CT during the interictal phase of migraine, yielding inconsistent findings. Indeed, compared to healthy controls, migraine patients' cortical GM was thinner, thicker, or even similar between attacks, according to earlier studies.

Datta et al.'s research, encompassing whole-brain and a priori specific region of interest (ROI)-based analyses, including the somatosensory cortex, sensorimotor cortex, V3A, and MT+ areas, revealed no significant anomalies in CT among migraine patients, nor any correlation between brain morphometric variables and the frequency or duration of migraine [39]. Magon et al. [40] gathered the MRI data from four distinct headache centers, employing varied sequences, and discovered that 131 migraine patients exhibited a thinner cortex in the bilateral central sulcus (encompassing its motor and somatosensory regions), the left middle frontal gyrus, the left visual cortices (both primary and secondary), and the right occipitotemporal gyrus, in contrast to 115 HCs. The frequency of migraine attacks and migraine history exhibited a negative correlation with CT in the left middle frontal gyrus and the left central sulcus [40]. Conversely, alternative ROI-based investigations indicated a greater CT in the somatosensory cortex, lacking a definitive association with clinical data [41], as well as in additional regions such as the superior frontal gyrus, paracentral gyrus, temporal pole, and precuneus [42], in comparison to HC. Further ad hoc research is necessary to ascertain whether thicker cortical regions are a consequence of plastic alterations associated with the persistent experience of severe migraine symptoms. Chong et al. discovered that migraine patients exhibiting interictal photosensitivity demonstrated heightened CT in the lingual gyrus and pericalcarine area, which are responsible for visual stimulus processing, as well as in the right isthmus cingulate, associated with emotional processing, and the left precentral, postcentral, and supramarginal regions [43]. Additionally, migraine patients exhibiting vestibular symptoms showed significantly reduced CT in the right superior parietal lobule, left middle temporal gyrus, and bilateral inferior temporal gyrus [44]. Using more permissive statistics (mapping threshold established at $p < 0.05$), another research group compared CT in 48 migraine patients to 48 HCs, again showing a decrease in CT. In this study, alterations were observed in the inferior frontal gyrus, posterior cingulate, bilateral cuneus, and middle temporal gyrus, all regions associated with the DMN [45]. Employing a more rigorous statistical threshold, a separate study analyzed 63 migraine patients (some on prophylactic medications) against 18 HCs and identified increased CT in the left temporo-occipital incisure and middle frontal cortex, alongside decreased CT in the left superior frontal cortex and precentral cortex in migraine patients relative to HCs [46]. Despite the identification of specific CT discrepancies between patient subgroups and controls, it is noteworthy that the mean CT abnormalities were unassociated with clinical variables and exhibited no variation across patients with and without white matter hyperintensities (WHs) [46]. Further ad hoc research with a larger cohort showed no statistically significant differences in CT and volume measurements among migraine patients with and without WHs compared to HCs [47].

Other studies have explored cortical plasticity in migraine by assessing whether migraine influences the typical age-related reduction in CT. A study demonstrated reduced age-related cortical thinning in the bilateral postcentral cortex, the right fusiform gyrus, and the right temporal pole in comparison to HCs [48]. Another independent research team corroborated that age showed a significant negative correlation with both thickness and volume of the frontal, parietal, temporal, occipital, and insula lobes among a larger cohort of female migraine patients [47]. In contrast to healthy individuals, female migraine patients exhibit a deficiency in insular thinning with age [42]. This is intriguing, as it implies that certain alterations in CT associated with migraine develop plastically over time rather than having enduring characteristics. This interpretation is corroborated by the discovery that, relative to younger patients, migraine sufferers over the age of 12 exhibited reduced CT in the superior and middle frontal gyri, pre- and postcentral cortex, paracentral lobule, superior and transverse temporal gyri, supramarginal gyrus, and posterior insula [49]. This indicates that decreasing the attack frequency, such as by preventive medicines, may influence the patterns of cortical alterations. In 15 patients with MO, spontaneous migraine attacks were accompanied by transient reduced CT and volume in pain-related areas (precentral, prefrontal, pericalcarine, hippocampus, and temporal pole), compared with the same patients scanned between attacks [50].

In conclusion, most studies conducted during the interictal phase of migraine have detected alterations in CT, with certain instances associated with accompanying symptoms. The thickness of the migraine cortex may either diminish or augment. This discrepancy among studies may be attributed to differences in statistical methodologies, the criteria applied, and the inclusion of patients undergoing preventative treatments. The imprecise timing of days between the last and subsequent attack may contribute to variability in findings, as some results could stem from ongoing plastic changes in the brain, contingent upon the stage of the migraine cycle during patient evaluation. Although other studies indicate potential trait abnormalities in the migraine-affected brain regions responsible for processing many multidimensional aspects of pain perception, certain pivotal findings suggest that these abnormalities may correlate with the duration of the disease.

5.2.3 *Diffusion Tensor Imaging (DTI)*

5.2.3.1 DTI Techniques to Study WM Microstructure in Migraine

DTI metrics include fractional anisotropy (FA), mean diffusivity (MD), axial diffusivity (AD), and radial diffusivity (RD). FA measures the magnitude of anisotropy and closely reflects the integrity of the membranes of WM axons as well as the directionality of water molecule movement [8]. MD, which comprises radial and axial diffusivity and typically changes inversely to FA, reflects the overall magnitude of water diffusion by indicating both cellular swelling and density [8]. AD and RD serve as in vivo surrogate markers of myelin and axonal damage, respectively. These metrics are closely associated with brain microstructural maturation processes and higher levels of cognitive function [51].

Tract-based spatial statistics (TBSS) is a tool that employs a tensor-fitting technique to produce various diffusion metrics. The method is fully automated and user-friendly, allowing for the reconstruction and examination of the WM structure of the entire brain without the need for prior specification or localization of regions or features of interest [52]. Another approach that can be used involves the quantification of the average values of FA, MD, AD, and RD in specific ROIs selected a priori or in WM tracts derived using an atlas-based approach [32, 53].

Numerous investigations have demonstrated alterations in WM microstructure during the interictal phase in individuals with migraine. Employing a hypothesis-driven methodology, the authors discovered that, in comparison to HCs, migraine patients exhibited altered DTI metrics in the thalami [54–56], hypothalamus [53, 57], trigeminal somatosensory pathway [41], genu/splenium and body of the corpus callosum [58–60], WM subjacent to areas V3A and MT+, left lateral geniculate nucleus [61], optic radiations [62], cerebellar vermis and peduncle tract, and spinal trigeminal nucleus [27]. Notably, certain researchers identified a significant reduction in AD in the right trigeminal nerve relative to the left nerve, as well as a decrease in FA in the left nerve compared to controls, independent of migraine history and clinical characteristics, with no differences observed in volume and cross-sectional area [63].

Whole-brain investigations have shown conflicting outcomes; specifically, both abnormal diffusivity metrics [34, 59, 64–69] and the absence of changes [68, 70–75] have been reported in MO patients relative to HCs. However, individuals with MO did not exhibit a negative association between DTI measures of the PAG and those of the trigeminal nerve, as shown in the HCs [76]. This data was viewed as a result of insufficient descending inhibition from the PAG on trigeminal activity.

Decreased FA in the genu and splenium of the corpus callosum, linked with diminished FC in the ACC, indicates structural and corresponding functional disturbances between the bilateral hemispheres [58]. In a separate investigation, elevated FA in the bilateral thalami exhibited a negative correlation with alterations in FC within the DMN, visuospatial system, and medial visual cortical regions [56]. Relative to HCs, interictal MO exhibited markedly elevated MD, AD, and RD values in the hypothalamus and its anterior and posterior sub-regions bilaterally, alongside reduced FA values in the posterior ROIs, independent of the connectivity with cortical networks [53]. During attacks, patients exhibited markedly changed diffusivity measurements in the hypothalamus, particularly in its posterior region, relative to HCs. The hypothalamic AD exhibited a positive correlation with migraine severity and the functional activity of the SN, while DTI measurements of the bilateral anterior hypothalamus were positively associated with the mean attack duration [57]. The authors proposed that the hypothalamus may have a multifaceted involvement in both the beginning and regulation of the duration and cessation of the attack. Another study showed that the integrated characteristics of diffusion metrics of the middle prefrontal cortex–amygdala pathways effectively distinguished between patients who improved after a placebo effect related to an 8-week sham acupuncture treatment and those who did not, achieving an accuracy of 84%. This suggests that the microstructural WM features of the prefrontal cortex–amygdala pathways may serve as imaging markers for identifying placebo responders in migraine patients [64].

Four studies investigated DTI measures during spontaneous migraine episodes [55, 57, 77]. No substantial variations in FA were observed in ten ictal patients with MO when compared to controls and non-self-matched interictal patients. A favorable connection was detected between the FA of the thalamus and the number of days since the last migraine attack when ictal and interictal individuals were mixed [55]. Furthermore, no substantial differences in thalamic DTI measurements between ictal MO and HCs were seen, nor was there any link with alterations in FC within the executive control network (ECN) and dorsoventral attention system [77].

Marciszewski et al. [78] conducted DTI analysis on 29 HCs and 36 individuals with migraine, revealing alterations in regional brainstem anatomy throughout the migraine cycle. They observed increased MD in the spinal trigeminal nucleus, dorsomedial/dorsolateral pons, and midbrain PAG/cuneiform nucleus between attacks, with MD normalization occurring during the 24-h period immediately preceding a migraine. The authors posited that these alterations facilitate the activation of the ascending trigeminal pathway, either by an elevation in basal activity or by sensitizing the trigeminal nuclei to external stimuli, which then culminates in the sense of the cephalic pain during a migraine episode [78].

Novel, more advanced approaches in the analysis of DTI images yield estimates of alternative parameters that may improve the understanding of the underlying microstructural changes in the brain. Among these new measures, the intracellular volume fraction (IVF) provides information regarding the proportion of the diffusion signal that arises from water inside the cells, while the orientation dispersion index (ODI) measures the degree of variability in the orientation of neurites [79].

Employing genome-wide association study data and Mendelian randomization, researchers identified that the FA of the left inferior fronto-occipital fasciculus and the ODI of the right posterior thalamic radiation have a significant causal relationship with migraine, while migraine significantly influences the orientation dispersion of the left superior cerebellar peduncle [80]. A bidirectional Mendelian randomization study involving 2.347 neuroimaging phenotypes combining both DTI and T1-weighted images revealed that altered IVF and ODI of the ACC, insula, and frontal and auditory areas were associated with an elevated risk of MA and MO, while increased CT and local gyrification index of the same areas were linked to a reduced risk of overall migraine, MA and MO [81].

In summary, research employing the DTI approach has revealed extensive involvement of WM characterized by the remodeling of neuronal connections via dendritic arborization, alterations in the quantity of local circuits, and variations in the prevalence of axonal membranes [8]. Evidence indicates that some microstructural abnormalities lead to the functional impairments of neurocognitive networks, which will be addressed in the subsequent section. Nonetheless, these aberrations seem to represent plastic alterations rather than permanent structural damage, arising in response to the recurrent migraine cycle.

5.2.3.2 DTI Techniques to Study Glymphatic System in Migraine

In 2012, the glymphatic system (GS) was discovered to eliminate solutes from brain interstitial fluid via perivascular clearance. The DTI analysis along the perivascular space (DTI-ALPS) approach was introduced to assess glymphatic function noninvasively [82]. This method involves the identification of an ROI within the cerebral WM region of interest that is generally situated on the left side, aligned with the upper lateral ventricles. The deep medullary veins run horizontally across the lateral ventricle and are typically aligned parallel to the perivascular space on the image slice. This structural configuration allows for the measurement of water diffusivity in the perivascular regions next to these veins, facilitating the calculation of the so-called DTI-ALPS index [83]. The GS has been hypothesized to play a role in the etiology of migraine. Two primary potential processes have been proposed: the inability to eliminate the buildup of proinflammatory chemicals, particularly calcitonin gene-related peptide (CGRP), and the excessive release of K+ following cortical spreading depression [84].

Most studies in patients with episodic MO showed no differences in terms of the DTI-ALPS index compared to HCs [85–88]. In one study, similar values of the DTI-ALPS index were found in migraine patients with and without WMHs [86]. In another study, the clinical manifestation of migraine was not associated with GS dysfunction, although increased perivascular spaces, a possible marker of GS dysfunction, was found to be an independent predictor of migraine [85]. A recent study confirmed the normal DTI-ALPS index in migraine patients but identified a significantly elevated diffusion kurtosis imaging ALPS index, an alternative promising method for assessing GS function, unrelated to the patients' clinical characteristics [89].

In conclusion, the existing methodologies for examining the glymphatic system revealed no anomalies in individuals with episodic migraine relative to HCs.

5.3 Functional Magnetic Resonance Imaging (fMRI) in Migraine

fMRI measures brain activity by detecting hemodynamic changes associated with blood flow, specifically the blood–oxygen-level dependent (BOLD) signal. fMRI can be utilized to identify BOLD responses resulting from tasks or stimuli, as well as to assess RS or negative-task states, which represent the participants' baseline BOLD variability. fMRI is based on the principle that an increase in BOLD corresponds to an increase in cerebral metabolic activity, although it is not possible to say whether this activity is inhibitory or excitatory. fMRI studies provide distinct measures, including functional connectivity, which refers to the direct temporal synchronization among cortical regions, and effective connectivity, which represents the causal influence that one brain area exerts on another, and measures such as infra-slow oscillatory activity, regional homogeneity, and amplitude of low-frequency fluctuations (ALFF) that assess spontaneous neural activity, offering valuable insights into brain function and network organization [90, 91].

5.3.1 Interictal Migraine

Numerous investigations were conducted on episodic migraine patients during interictal periods utilizing fMRI to assess responses to noxious stimuli applied to trigeminal or extratrigeminal regions. They exhibited an augmented BOLD response in brain regions associated with nociception/antinociception, as well as the affective and cognitive dimensions of pain processing, including the insula, middle cingulate cortex, ACC, secondary somatosensory cortex, amygdala, cerebellum, caudate nuclei, motor and premotor areas, temporal pole, lentiform nuclei, posterior thalamus, fusiform gyrus, subthalamic nucleus, pre- and postcentral gyrus, hippocampus, parahippocampal gyrus, dorsolateral prefrontal cortex (DLPFC), and perigenual ACC. Meanwhile, they demonstrated diminished BOLD activation in the brainstem, specifically the trigeminal nucleus caudalis and nucleus cuneiformis [5, 92–98]. Moreover, these pain-induced BOLD signal alterations were not associated with the presence of depression or anxiety [94]. Conversely, the interval to the subsequent attack exhibited a positive correlation with activation strength in the trigeminal nuclei in one study [5]. Headache intensity was negatively associated with the middle prefrontal cortex and PCC, but positively correlated with bilateral insula activation [95]. Attack frequency was linked to activation strength in several brain regions, including the middle cingulate, insula, fusiform gyrus, hippocampus, DLPFC, and precentral gyrus [92, 94, 95]. Additionally, the duration of migraine history was positively correlated with activation strength in the fusiform gyrus [94] and negatively correlated with the superior temporal gyrus [95]. In non-pain-related fMRI studies, such as those involving visual tasks, research has shown conflicting results: either no difference between patients with MO and HCs [99] or an increased BOLD signal in the occipital cortex following continuous stimulation [100].

Numerous fMRI research on migraine evaluated resting-state FC across various brain networks, indicating a linked between migraine and functional brain changes (Fig. 5.2). Research conducted by multiple independent groups has demonstrated that the intrinsic connectivity among brain regions associated with the DMN, which is implicated in self-referential orientation and monitoring, is diminished during the interictal period in MO patients when compared to HCs [101–107]. Furthermore, the DMN exhibited modified dynamic activity [107] and showed increased FC with the ECN and the insula [108], while showing reduced FC with the prefrontal and temporal areas [101] and the visuospatial system [56]. The intra-regional FC of the ECN was reduced [105, 106, 109, 110], yet exhibited heightened dynamic activity in interictal migraine [107], whereas the ECN demonstrated diminished interconnectivity with the middle frontal gyrus, the dorsal ACC [111], and the precuneus [112]. Visual regions are significantly implicated in migraine pathophysiology, exhibiting diminished intrinsic FC [103, 113], particularly within the visuospatial [102] and dorsal attention [106] systems. The latter demonstrates reduced interconnectivity with the DMN [56] and the ECN [109] in patients with MO. Compared to HCs, regions within the sensorimotor [102, 103, 106], auditory [103, 106], and

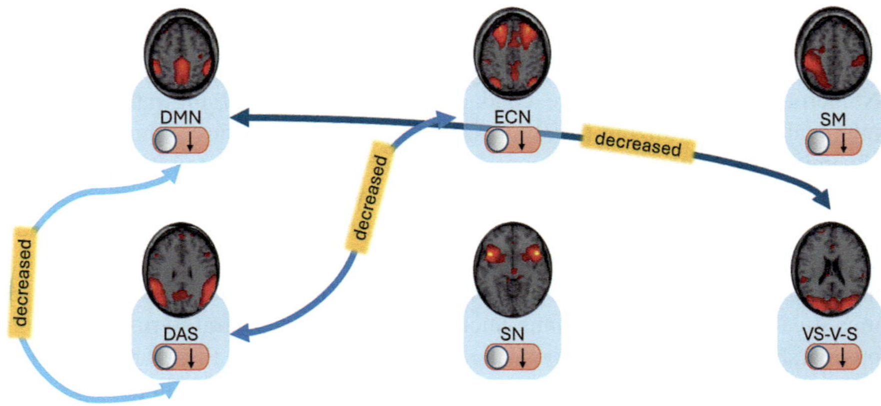

Fig. 5.2 Schematic representation of the results obtained by recording functional MRI activity at rest in patients with episodic migraine without aura between attacks. Low functional connectivity (FC) was found within the default mode network (DMN), executive control network (ECN), sensorimotor network (SM), dorsal attention system (DAS), salience network (SN), and visual networks, including the visuospatial network (VS-V-S). Between-network connectivity analysis revealed decreased FC between the DMN and the visual and attentive networks (VS-V-S and DAS) and between the attentive (DAS) and executive (ECN) networks

cingulo-opercular [106] networks exhibited reduced FC in patients with MO. Regions associated with the SN, primarily engaged in the detection and integration of prominent sensory stimuli, had diminished FC in MO patients compared to HCs [106]. The limbic system, which facilitates several activities such as emotion, behavior, motivation, and long-term memory, exhibited greater connectivity in patients with episodic MO compared to HCs [114]. Compared to controls, individuals with MO exhibited significant elevations in fractional amplitude of low-frequency hemodynamic fluctuations (fALFF) in the bilateral ventral posteromedial thalamus and the brainstem, encompassing the rostral ventromedial medulla and trigeminocervical complex [115]. In a study with a larger cohort of 143 patients with migraine and 100 healthy controls, researchers determined that the aberrant inter-network connectivity was predominantly influenced by thalamic dysfunction in migraine patients [116]. In a separate investigation, patients with MO demonstrated markedly diminished connection from the left thalamus to the left brainstem, and from the left brainstem to the contralateral insula, in comparison to HCs. All these investigations emphasize that interictal thalamic dysfunction may underlie cortical dysfunction in migraine and may be associated with aberrant control by the brainstem [117].

Patients with MO had increased FC from the right lateral cingulate to the left lingual and calcarine sulcus, as well as to the right frontal medial gyrus/orbital area, relative to HCs [118]. Furthermore, the PAG, a critical area in descending pain modulation, exhibited diminished (rostral anterior cingulate cortex/medial prefrontal cortex) and enhanced (cingulate gyrus, pre-postcentral gyri, superior frontal gyrus, caudate, and middle occipital gyrus) effective connections with multiple brain regions associated with pain perception and emotion in interictal patients relative to healthy controls [119–121].

To elucidate the impact of migraine clinical characteristics on alterations in FC, many authors conducted regression analyses within patient cohorts.

In episodic migraine patients during interictal periods, average pain intensity exhibited a negative correlation with the FC between the right ACC and PCC in MO [105], with abnormal inflows to the right posterior thalamus from the right DLPFC [122], with diminished connectivity within the middle frontal gyrus [111], and with alterations in connectivity between the anterior insula and occipital regions [123]. The duration of migraine disease exhibited a negative correlation with the strength of both intrinsic connectivity and causal influences from the frontoinsular cortex to the ACC [66, 105], as well as with insular sub-regions [124], and with FC values in the prefrontal cortex, putamen, right nucleus accumbens, and bilateral caudate [125, 126]. The duration of migraine disease exhibited a positive correlation with the FC of the bilateral PAG to the bilateral thalamus (notably the ventral posteromedial region), brainstem, putamen, left pallidum, and right medial OFC [115, 127]. Additionally, there was enhanced FC between the dorsal ACC and the DLPFC/OFC [30], increased connectivity between the DMN/ECN and the insula [108], as well as elevated average regional homogeneity values in the thalamus, brainstem, and temporal pole [128]. The mean monthly frequency of migraine attacks exhibited a negative correlation with the enhanced causal influences from the right frontal inferior cortex to the right DLPFC [105], and a positive correlation with the connectivity between the left middle frontal gyrus and the medial prefrontal cortex (PFC) [123], as well as with the FC between the bilateral caudate and left insula [126], and with the connectivity between the PAG and various cortical regions primarily associated with nociception and somatosensory processing, including the dorsomedial PFC, primary somatosensory cortex, primary motor cortex, ACC, parahippocampal gyrus, amygdala, DLPFC, angular gyrus, and medial thalamus [129]. The time interval preceding the next migraine attack was positively connected with the connection between the left middle frontal gyrus and the medial prefrontal cortex in MO.

5.3.2 Peri-ictal and Ictal Migraine

Functional anomalies in the brain regions were also found during migraine attacks. An augmented BOLD signal in relation to noxious stimuli was detected throughout the temporal lobe structures [92] and in the dorsal regions of the pons [5]. The activation of the spinal trigeminal nucleus appears to vary throughout the migraine cycle: it is marginally elevated in the preictal phase relative to healthy individuals, but significantly increased compared to interictal scans, while it diminishes during an acute attack when compared to both healthy controls and migraine patients assessed during the preictal period [5].

Certain researchers conducted a longitudinal daily scan of a migraine patient for 30 days, utilizing olfactory stimuli (gaseous ammonia) as a functional task in the

MRI during the ictal phase, in comparison to the preictal and interictal phases [98]. The hypothalamus in this patient had markedly increased activity just prior to the headache phase, demonstrating the highest FC with the spinal trigeminal nuclei. In the ictal state, the hypothalamus exhibited functional coupling with the dorsal rostral pons [98]. This conclusion was supported by two additional studies from the same research group, which also indicated that ROI-to-voxel analysis showed heightened connectivity between the dopaminergic right accumbens and the dorsal rostral pons during the preictal phase relative to the interictal phase [130, 131]. Significantly, pain-related fMRI indicates that the posterior hypothalamus shows increased activation during the acute pain phase, whereas the anterior area appears to play a role in the onset of attacks [132].

Limited research has investigated the brains of migraine sufferers during attacks with RS fMRI (Fig. 5.3). Coppola et al. [77] observed that during the first 6 h of a spontaneous migraine attack, the ECN and the dorsoventral attention system exhibited considerably reduced interconnectivity. In healthy individuals, a stronger dorsoventral attention system correlates with lower bilateral thalamic diffusivity values; conversely, in patients, a stronger strength of ECN FC is associated with fewer monthly migraine days [77]. In a related study by the same researchers, ictal patients exhibited enhanced FC among brain regions associated with the DMN, specifically between the MPFC and the PCC, as well as between the MPFC and bilateral insula. Additionally, it was noted that the strength of MPFC-to-insula connectivity was inversely correlated with pain intensity [133]. Amin and

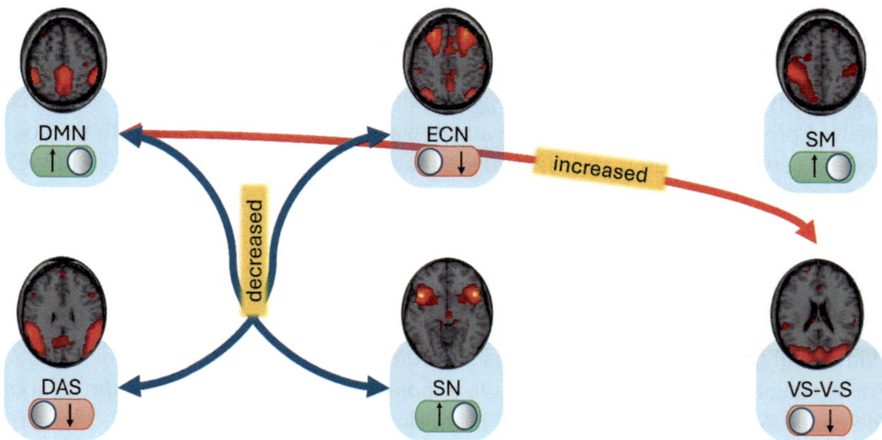

Fig. 5.3 Schematic representation of the results obtained by recording resting-state functional MRI activity during attacks of migraine without aura. Increased functional connectivity (FC) was detected within the default mode network (DMN), sensorimotor network (SM), and salience network (SN). In contrast, low FC was detected in the executive control network (ECN), dorsal attention system (DAS), and visual networks (VS-V-S). Between-network connectivity analysis revealed increased FC between the DMN and the visual networks and decreased FC between the DMN and the DAS and between the SN and the ECN

associates investigated cerebral RS FC during the initial phase before a migraine-like headache triggered by the administration of pituitary adenylate cyclase-activating polypeptide-38 (PACAP38) [134]. During the initial headache phase, PACAP38 altered the FC patterns in the preselected SN, sensorimotor network, and DMN, but vasoactive intestinal polypeptide, which does not elicit attacks, did not exhibit such changes [134]. During spontaneous migraine attacks, the authors identified abnormal brain network connectivity between the thalamus and various pain-modulating and pain-encoding cortical regions, including the superior parietal lobule, insular cortex, primary motor and premotor cortices, supplementary motor area, and OFC [135]. Some authors examined a cohort of patients with MO and MA after the injection of nitroglycerin or placebo. During the premonitory phase of induced migraine, researchers observed a positive functional coupling between the bilateral thalami and the right precuneus/cuneus, as well as a negative coupling between the pons and the limbic lobe. During the headache phase, a negative correlation was noted between the pons and the cingulate and frontal cortices, while a positive correlation was detected between the pons, cerebellar tonsils, and medulla [136].

An fMRI study revealed an increase in infra-slow oscillatory activity, FC, and regional homogeneity in hypothalamic and brainstem regions, particularly the spinal trigeminal nucleus, dorsal pons, and hypothalamus, immediately prior to a migraine, which also display altered activity during the migraine episode. Significantly, these modifications in oscillatory activity and FC did not occur immediately prior to or during migraine episodes and were distinctly different from those of HCs [137]. In seven ictal patients, the bilateral hypothalamus had diminished FC with the visual cortex, although the intrinsic connectivity of the trigeminocervical complex was elevated relative to both interictal patients and HCs [138, 139]. The same seven individuals showed decreased activity from the bilateral hypothalamus to the right inferior parietal gyrus relative to healthy controls [138]. During a spontaneous migraine attack, patients displayed increased activity in the pain-inhibitory left frontal pole and OFC while performing a verbal working memory task, alongside decreased FC in sensorimotor and insular regions, which are associated with nociception and autonomic responses, compared to the interictal phase [140, 141].

In summary, the findings from task-related and RS FC investigations indicate a comprehensive engagement of both internalizing and externalizing cortical networks in migraine, regardless of the occurrence of headache pain. Noteworthy is the pivotal role of certain truncal structures with diverse functions, including the spinal trigeminal nucleus and the PAG, alongside specific diencephalic structures that facilitate the processing and categorization of sensory information, both pain-related and non-pain-related, as well as the stress response, exemplified by the hypothalamus. The intricate cortico-subcortical engagement evident in migraine may stem from a multifaceted interaction of several cerebral components in reaction to pain; nevertheless, the anatomical and functional basis for the recurrence of attacks has yet to be established.

5.4 Arterial Spin Labelling (ASL) in Migraine

ASL is an MRI technique utilized to assess cerebral blood perfusion by labelling blood water during its circulation in the brain, hence obviating the need for gadolinium contrast. However, major limitation of the ASL is that signal-to-noise ratio and temporal resolution are inherently low, resulting in a reduced contrast-to-noise ratio [142].

Several studies have examined the interictal phase of migraine sufferers without aura using ASL. Employing a more permissive statistic, one study identified an elevation in cerebral blood flow (CBF) within the superior temporal gyrus [143], while another study observed an increase in the bilateral primary somatosensory cortices and the left primary motor cortex in patients relative to healthy individuals [144]. In a study with a larger cohort, some authors observed an increase in regional CBF (rCBF) in the OFC and right medial frontal gyrus and a decrease in the cerebellar vermis in patients relative to healthy people [145]. The same authors conducted a correlation analysis of CBF regions and identified diminished connection of the right OFC with the putamen, caudate, right angular gyrus, and left superior frontal gyrus, whereas enhanced connectivity was noted with the left visual cortex [145]. In comparison to HCs, individuals with menstrual migraine had increased CBF in the left insula and right supplementary motor region [146]. The occurrence of rCBF abnormalities was consistent regardless of the presence of WMHs in patients with MO [147]. A study examining variations in rCBF comparing migraine patients with and without tinnitus revealed a reduction in CBF in the superior frontal gyrus and the right middle frontal gyrus among those with both migraine and tinnitus comorbidity [148]. A study assessed the alterations in CBF and BOLD signals in response to inhalation of 5% carbon dioxide to evaluate cerebrovascular reactivity, revealing comparable results between patients and controls [149].

Certain investigations indicated variations in rCBF and other connectivity metrics between those experiencing migraine with aura and those without, with inconclusive results [147, 150–154].

Most of the research that longitudinally examined the behavior of rCBF during the migraine cycle yielded some significant results [155–158], except for one negative study [159].

Certain authors discovered that less than 24 h before a spontaneous migraine episode, the CBF in migraine sufferers decreased in the right hypothalamus, right retrosplenial brain, and left visual areas compared to HCs [155]. A gradual hyperperfusion in the nucleus accumbens, insula, and right precentral gyrus was noted throughout the days between two spontaneous migraine episodes. In a double-blind randomized placebo-controlled fMRI study, patients exhibiting premonitory symptoms induced by NTG administration demonstrated a significant increase in CBF in the ACC, caudate, midbrain, lentiform nucleus, amygdala, and hippocampus, along with an additional increase in regional CBF of the hypothalamic region of interest [158]. In a separate investigation where migraine was induced by the administration of CGRP and sildenafil, only patients in whom an attack was successfully elicited exhibited an increase in rCBF in the dorsolateral pons ipsilateral to the pain site [157].

The rCBF in the bilateral somatosensory cortices, left primary cortex, and right OFC increased with an increase in attack frequency [144, 145], whereas the rCBF in the right supplementary motor area exhibited a positive correlation with disease duration [146]. Additionally, the rCBF level in the superior temporal gyrus positively correlated with the Hamilton Depression Scale [143], while the rCBF in the right OFC correlated with the Visual Light Sensitivity Questionnaire (VSLQ-8) [145].

In summary, the ASL studies exhibited contradictory findings, with no commonality in the regions of altered rCBF across studies, indicating that this method, due to its limited signal-to-noise ratio and spatial resolution, is likely less effective than others in identifying hemodynamic abnormalities in migraine.

5.5 Conclusions

Analysis of MRI studies employing diverse structural and functional methodologies illustrates a complex engagement of both WM and GM in episodic migraine patients.

The macrostructure of the GM frequently exhibits subtle volumetric variations in regions associated with multimodal information processing including nociception and antinociception. These morphological abnormalities seem to be dynamic, influenced by the migraine cycle (ictal/interictal) and varying longitudinally with illness burden and pharmaceutical treatment.

The microstructure of the WM appears to exhibit similar behavior to that of the GM. Various regions and fiber bundles of the WM exhibit differences in migraine patients relative to HCs. The changes are fundamentally due to the reorganization of synaptic connections, dendritic spines, and their branching, resulting in modifications to both local and extensive brain circuit physiology. The nuclei of the GM exhibit variations in certain DTI metrics, including those of the thalamus and hypothalamus, possibly due to their composition of sub-nuclei interconnected by fiber bundles, as well as the metrics reflecting cellular swelling and membrane activity. Similar to GM volume, DTI measurements are dynamic and seem to fluctuate based on the recurrence of the migraine cycle and the interval between attacks, potentially predisposing individuals to subsequent episodes. This phenomenon is frequently noted in critical regions pertinent to migraine pathophysiology, including the thalamus, PAG, spinal trigeminal nucleus, hypothalamus, and the dorsolateral pontine area, with the latter regarded as the generators of migraine.

Currently, both the glymphatic system assessed with DTI-ALPS and cerebral perfusion confirmed through ALS appear to be unreliable procedures. This is likely due to the DTI-ALPS approach being unpolished and its efficacy in studying the glymphatic system remaining unknown. Conversely, ALS is a method characterized by an inherently low signal-to-noise ratio and diminished spatial resolution.

Nonetheless, longitudinal analysis of the ALS data indicates that the hypothalamus and some other brain regions are implicated prior to the beginning of a migraine attack.

The engagement of our stress response system, specifically the hypothalamus, is corroborated by longitudinal fMRI data, both during tasks and at rest. The fMRI results indicate a dynamic trend in cerebral hemodynamics, influenced by the recurrence and frequency of attacks (ictal/interictal) and the severity of the disease's clinical manifestations. The analysis of independent components at rest indicates significant engagement of internalizing and externalizing neurocognitive networks. Multiple evidences indicate a hypofunction of all cerebral networks, including the DMN, ECN, SN, sensorimotor, visual, and attentional networks, during the interictal phase, which partially reactivate during the attack, particularly the DMN, while the connectivity of the dorsoventral attentional system diminishes at the expense of the ECN, likely attempting to induce analgesia. This implies that alterations in the functional connection are just a cognitive physiological reaction of our nervous system attempting to mitigate the unidentified element likely responsible for migraine headaches, which remains mostly enigmatic. The thalamus appears to play a significant role, since it has consistently demonstrated FC and disconnection with cortical regions and networks throughout the migraine cycle.

Notably, some of this evidence is derived from research employing a multimodal approach to MR image analysis, including DTI and fMRI or VBM and fMRI. We believe that this area of multimodal research should be promoted, as modern models of human brain organization increasingly demonstrate the significant influence of anatomical structure on brain function and vice versa: our identity is shaped by our anatomy, which evolves based on its utilization.

Nonetheless, additional longitudinal research tracking migraine sufferers from youth to maturity, examining morpho-functional changes across life stages—particularly in women—comparing various migraine phenotypes and comorbidities, may elucidate illness causes.

This multifaceted approach may provide answers to the 'universal' inquiries posed by our patients daily: what causes my migraine? How does it occur? And why does it happen?.

References

1. Burstein R, Cutrer MF, Yarnitsky D. The development of cutaneous allodynia during a migraine attack clinical evidence for the sequential recruitment of spinal and supraspinal nociceptive neurons in migraine. Brain. 2000;123:1703–9.
2. Olesen J. Personal view: modelling pain mechanisms of migraine without aura. Cephalalgia. 2022;42:1425–35. https://doi.org/10.1177/03331024221111529.
3. Weiller C, May A, Limmroth V, et al. Brain stem activation in spontaneous human migraine attacks. Nat Med. 1995;1:658–60.
4. Bahra A, Matharu MS, Buchel C, et al. Brainstem activation specific to migraine headache. Lancet. 2001;357:1016–7.

5. Stankewitz A, Aderjan D, Eippert F, May A. Trigeminal nociceptive transmission in migraineurs predicts migraine attacks. J Neurosci. 2011;31:1937–43.
6. Coppola G, Parisi V, Di Renzo A, Pierelli F. Cortical pain processing in migraine. J Neural Transm. 2020;127:551–66. https://doi.org/10.1007/s00702-019-02089-7.
7. Winkler AM, Kochunov P, Blangero J, et al. Cortical thickness or grey matter volume? The importance of selecting the phenotype for imaging genetics studies. NeuroImage. 2010;53:1135–46. https://doi.org/10.1016/J.NEUROIMAGE.2009.12.028.
8. Beaulieu C. The basis of anisotropic water diffusion in the nervous system – a technical review. NMR Biomed. 2002;15:435–55. https://doi.org/10.1002/nbm.782.
9. Hougaard A, Amin FM, Hoffmann MB, et al. Structural gray matter abnormalities in migraine relate to headache lateralization, but not aura. Cephalalgia. 2015;35:3–9. https://doi.org/10.1177/0333102414532378.
10. Li Z, Zhou J, Lan L, et al. Concurrent brain structural and functional alterations in patients with migraine without aura: an fMRI study. J Headache Pain. 2020;21:141. https://doi.org/10.1186/s10194-020-01203-5.
11. Coppola G, Petolicchio B, Di Renzo A, et al. Cerebral gray matter volume in patients with chronic migraine: correlations with clinical features. J Headache Pain. 2017;18:115. https://doi.org/10.1186/s10194-017-0825-z.
12. Masson R, Demarquay G, Meunier D, et al. Is migraine associated to brain anatomical alterations? New data and coordinate-based meta-analysis. Brain Topogr. 2021;34:384–401. https://doi.org/10.1007/s10548-021-00824-6.
13. Maleki N, Becerra L, Brawn J, et al. Common hippocampal structural and functional changes in migraine. Brain Struct Funct. 2013;218:903–12. https://doi.org/10.1007/s00429-012-0437-y.
14. Kim JH, Suh S-I, Seol HY, et al. Regional grey matter changes in patients with migraine: a voxel-based morphometry study. Cephalalgia. 2008;28:598–604. https://doi.org/10.1111/j.1468-2982.2008.01550.x.
15. Matharu MS, Good CD, May A, et al. No change in the structure of the brain in migraine: a voxel-based morphometric study. Eur J Neurol. 2003;10:53–7. https://doi.org/10.1046/j.1468-1331.2003.00510.x.
16. Husøy AK, Håberg AK, Rimol LM, et al. Cerebral cortical dimensions in headache sufferers aged 50 to 66 years: a population-based imaging study in the Nord-Trøndelag Health Study (HUNT-MRI). Pain. 2019;160:1634–43. https://doi.org/10.1097/j.pain.0000000000001550.
17. Zhang X, Zhou J, Guo M, et al. A systematic review and meta-analysis of voxel-based morphometric studies of migraine. J Neurol. 2023;270:152–70. https://doi.org/10.1007/s00415-022-11363-w.
18. Rocca MA, Ceccarelli A, Falini A, et al. Brain gray matter changes in migraine patients with T2-visible lesions: a 3-T MRI study. Stroke. 2006;37:1765–70. https://doi.org/10.1161/01.STR.0000226589.00599.4d.
19. Dai Z, Zhong J, Xiao P, et al. Gray matter correlates of migraine and gender effect: a meta-analysis of voxel-based morphometry studies. Neuroscience. 2015;299:88–96. https://doi.org/10.1016/j.neuroscience.2015.04.066.
20. Mehnert J, May A. Functional and structural alterations in the migraine cerebellum. J Cereb Blood Flow Metab. 2019;39:730–9. https://doi.org/10.1177/0271678X17722109.
21. Hougaard A, Amin FM, Ashina M. Migraine and structural abnormalities in the brain. Curr Opin Neurol. 2014;27:309–14. https://doi.org/10.1097/WCO.0000000000000086.
22. Messina R, Rocca MA, Colombo B, et al. Gray matter volume modifications in migraine: a cross-sectional and longitudinal study. Neurology. 2018;91:e280–92. https://doi.org/10.1212/WNL.0000000000005819.
23. Zhang J, Wu Y-L, Su J, et al. Assessment of gray and white matter structural alterations in migraineurs without aura. J Headache Pain. 2017;18:74. https://doi.org/10.1186/s10194-017-0783-5.

24. Liu H-Y, Lee P-L, Chou K-H, et al. The cerebellum is associated with 2-year prognosis in patients with high-frequency migraine. J Headache Pain. 2020;21:29. https://doi.org/10.1186/s10194-020-01096-4.
25. Yin T, Lan L, Tian Z, et al. Parahippocampus hypertrophy drives gray matter morphological alterations in migraine patients without aura. J Headache Pain. 2023;24:53. https://doi.org/10.1186/s10194-023-01588-z.
26. Cao Z, Yu W, Zhang Z, et al. Decreased gray matter volume in the frontal cortex of migraine patients with associated functional connectivity alterations: a VBM and rs-FC study. Pain Res Manag. 2022;2022:2115956. https://doi.org/10.1155/2022/2115956.
27. Qin Z, He X-W, Zhang J, et al. Structural changes of cerebellum and brainstem in migraine without aura. J Headache Pain. 2019;20:93. https://doi.org/10.1186/s10194-019-1045-5.
28. Palm-Meinders IH, Arkink EB, Koppen H, et al. Volumetric brain changes in migraineurs from the general population. Neurology. 2017;89:2066–74. https://doi.org/10.1212/WNL.0000000000004640.
29. Maleki N, Becerra L, Brawn J, et al. Concurrent functional and structural cortical alterations in migraine. Cephalalgia. 2012;32:607–20. https://doi.org/10.1177/0333102412445622.
30. Jin C, Yuan K, Zhao L, et al. Structural and functional abnormalities in migraine patients without aura. NMR Biomed. 2013;26:58–64. https://doi.org/10.1002/nbm.2819.
31. Messina R, Goadsby PJ, Filippi M. Editorial: functional and structural brain alterations in headache: a trait or a state? Front Neurol. 2020;11:859. https://doi.org/10.3389/fneur.2020.00859.
32. Messina R, Rocca MA, Colombo B, et al. White matter microstructure abnormalities in pediatric migraine patients. Cephalalgia. 2015;35:1278–86. https://doi.org/10.1177/0333102415578428.
33. Rocca MA, Messina R, Colombo B, et al. Structural brain MRI abnormalities in pediatric patients with migraine. J Neurol. 2014;261:350–7. https://doi.org/10.1007/s00415-013-7201-y.
34. Schmitz N, Admiraal-Behloul F, Arkink EB, et al. Attack frequency and disease duration as indicators for brain damage in migraine. Headache. 2008;48:1044–55. https://doi.org/10.1111/j.1526-4610.2008.01133.x.
35. Messina R, Rocca MA, Valsasina P, et al. Clinical correlates of hypothalamic functional changes in migraine patients. Cephalalgia. 2021. https://doi.org/10.1177/03331024211046618.
36. Coppola G, Di Renzo A, Tinelli E, et al. Evidence for brain morphometric changes during the migraine cycle: a magnetic resonance-based morphometry study. Cephalalgia. 2015;35:783–91. https://doi.org/10.1177/0333102414559732.
37. Chen W-T, Chou K-H, Lee P-L, et al. Comparison of gray matter volume between migraine and "strict-criteria" tension-type headache. J Headache Pain. 2018;19:4. https://doi.org/10.1186/s10194-018-0834-6.
38. Schwedt TJ, Si B, Li J, et al. Migraine subclassification via a data-driven automated approach using multimodality factor mixture modeling of brain structure measurements. Headache. 2017;57:1051–64. https://doi.org/10.1111/head.13121.
39. Datta R, Detre JA, Aguirre GK, Cucchiara B. Absence of changes in cortical thickness in patients with migraine. Cephalalgia. 2011;31:1452–8.
40. Magon S, May A, Stankewitz A, et al. Cortical abnormalities in episodic migraine: a multi-center 3T MRI study. Cephalalgia. 2019;39:665–73. https://doi.org/10.1177/0333102418795163.
41. DaSilva AFM, Granziera C, Snyder J, Hadjikhani N. Thickening in the somatosensory cortex of patients with migraine. Neurology. 2007;69:1990–5. https://doi.org/10.1212/01.wnl.0000291618.32247.2d.
42. Maleki N, Barmettler G, Moulton EA, et al. Female migraineurs show lack of insular thinning with age. Pain. 2015;156:1232–9. https://doi.org/10.1097/J.PAIN.0000000000000159.

43. Chong CD, Starling AJ, Schwedt TJ. Interictal photosensitivity associates with altered brain structure in patients with episodic migraine. Cephalalgia. 2016;36:526–33. https://doi.org/10.1177/0333102415606080.
44. Zhe X, Chen L, Zhang D, et al. Cortical areas associated with multisensory integration showing altered morphology and functional connectivity in relation to reduced life quality in vestibular migraine. Front Hum Neurosci. 2021;15. https://doi.org/10.3389/FNHUM.2021.717130.
45. Yu ZB, Peng J, Lv YB, et al. Different mean thickness implicates involvement of the cortex in migraine. Medicine. 2016;95. https://doi.org/10.1097/MD.0000000000004824.
46. Messina R, Rocca MA, Colombo B, et al. Cortical abnormalities in patients with migraine: a surface-based analysis. Radiology. 2013;268:170–80. https://doi.org/10.1148/radiol.13122004.
47. Komáromy H, He M, Perlaki G, et al. Influence of hemispheric white matter lesions and migraine characteristics on cortical thickness and volume. J Headache Pain. 2019;20. https://doi.org/10.1186/s10194-019-0959-2.
48. Chong CD, Dodick DW, Schlaggar BL, Schwedt TJ. Atypical age-related cortical thinning in episodic migraine. Cephalalgia. 2014;34:1115–24. https://doi.org/10.1177/0333102414531157/ASSET/IMAGES/LARGE/10.1177_0333102414531157-FIG3.JPEG.
49. Guarnera A, Bottino F, Napolitano A, et al. Early alterations of cortical thickness and gyrification in migraine without aura: a retrospective MRI study in pediatric patients. J Headache Pain. 2021;22:79. https://doi.org/10.1186/s10194-021-01290-y.
50. Amin FM, De Icco R, Al-Karagholi MA-M, et al. Investigation of cortical thickness and volume during spontaneous attacks of migraine without aura: a 3-Tesla MRI study. J Headache Pain. 2021;22:98. https://doi.org/10.1186/s10194-021-01312-9.
51. Alexander AL, Lee JE, Lazar M, Field AS. Diffusion tensor imaging of the brain. Neurotherapeutics. 2007;4:316–29.
52. Smith SM, Jenkinson M, Johansen-Berg H, et al. Tract-based spatial statistics: voxelwise analysis of multi-subject diffusion data. NeuroImage. 2006;31:1487–505. https://doi.org/10.1016/j.neuroimage.2006.02.024.
53. Porcaro C, Di Renzo A, Tinelli E, et al. Hypothalamic structural integrity and temporal complexity of cortical information processing at rest in migraine without aura patients between attacks. Sci Rep. 2021;11:1–11. https://doi.org/10.1038/s41598-021-98213-3.
54. Granziera C, Daducci A, Romascano D, et al. Structural abnormalities in the thalamus of migraineurs with aura: a multiparametric study at 3 T. Hum Brain Mapp. 2014;35:1461–8. https://doi.org/10.1002/hbm.22266.
55. Coppola G, Tinelli E, Lepre C, et al. Dynamic changes in thalamic microstructure of migraine without aura patients: a diffusion tensor magnetic resonance imaging study. Eur J Neurol. 2014;21:287-e13. https://doi.org/10.1111/ene.12296.
56. Coppola G, Di Renzo A, Tinelli E, et al. Thalamo-cortical network activity between migraine attacks: insights from MRI-based microstructural and functional resting-state network correlation analysis. J Headache Pain. 2016;17:100. https://doi.org/10.1186/s10194-016-0693-y.
57. Porcaro C, Di Renzo A, Tinelli E, et al. A hypothalamic mechanism regulates the duration of a migraine attack: insights from microstructural and temporal complexity of cortical functional networks analysis. Int J Mol Sci. 2022;23:13238. https://doi.org/10.3390/ijms232113238.
58. Yuan K, Qin W, Liu P, et al. Reduced fractional anisotropy of corpus callosum modulates inter-hemispheric resting state functional connectivity in migraine patients without aura. PLoS One. 2012;7:10.
59. Russo A, Silvestro M, Trojsi F, et al. Cognitive networks disarrangement in patients with migraine predicts cutaneous allodynia. Headache. 2020;60:1228–43. https://doi.org/10.1111/head.13860.

60. Tantik Pak A, Nacar Dogan S, Sengul Y. Structural integrity of corpus callosum in patients with migraine: a diffusion tensor imaging study. Acta Neurol Belg. 2023;123:385–90. https://doi.org/10.1007/s13760-021-01863-3.
61. Granziera C, DaSilva AFM, Snyder J, et al. Anatomical alterations of the visual motion processing network in migraine with and without aura. PLoS Med. 2006;3:e402. https://doi.org/10.1371/journal.pmed.0030402.
62. Rocca MA, Pagani E, Colombo B, et al. Selective diffusion changes of the visual pathways in patients with migraine: a 3-T tractography study. Cephalalgia. 2008;28:1061–8. https://doi.org/10.1111/j.1468-2982.2008.01655.x.
63. Mungoven TJ, Meylakh N, Marciszewski KK, et al. Microstructural changes in the trigeminal nerve of patients with episodic migraine assessed using magnetic resonance imaging. J Headache Pain. 2020;21:59. https://doi.org/10.1186/s10194-020-01126-1.
64. Liu J, Mu J, Chen T, et al. White matter tract microstructure of the mPFC-amygdala predicts interindividual differences in placebo response related to treatment in migraine patients. Hum Brain Mapp. 2019;40:284–92. https://doi.org/10.1002/hbm.24372.
65. Yu D, Yuan K, Qin W, et al. Axonal loss of white matter in migraine without aura: a tract-based spatial statistics study. Cephalalgia. 2013;33:34–42.
66. Yu D, Yuan K, Zhao L, et al. Regional homogeneity abnormalities in patients with interictal migraine without aura: a resting-state study. NMR Biomed. 2012;25:806–12.
67. Yu D, Yuan K, Zhao L, et al. White matter integrity affected by depressive symptoms in migraine without aura: a tract-based spatial statistics study. NMR Biomed. 2013;26:1103–12.
68. Planchuelo-Gómez Á, García-Azorín D, Guerrero ÁL, et al. White matter changes in chronic and episodic migraine: a diffusion tensor imaging study. J Headache Pain. 2020;21:1. https://doi.org/10.1186/s10194-019-1071-3.
69. Chong CD, Schwedt TJ. Migraine affects white-matter tract integrity: a diffusion-tensor imaging study. Cephalalgia. 2015. https://doi.org/10.1177/0333102415573513.
70. Szabó N, Kincses ZT, Párdutz A, et al. White matter microstructural alterations in migraine: a diffusion-weighted MRI study. Pain. 2012;153:651–6.
71. Tedeschi G, Russo A, Conte F, et al. Increased interictal visual network connectivity in patients with migraine with aura. Cephalalgia. 2016;36:139–47. https://doi.org/10.1177/0333102415584360.
72. Szabó N, Faragó P, Király A, et al. Evidence for plastic processes in migraine with aura: a diffusion weighted MRI study. Front Neuroanat. 2018;11:138. https://doi.org/10.3389/fnana.2017.00138.
73. Coppola G, Di Renzo A, Tinelli E, et al. Patients with chronic migraine without history of medication overuse are characterized by a peculiar white matter fiber bundle profile. J Headache Pain. 2020;21. https://doi.org/10.1186/s10194-020-01159-6.
74. Yang Y, Xu H, Deng Z, et al. Functional connectivity and structural changes of thalamic subregions in episodic migraine. J Headache Pain. 2022;23:119. https://doi.org/10.1186/s10194-022-01491-z.
75. Neeb L, Bastian K, Villringer K, et al. No microstructural white matter alterations in chronic and episodic migraineurs: a case-control diffusion tensor magnetic resonance imaging study. Headache. 2015;55:241–51. https://doi.org/10.1111/head.12496.
76. Mungoven TJ, Meylakh N, Macefield VG, et al. Alterations in brain structure associated with trigeminal nerve anatomy in episodic migraine. Front Pain Res (Lausanne). 2022;3:951581. https://doi.org/10.3389/fpain.2022.951581.
77. Coppola G, Di Renzo A, Tinelli E, et al. Thalamo-cortical network activity during spontaneous migraine attacks. Neurology. 2016;87:2154–60. https://doi.org/10.1212/WNL.0000000000003327.
78. Marciszewski KK, Meylakh N, Pietro FD, et al. Fluctuating regional brainstem diffusion imaging measures of microstructure across the migraine cycle. eNeuro, ENEURO.0005-19.2019. 2019;64. https://doi.org/10.1523/ENEURO.0005-19.2019.

79. Zhang H, Schneider T, Wheeler-Kingshott CA, Alexander DC. NODDI: practical in vivo neurite orientation dispersion and density imaging of the human brain. NeuroImage. 2012;61:1000–16. https://doi.org/10.1016/J.NEUROIMAGE.2012.03.072.
80. Zhao L, Zhao W, Anttila V, et al. Causal relationships between migraine and microstructural white matter: a Mendelian randomization study. J Headache Pain. 2023;24:10. https://doi.org/10.1186/s10194-023-01550-z.
81. Sun Z, Liu M, Zhao G, et al. Causal relationships between cortical brain structural alterations and migraine subtypes: a bidirectional Mendelian randomization study of 2,347 neuroimaging phenotypes. J Headache Pain. 2024;25:186. https://doi.org/10.1186/s10194-024-01896-y.
82. Taoka T, Masutani Y, Kawai H, et al. Evaluation of glymphatic system activity with the diffusion MR technique: diffusion tensor image analysis along the perivascular space (DTI-ALPS) in Alzheimer's disease cases. Jpn J Radiol. 2017;35:172–8. https://doi.org/10.1007/s11604-017-0617-z.
83. Ringstad G. Glymphatic imaging: a critical look at the DTI-ALPS index. Neuroradiology. 2024;66:157–60. https://doi.org/10.1007/S00234-023-03270-2/FIGURES/2.
84. Vittorini MG, Sahin A, Trojan A, et al. The glymphatic system in migraine and other headaches. J Headache Pain. 2024;25:1–12. https://doi.org/10.1186/S10194-024-01741-2.
85. Yuan Z, Li W, Tang H, et al. Enlarged perivascular spaces in patients with migraine: a case-control study based on 3T MRI. Ann Clin Transl Neurol. 2023;10:1160–9. https://doi.org/10.1002/ACN3.51798.
86. Lee DA, Lee H-J, Park KM. Normal glymphatic system function in patients with migraine: a pilot study. Headache. 2022;62:718–25. https://doi.org/10.1111/head.14320.
87. Zhang X, Wang W, Bai X, et al. Increased glymphatic system activity in migraine chronification by diffusion tensor image analysis along the perivascular space. J Headache Pain. 2023;24. https://doi.org/10.1186/S10194-023-01673-3.
88. Wu CH, Chang FC, Wang YF, et al. Impaired glymphatic and meningeal lymphatic functions in patients with chronic migraine. Ann Neurol. 2024;95:583–95. https://doi.org/10.1002/ANA.26842.
89. Cao Y, Huang M, Fu F, et al. Abnormally glymphatic system functional in patients with migraine: a diffusion kurtosis imaging study. J Headache Pain. 2024;25:118. https://doi.org/10.1186/s10194-024-01825-z.
90. Lv H, Wang Z, Tong E, et al. Resting-state functional MRI: everything that nonexperts have always wanted to know. AJNR Am J Neuroradiol. 2018;39:1390–9. https://doi.org/10.3174/ajnr.A5527.
91. Chen JE, Glover GH. Functional magnetic resonance imaging methods. Neuropsychol Rev. 2015;25:289–313. https://doi.org/10.1007/s11065-015-9294-9.
92. Moulton EA, Becerra L, Maleki N, et al. Painful heat reveals hyperexcitability of the temporal pole in interictal and ictal migraine states. Cerebral cortex (New York, NY: 1991). 2011;21:435–48.
93. Stankewitz A, Schulz E, May A. Neuronal correlates of impaired habituation in response to repeated trigemino-nociceptive but not to olfactory input in migraineurs: an fMRI study. Cephalalgia. 2013;33:256–65.
94. Schwedt TJ, Chong CD, Chiang C-C, et al. Enhanced pain-induced activity of pain-processing regions in a case-control study of episodic migraine. Cephalalgia. 2014;34:947–58. https://doi.org/10.1177/0333102414526069.
95. Mathur VA, Moayedi M, Keaser ML, et al. High frequency migraine is associated with lower acute pain sensitivity and abnormal insula activity related to migraine pain intensity, attack frequency, and pain catastrophizing. Front Hum Neurosci. 2016;10:489. https://doi.org/10.3389/fnhum.2016.00489.
96. Russo A, Tessitore A, Esposito F, et al. Functional changes of the perigenual part of the anterior cingulate cortex after external trigeminal neurostimulation in migraine patients. Front Neurol. 2017;8:282. https://doi.org/10.3389/fneur.2017.00282.

97. Russo A, Tessitore A, Bruno A, et al. Migraine does not affect pain intensity perception: a cross-sectional study. Pain Med. 2017. https://doi.org/10.1093/pm/pnx174.
98. Schulte LH, May A. The migraine generator revisited: continuous scanning of the migraine cycle over 30 days and three spontaneous attacks. Brain. 2016;139:1987–93. https://doi.org/10.1093/brain/aww097.
99. Datta R, Aguirre GK, Hu S, et al. Interictal cortical hyperresponsiveness in migraine is directly related to the presence of aura. Cephalalgia. 2013;33:365–74.
100. Martín H, Sánchez del Rio M, de Silanes C, et al. Photoreactivity of the occipital cortex measured by functional magnetic resonance imaging-blood oxygenation level dependent in migraine patients and healthy volunteers: pathophysiological implications. Headache. 2011;51:1520–8.
101. Tessitore A, Russo A, Giordano A, et al. Disrupted default mode network connectivity in migraine without aura. J Headache Pain. 2013;14:89.
102. Hubbard CS, Khan SA, Keaser ML, et al. Altered brain structure and function correlate with disease severity and pain catastrophizing in migraine patients. eNeuro. 2014;1:e20.14. https://doi.org/10.1523/ENEURO.0006-14.2014.
103. Hodkinson DJ, Veggeberg R, Kucyi A, et al. Cortico–cortical connections of primary sensory areas and associated symptoms in migraine. eNeuro. 2016;3:ENEURO.0163-16.2016. https://doi.org/10.1523/ENEURO.0163-16.2016.
104. Faragó P, Tuka B, Tóth E, et al. Interictal brain activity differs in migraine with and without aura: resting state fMRI study. J Headache Pain. 2017;18:8. https://doi.org/10.1186/s10194-016-0716-8.
105. Yu D, Yuan K, Luo L, et al. Abnormal functional integration across core brain networks in migraine without aura. Mol Pain. 2017;13:174480691773746. https://doi.org/10.1177/1744806917737461.
106. Yang F-C, Chou K-H, Hsu A-L, et al. Altered brain functional connectome in migraine with and without restless legs syndrome: a resting-state functional MRI study. Front Neurol. 2018;9:25. https://doi.org/10.3389/fneur.2018.00025.
107. Wang X, Zhang Y, Qi W, et al. Alteration in functional magnetic resonance imaging signal complexity across multiple time scales in patients with migraine without aura. Front Neurosci. 2022;16:825172. https://doi.org/10.3389/fnins.2022.825172.
108. Xue T, Yuan K, Zhao L, et al. Intrinsic brain network abnormalities in migraines without aura revealed in resting-state fMRI. PLoS One. 2012;7:10.
109. Zhou Y, Gong L, Yang Y, et al. Spatio-temporal dynamics of resting-state brain networks are associated with migraine disability. J Headache Pain. 2023;24:13. https://doi.org/10.1186/s10194-023-01551-y.
110. Cui W-Q, Zhang S-S, Xu F, et al. A resting-state functional magnetic resonance imaging study of abnormal frontoparietal network function in migraine without aura. Med Sci Monit. 2022;28:e934975. https://doi.org/10.12659/MSM.934975.
111. Russo A, Tessitore A, Giordano A, et al. Executive resting-state network connectivity in migraine without aura. Cephalalgia. 2012;32:1041–8.
112. Li Z, Lan L, Zeng F, et al. The altered right frontoparietal network functional connectivity in migraine and the modulation effect of treatment. Cephalalgia. 2017;37:161–76. https://doi.org/10.1177/0333102416641665.
113. Wei H-L, Tian T, Zhou G-P, et al. Disrupted dynamic functional connectivity of the visual network in episodic patients with migraine without aura. Neural Plast. 2022;2022:9941832. https://doi.org/10.1155/2022/9941832.
114. Chen Z, Chen X, Liu M, et al. Altered functional connectivity architecture of the brain in medication overuse headache using resting state fMRI. J Headache Pain. 2017;18:25. https://doi.org/10.1186/s10194-017-0735-0.
115. Kim YE, Kim MK, Suh S-I, Kim JH. Altered trigeminothalamic spontaneous low-frequency oscillations in migraine without aura: a resting-state fMRI study. BMC Neurol. 2021;21:342. https://doi.org/10.1186/s12883-021-02374-7.

116. Quan S, Wang C, Huang J, et al. Abnormal thalamocortical network dynamics in patients with migraine and its relationship with electroacupuncture treatment response. Brain Imaging Behav. 2024. https://doi.org/10.1007/s11682-024-00938-y.
117. Qin Z, Qu H, Liang H-B, et al. Altered resting-state effective connectivity of trigeminal vascular system in migraine without aura: a spectral dynamic causal modeling study. Headache. 2023;63:1119–27. https://doi.org/10.1111/head.14602.
118. Shen B, Cheng J, Zhang X, et al. The abnormally increased functional connectivity of the locus coeruleus in migraine without aura patients. BMC Res Notes. 2024;17:330. https://doi.org/10.1186/s13104-024-06991-6.
119. Liu K, Cheng J, Cao Y, et al. Abnormally increased effective connectivity of the periaqueductal gray in migraine without aura patients. Clin J Pain. 2023;39:175–9. https://doi.org/10.1097/AJP.0000000000001099.
120. Li Z, Liu M, Lan L, et al. Altered periaqueductal gray resting state functional connectivity in migraine and the modulation effect of treatment. Sci Rep. 2016;6:20298. https://doi.org/10.1038/srep20298.
121. Gecse K, Dobos D, Aranyi CS, et al. Association of plasma tryptophan concentration with periaqueductal gray matter functional connectivity in migraine patients. Sci Rep. 2022;12:739. https://doi.org/10.1038/s41598-021-04647-0.
122. Wang T, Zhan W, Chen Q, et al. Altered resting-state ascending/descending pathways associated with the posterior thalamus in migraine without aura. Neuroreport. 2016;27:257–63. https://doi.org/10.1097/WNR.0000000000000529.
123. Niddam DM, Lai K-L, Fuh J-L, et al. Reduced functional connectivity between salience and visual networks in migraine with aura. Cephalalgia. 2016;36:53–66. https://doi.org/10.1177/0333102415583144.
124. Yu Z, Lv Y, Song L, et al. Functional connectivity differences in the insular sub-regions in migraine without aura: a resting-state functional magnetic resonance imaging study. Front Behav Neurosci. 2017;11:124. https://doi.org/10.3389/fnbeh.2017.00124.
125. Gao Q, Xu F, Jiang C, et al. Decreased functional connectivity density in pain-related brain regions of female migraine patients without aura. Brain Res. 2016;1632:73–81. https://doi.org/10.1016/j.brainres.2015.12.007.
126. Yuan K, Zhao L, Cheng P, et al. Altered structure and resting-state functional connectivity of the basal ganglia in migraine patients without aura. J Pain. 2013;14:836–44.
127. Chen Z, Chen X, Liu M, et al. Disrupted functional connectivity of periaqueductal gray subregions in episodic migraine. J Headache Pain. 2017;18:36. https://doi.org/10.1186/s10194-017-0747-9.
128. Zhao L, Liu J, Dong X, et al. Alterations in regional homogeneity assessed by fMRI in patients with migraine without aura stratified by disease duration. J Headache Pain. 2013;14:85.
129. Mainero C, Boshyan J, Hadjikhani N. Altered functional magnetic resonance imaging resting-state connectivity in periaqueductal gray networks in migraine. Ann Neurol. 2011;70:838–45.
130. Schulte LH, Mehnert J, May A. Longitudinal neuroimaging over 30 days: temporal characteristics of migraine. Ann Neurol. 2020;87:646–51. https://doi.org/10.1002/ana.25697.
131. Schulte LH, Menz MM, Haaker J, May A. The migraineur's brain networks: continuous resting state fMRI over 30 days. Cephalalgia. 2020. https://doi.org/10.1177/0333102420951465.
132. Schulte LH, Allers A, May A. Hypothalamus as a mediator of chronic migraine. Neurology. 2017;88:2011–6. https://doi.org/10.1212/WNL.0000000000003963.
133. Coppola G, Di Renzo A, Tinelli E, et al. Resting state connectivity between default mode network and insula encodes acute migraine headache. Cephalalgia. 2018;38:846–54. https://doi.org/10.1177/0333102417715230.
134. Amin FM, Hougaard A, Magon S, et al. Change in brain network connectivity during PACAP38-induced migraine attacks: a resting-state functional MRI study. Neurology. 2016;86:180–7.

135. Amin FM, Hougaard A, Magon S, et al. Altered thalamic connectivity during spontaneous attacks of migraine without aura: a resting-state fMRI study. Cephalalgia. 2018;38:1237–44. https://doi.org/10.1177/0333102417729113.
136. Karsan N, Bose PR, O'Daly O, et al. Alterations in functional connectivity during different phases of the triggered migraine attack. Headache. 2020;60:1244–58. https://doi.org/10.1111/HEAD.13865.
137. Meylakh N, Marciszewski KK, Di Pietro F, et al. Deep in the brain: changes in subcortical function immediately preceding a migraine attack. Hum Brain Mapp. 2018;39:2651–63. https://doi.org/10.1002/hbm.24030.
138. Zhang L, Yu W, Xu M, et al. The hypothalamus may mediate migraine and ictal photophobia: evidence from granger causality analysis. Neurol Sci. 2022;43:6021–30. https://doi.org/10.1007/s10072-022-06245-y.
139. Zhang L, Yu W, Zhang Z, et al. Altered brain activity and functional connectivity in migraine without aura during and outside attack. Neurol Res. 2023;45:603–9. https://doi.org/10.1080/01616412.2023.2170938.
140. Ruiz-Tagle A, Figueiredo P, Pinto J, et al. Working memory during spontaneous migraine attacks: an fMRI study. Neurol Sci. 2024;45:1201–8. https://doi.org/10.1007/s10072-023-07120-0.
141. Araújo RP, Figueiredo P, Pinto J, et al. Altered functional connectivity in a sensorimotor-insular network during spontaneous migraine attacks: a resting-state FMRI study. Brain Res. 2023;1818. https://doi.org/10.1016/J.BRAINRES.2023.148513.
142. Petcharunpaisan S, Ramalho J, Castillo M. Arterial spin labeling in neuroimaging. World J Radiol. 2010;2:384. https://doi.org/10.4329/WJR.V2.I10.384.
143. Chen Z, Chen X, Liu M, et al. Evaluation of gray matter perfusion in episodic migraine using voxel-wise comparison of 3D pseudo-continuous arterial spin labeling. J Headache Pain. 2018;19:36. https://doi.org/10.1186/s10194-018-0866-y.
144. Hodkinson DJ, Veggeberg R, Wilcox SL, et al. Primary somatosensory cortices contain altered patterns of regional cerebral blood flow in the Interictal phase of migraine. PLoS One. 2015;10:e0137971. https://doi.org/10.1371/journal.pone.0137971.
145. Zhang D, Huang X, Mao C, et al. Assessment of normalized cerebral blood flow and its connectivity with migraines without aura during interictal periods by arterial spin labeling. J Headache Pain. 2021;22:72. https://doi.org/10.1186/s10194-021-01282-y.
146. Li X, Khan A, Li Y, et al. Hyperconnection and hyperperfusion of overlapping brain regions in patients with menstrual-related migraine: a multimodal neuroimaging study. Neuroradiology. 2021;63:741–9. https://doi.org/10.1007/s00234-020-02623-5.
147. Zhang Q, Datta R, Detre JA, Cucchiara B. White matter lesion burden in migraine with aura may be associated with reduced cerebral blood flow. Cephalalgia. 2017;37:517–24. https://doi.org/10.1177/0333102416649760.
148. Xu Z-G, Xu J-J, Chen Y-C, et al. Aberrant cerebral blood flow in tinnitus patients with migraine: a perfusion functional MRI study. J Headache Pain. 2021;22:61. https://doi.org/10.1186/s10194-021-01280-0.
149. Hoogeveen ES, Pelzer N, Ghariq E, et al. Cerebrovascular reactivity to hypercapnia in patients with migraine: a dual-echo arterial spin labeling MRI study. Headache. 2024;64:276–84. https://doi.org/10.1111/head.14680.
150. Michels L, Villanueva J, O'Gorman R, et al. Interictal hyperperfusion in the higher visual cortex in patients with episodic migraine. Headache: the journal of head and face. Pain. 2019;59:1808–20. https://doi.org/10.1111/head.13646.
151. Zhang C, Detre JA, Kasner SE, Cucchiara B. Basilar artery lateral displacement may be associated with migraine with aura. Front Neurol. 2018;9:80. https://doi.org/10.3389/fneur.2018.00080.
152. Fu T, Liu L, Huang X, et al. Cerebral blood flow alterations in migraine patients with and without aura: an arterial spin labeling study. J Headache Pain. 2022;23:131. https://doi.org/10.1186/s10194-022-01501-0.

153. Park S, Lee DA, Lee HJ, et al. Brain networks in migraine with and without aura: an exploratory arterial spin labeling MRI study. Acta Neurol Scand. 2022;145:208–14. https://doi.org/10.1111/ANE.13536.
154. Silvestro M, Esposito F, De Rosa AP, et al. Reduced neurovascular coupling of the visual network in migraine patients with aura as revealed with arterial spin labeling MRI: is there a demand-supply mismatch behind the scenes? J Headache Pain. 2024;25:180. https://doi.org/10.1186/s10194-024-01885-1.
155. Meylakh N, Marciszewski KK, Di Pietro F, et al. Altered regional cerebral blood flow and hypothalamic connectivity immediately prior to a migraine headache. Cephalalgia. 2020;40:448–60. https://doi.org/10.1177/0333102420911623.
156. Stankewitz A, Keidel L, Rehm M, et al. Migraine attacks as a result of hypothalamic loss of control. Neuroimage Clin. 2021;32:102784. https://doi.org/10.1016/j.nicl.2021.102784.
157. Younis S, Christensen CE, Vestergaard MB, et al. Glutamate levels and perfusion in pons during migraine attacks: a 3T MRI study using proton spectroscopy and arterial spin labeling. J Cereb Blood Flow Metab. 2021;41:604–16. https://doi.org/10.1177/0271678X20906902.
158. Karsan N, Bose RP, O'Daly O, et al. Regional cerebral perfusion during the premonitory phase of triggered migraine: a double-blind randomized placebo-controlled functional imaging study using pseudo-continuous arterial spin labeling. Headache. 2023;63:771–87. https://doi.org/10.1111/head.14538.
159. Gil-Gouveia R, Pinto J, Figueiredo P, et al. An arterial spin labeling MRI perfusion study of migraine without aura attacks. Front Neurol. 2017;8:280. https://doi.org/10.3389/fneur.2017.00280.

Chapter 6
Neuroimaging Studies of Migraine with Aura

Igor Petrušić and Nouchine Hadjikhani

6.1 Introduction

Migraine with aura (MwA) is a type of migraine that can be manifested very heterogeneously [1]. According to the manifestation of aura symptoms, MwA is primarily divided into migraine with typical aura (MwTA), migraine with brainstem aura, hemiplegic migraine (HM), and retinal migraine [1]. Considering that MwTA could be manifested with a plethora of symptoms, including visual, somatosensory, language, and memory disturbances, it could be further subdivided into groups of patients who suffer from only migraine with pure visual aura (MwPVA) and those who, in some or most of the migraine with typical aura attacks, suffer from somatosensory and/or higher cortical dysfunctions (MwVSD) [2, 3]. Furthermore, HM, a rare autosomal dominant form of migraine that is characterized by a motor aura [1], is influenced by specific genetic mutations, which should be considered separately when neuroimaging studies are designed.

Although MwA is prevalent in the general population, approximately 4.5% of the global population has experienced MwA attacks during their lifetime [2]; there are no validated neuroimaging biomarkers, although numerous studies proposed specific findings in neuroimaging studies related to MwA or their subtypes [3–16].

I. Petrušić (✉)
Laboratory for Advanced Analysis of Neuroimages, Faculty of Physical Chemistry, University of Belgrade, Belgrade, Serbia

N. Hadjikhani
Gillberg Neuropsychiatry Centre, Institute of Neuroscience and Physiology, University of Gothenburg, Gothenburg, Sweden

Athinoula A. Martinos Center for Biomedical Imaging, Massachusetts General Hospital, Harvard Medical School, Boston, MA, USA

I. Petrušić, Y. Wang (eds.), *Neuroimaging of Headache Disorders*, Headache,
https://doi.org/10.1007/978-3-031-85402-6_6

Cortical spreading depolarization followed by cortical spreading depression is a widely accepted model that explains the pathogenesis of migraine aura [16]. However, it is not well understood whether cortical spreading depolarization always originates in the same area (i.e., occipital cortex) and spreads always in a given direction, as well as it is unifocal or multifocal [17]. Understanding the neuroimaging features of MwA and its subtypes is crucial for advancing diagnostic methods and treatment strategies in migraine disorders. Herewith, we presented the key findings associated with MwA during the interictal and ictal phases investigated by various neuroimaging modalities.

6.2 Neuroimaging Studies of Migraine with Typical Aura

6.2.1 Neuroimaging Studies of Migraine with Typical Aura During the Interictal Phase

6.2.1.1 Structural Magnetic Resonance Imaging (MRI) Studies of Migraine with Typical Aura During the Interictal Phase

Advanced post-processing MRI techniques [18–20] have enabled detailed analyses of brain structure during the interictal phase in MwA patients, facilitating comparisons between MwA, migraine without aura, and healthy controls (HCs). Examining the findings, implications, and limitations of these structural MRI studies, particularly those focusing on MwTA patients in the interictal phase (the symptom-free period between migraine attacks), can enhance our understanding of the condition. Given that visual symptoms are predominant in MwTA, structural characteristics of the visual cortex were investigated in several studies that showed increased cortical thickness and volume in visual cortical areas in MwA compared to HCs [7, 21], suggesting also a positive correlation between the complexity of migraine aura, in terms of additional nonvisual symptoms, and cortical thickness of the visual cortex [9, 22]. However, increased cortical thickness in the V3A area of the visual cortex has been demonstrated in both migraine with and without aura [23], precluding visual cortex thickness as a specific marker for MwA. Similar findings were shown for the somatosensory region [24, 25], also pointing toward a positive correlation between the complexity of migraine aura, determined by the Migraine Aura Complexity Score (MACS), and cortical thickness of the somatosensory cortex [22]. However, there were also studies with opposing findings regarding the investigation of the somatosensory cortex [26], overall suggesting the need for further investigation using a high-quality design approach, including advanced, standardized, and reproducible MRI protocols for image acquisition and post-processing, and carefully selected MwA patients which constitute a clinically homogenous group.

Additionally, other studies have demonstrated differences in cortical thickness and other cortical features in areas outside of the visual and somatosensory cortex in subjects with MwA compared to HCs, including the middle temporal cortex [23, 25], right insula, bilateral supramarginal gyrus and left inferior temporal gyrus [27], and left temporal pole, fusiform gyrus, and pars opercularis [3, 28]. In addition, MwVSD patients have reduced cortical surface area of the left rostral middle frontal cortex and increased cortical thickness in the bilateral primary, secondary and V5/MT visual cortical areas, as well as left pericalcarine gyrus and left pars opercularis, compared with MwPVA group [3, 9, 28]. In contrast, other study show decreased cortical thickness in the inferior, middle, superior, and lingual gyri, as well as in several regions in the temporal and frontal lobes, in MwVSD patients compared to MwVSD [25]. Therefore, whether MwA and its subtypes are truly associated with cortical thickness alterations is still argued [29]. Many potential confounders, such as underpowered sample size, heterogeneous patient selection criteria, heterogeneous clinical manifestation of MwTA, and differences in imaging collection and post-processing techniques, may contribute to the inconsistencies of cortical thickness investigation. Furthermore, factors such as medication use, comorbid conditions, and attack frequency can influence brain structure and must be carefully controlled in studies to ensure an accurate interpretation of the results. Thus, longitudinal population-based multimodal neuroimaging studies at different migraine phases that subtype homogeneous patients with well-powered sample sizes using standardized imaging collection protocols and well-validated processing and analysis pipelines are required to improve the reliability of the results that characterize cortical thickness alterations in MwTA [29, 30]. Significant findings of structural magnetic resonance imaging studies of MwTA during the interictal phase are shown in Table 6.1.

Very few studies specifically investigated subcortical nuclei volumes between MwA and compared them to HCs. One study demonstrated reduced volumes in the putamen and globus pallidus in MwA compared to HCs [32]. In addition, other study demonstrated larger brainstem volumes in MwA [33], suggesting that deep subcortical brain nuclei and brainstem structures may be altered in MwA.

White matter changes are commonly observed in MwTA individuals during the interictal phase. These changes can be detected through various techniques, such as the identification of white matter hyperintensities, bright spots visible on T2-weighted MRI scans, and diffusion tensor imaging studies. Previous studies demonstrated that white matter hyperintensities were more common in those with MwA, particularly in the posterior circulation [34]. A subsequent 9-year follow-up study showed no other progressive structural brain changes and no cognitive impact of the white matter hyperintensities [35]. Furthermore, a subsequent meta-analysis of 19 studies has confirmed the suggestion of an increased risk of white matter hyperintensities in MwA compared to HCs and those with migraine without aura; however, there was no association between MwA and silent brain infarcts [36–38]. Studies have shown lower fractional anisotropy (FA) in the ventral trigeminothalamic tract and increased FA in the left parieto-occipital white matter in MwA patients compared to those without aura [39, 40]. Additionally, broad microstructural alterations in the thalamus, observed in MwA patients relative to both healthy controls (HCs) and those without aura, suggest increased iron deposition and higher

Table 6.1 Structural magnetic resonance imaging studies of MwTA during the interictal phase—significant findings

Authors, years	Subjects	Type of measurements	Main findings
Granziera et al. [23]	12 MwA 12 MwoA 15 HCs	Cortical thickness	Increased cortical thickness of the V3A and middle temporal cortex in MwA and MwoA compared to HCs
DaSilva [24]	12 MwA 12 MwoA 12 HCs	Cortical thickness	Increased cortical thickness of the somatosensory cortex in MwA and MwoA compared to HCs
Messina et al. [27]	32 MwA 31 MwoA 18 HCs	Cortical thickness, cortical surface area	Compared with HCs and MwoA, MwA patients had an increased cortical thickness of the bilateral supramarginal gyrus and a decreased cortical thickness of the right central sulcus and right insula. Also, MwA had an increased cortical surface area of the left lingual gyrus and left pericallosal sulcus and a decreased cortical surface area of the left inferior temporal gyrus
Gaist et al. [7]	165 MwA 137 HCs	Cortical thickness	MwA patients had thicker cortex in areas V2 and V3A
Petrusic et al. [22]	23 MwA	Cortical thickness	The MACS exhibited positive correlations with cortical thickness in MwA patients (the left and right lateral occipital, right cuneus, right precuneus, left postcentral, and left and right superior parietal cortices)
Petrusic et al. [28]	48 MwA 30 HCs	Cortical thickness, cortical surface area, and other cortical morphometry	MwA patients had significantly reduced volume of the left fusiform gyrus relative to HCs
Petrusic et al. [9]	32 MwA	Cortical thickness	Patients with higher MACS had thicker cortex in several visual and somatosensory cortical regions
Mitrović et al. [3]	46 MwA 32 HCs	Cortical thickness, cortical surface area, and other cortical morphometry	Left temporal pole thickness, right lingual gyrus thickness, and left pars opercularis thickness are the most significant features in recognizing MwA

(continued)

Table 6.1 (continued)

Authors, years	Subjects	Type of measurements	Main findings
Mitrović et al. [31]	40 MwA	Cortical thickness, cortical surface area, and other cortical morphometry	Advanced machine learning algorithms for increased MACS prediction pointed to various cortical features spread out throughout a whole-brain network affecting predominately parietal and temporal regions
Niddam et al. [21]	50 MwA 50 MwoA 50 HCs	Cortical volume, functional connectivity	Increased gray matter volume was found in the medial visual cortex and the middle frontal cortex. A multivariate pattern of gray matter voxels within a functionally defined ventral medial visual network contains significant information related to the diagnosis of MwA

MwA migraine with aura, *MwoA* migraine without aura, *HCs* healthy controls

myelin content or cellularity [41]. However, subsequent diffusion tensor imaging studies found no significant differences in FA, mean diffusivity (MD), radial diffusivity (RD), or axial diffusivity (AD) between HCs and MwTA patients, nor among MwTA subtypes [25, 42].

In summary, structural MRI studies have provided valuable insights into the neurobiology of MwTA during the interictal phase; however, it should be noted that MwTA is a heterogeneous disorder, and not all individuals exhibit the same structural alterations. Currently, this variability can make it challenging to draw definitive conclusions and generalize findings. Future research, particularly longitudinal studies and those combining structural and functional imaging techniques, will be crucial in unraveling the relationship between brain structure, migraine pathophysiology, and clinical symptoms. As our understanding grows, these insights may pave the way for improved diagnostic and therapeutic approaches for individuals suffering from MwTA.

6.2.1.2 Functional MRI Studies of Migraine with Typical Aura During the Interictal Phase

MwA is likely mediated by widespread interictal brain dysfunction in areas involving, but not limited to, the visual, extrastriate, somatosensory, and insular cortex and thalamus [15]. Tedeschi and colleagues revealed that MwA patients have altered resting-state visual network connectivity compared to those with migraine without aura and HCs [5], as well as increased connectivity in the left angular and supramarginal gyri, right precentral and postcentral gyri, and right insular cortex [43]. Increased glutamate levels in the visual cortex interictally have also been demonstrated in MwA patients [44]. Also, it was shown that MwA patients have reduced connectivity between the anterior insular and V3A regions, which correlates with headache severity [45]. Furthermore, Datta and colleagues found a greater response to visual stimulation within the primary visual cortex in MwA patients compared to those with migraine without aura and HCs [46]. Additionally, Hougaard and colleagues demonstrated a greater response to visual stimulation in the symptomatic hemisphere, in particular parietal and frontal regions, of patients who suffer from MwA compared to HCs [47]. Moreover, magnetic resonance spectroscopy imaging study revealed differences in the mitochondrial function of neurons in the visual cortex after photic stimulation manifested as increased lactate and significantly more decreased N-acetyl aspartate peak in MwA patients compared to those without aura and HCs [48]. In addition, increased blood–oxygenation level-dependent (BOLD) response to trigeminal noxious stimulation in the lingual gyrus, inferior parietal lobule, frontal gyri, and cerebellum was shown in MwA patients compared to those with migraine without aura and HCs [49]. Moreover, Bridge and colleagues noted reduced gamma-aminobutyric acid levels in MwA patients, suggesting reduced inhibition in the occipital cortex consistent with occipital hyperexcitability [4]. Additionally, the same study demonstrated a positive correlation between glutamate levels and BOLD activation in the visual cortex during visual stimulation, indicating enhanced glutamate activation and abnormal excitation–inhibition coupling [4]. Furthermore, using magnetic resonance spectroscopic imaging with 8-Hz checkerboard visual stimulation, an increased lactate concentration was noted in the visual cortex in MwVSD patients compared to those who have MwPVA and HCs [50]. In contrast, MwPVA was characterized by increased lactate concentration in the visual cortex during resting and without further increase during visual stimulation [50]. Authors interpreted these findings as a consequence of dishabituation and a predominant mitochondrial dysfunction in MwVSD [50]. In addition, Fu and colleagues demonstrated higher cerebral blood flow in regions such as the bilateral superior frontal gyrus, bilateral postcentral gyrus, and cerebellum and lower cerebral blood flow in the bilateral middle frontal gyrus, thalamus, and medioventral occipital cortex, when patients who have MwA are compared with those without aura and HCs [13, 51]. In contrast, hypoperfusion in the postcentral gyrus and inferior temporal gyrus was demonstrated in MwA patients [52].

Another study demonstrated a disrupted executive control network functional connectivity in migraine patients, including those who have MwTA [53]. Additionally, functional connectivity between the default mode network and dorsal attention system is disrupted in MwA patients compared to HCs [10]. The same authors investigated the influence of visual stimulation in MwTA patients and demonstrated improved connectivity between the default mode network, salience network, and executive control network, suggesting a stronger cognitive impact of visual stimulation on MwTA patients compared to HCs [11]. Additionally, it was found that amygdala connectivity in both groups with migraine with and without aura was increased to the visceroceptive insula relative to trigeminal neuralgia, carpal tunnel syndrome, and healthy control groups [54]. Moreover, resting-state BOLD signal fluctuation in the cingulate cortex, superior parietal lobule, cerebellum, and bilateral frontal regions was higher in MwTA patients compared to those without aura and HCs [55]. In addition, the same study demonstrated an increased amplitude of activity in all resting-state networks in MwTA patients [8, 55]. Increased fluctuation of connectivity within the salience network was also noted in

MwA patients [56]. In addition, Silvestro and colleagues suggested that higher extrastriate brain changes may lead to the propagation of aura from simple visual symptoms to more complex phenotypes [14]. However, some studies did not find any difference in terms of functional connectivity between MwA patients and HCs [57]. Hougaard and colleagues suggested that the previously reported increased cortical hyperresponsivity in the interictal phase of MwA is unlikely to be caused by abnormalities of intrinsic brain connectivity. In addition, they concluded that the interictal migraine aura brain may be abnormally functioning only during exposure to external stimuli [57, 58]. Significant findings of functional magnetic resonance imaging studies of MwTA during the interictal phase are shown in Table 6.2.

Considering all of the abovementioned, there is a great need for the formation of an expert consortium that will recommend best practices in functional neuroimaging research of MwA. Among others, the primary goal would be to reduce sources of heterogeneity in the selection of MwA patients and HCs, as well as the variability in analysis methods for functional MRI datasets [30].

6.2.1.3 Ultrasound Studies of Migraine with Typical Aura During the Interictal Phase

Cerebrovascular reactivity and blood flow velocity in MwTA individuals have been previously examined using different techniques [59–62]. However, knowledge about the cerebral blood flow difference between MwTA individuals and HCs, as well as the correlation between the clinical presentation of MwA and cerebral blood flow parameters, remains insufficient. Ornello and colleagues systematically investigated literature regarding the cerebrovascular reactivity to hypercapnia or hypocapnia in migraine patients, and the results were conflicting [63]. However, meta-analyses of transcranial Doppler ultrasound studies revealed higher resting mean blood flow velocity in the anterior circulation to be more evident in MwA individuals [62], supporting furthermore the literature data that increased cerebrovascular reactivity is a feature of MwA [60]. Moreover, Reinhard and colleagues reported that MwA patients have poorer autoregulation in the cerebellar circulation than HCs [64]. In addition, another study's findings revealed increased arterial stiffness as indicated by a higher pulsatility index in the middle and anterior parts of the Willis circle in female patients who have MwA relative to HCs [65]. Future multimodal studies that include functional MRI, evoked potentials, and transcranial Doppler ultrasound examination performed on a clinically homogenized group of MwTA patients may allow definitive conclusions.

It is worth noting that there is still an undergoing debate about the influence of right-to-left shunt on MwA patients, although several studies demonstrated that closure of a patent foramen ovale failed to show a reduction in days with migraine [66]; however, it is showed that a patent foramen ovale may influence the pathophysiology of MwA [67]. Furthermore, Shin and colleagues proposed that microemboli can play a pivotal role in the development of migraine attacks [68]. Interestingly, Petrusic and colleagues demonstrated that MwVSD patients more frequently

Table 6.2 Functional magnetic resonance imaging studies of migraine with typical aura during the interictal phase—significant findings

Authors, years	Subjects	Main findings
Datta et al. [46]	25 MwA 25 MwoA 25 HCs	Increased response to visual stimulation within the primary visual cortex
Hougaard et al. [47]	20 MwA (unilateral side-fixed visual aura) 20 HCs	Increased response to visual stimulation in the symptomatic hemisphere, in particular, parietal and frontal regions
Tessitore et al. [53]	20 MwA 20 MwoA 20 HCs	Disrupted executive control network functional connectivity in MwA and migraine without aura
Tedeschi et al. [5]	20 MwA 20 MwoA 20 HCs	Increased functional connectivity in the right lingual gyrus within the resting-state visual network
Niddam et al. [45]	26 MwA 26 MwoA 26 HCs	Reduced connectivity between anterior insular and V3A regions
Faragó et al. [55]	18 MwA 35 MwoA 32 HCs	Increased BOLD signal fluctuation in the cingulate cortex, superior parietal lobule, cerebellum, and bilateral frontal regions. Increased amplitude of activity in all resting-state networks
Lo Buono et al. [43]	14 MwA 14 MwoA 14 HCs	Increased connectivity in the left angular and supramarginal gyri, right precentral and postcentral gyri, and right insular cortex
Russo et al. [49]	17 MwA 18 MwoA 15 HCs	Increased BOLD response to trigeminal noxious stimulation in the lingual gyrus, inferior parietal lobule, frontal gyri, and cerebellum
Veréb et al. [56]	20 MwA 37 MwoA 32 HCs	Increased fluctuation of connectivity within the salience network
Coppola et al. [10]	35 MwA 19 HCs	Disrupted functional connectivity between the default mode network and dorsal attention system

MwA migraine with aura, *MwoA* migraine without aura, *HCs* healthy controls, *BOLD* blood–oxygenation level-dependent

exhibited microemboli signals detected by transcranial Doppler ultrasound compared to MwPVA and HCs [69]. The exact pathophysiological mechanism of these findings is not clear and thus requires additional research.

6.2.1.4 Magnetoencephalography and Electroencephalography Studies of Migraine with Typical Aura During the Interictal Phase

It is well known that the cerebral cortex plays a key role in MwA attacks; however, its neural mechanism is poorly understood. Nonetheless, evoked cortical potential and nociceptive blink reflex studies demonstrate that lack of habituation during repetitive stimulation is a reproducible central nervous system dysfunction interictally in MwA [70].

The chapter "Neurophysiology of Migraine with Aura" by Ambrosini and Coppola, featured in the book *Neurophysiology of the Migraine Brain* (part of the "Headache" series), provides a comprehensive exploration of the use of electroencephalography, evoked potentials, and neuromodulation techniques in investigating the underlying mechanisms and neurophysiological changes associated with MwA [71]. In addition, more recent studies also provided new evidence of subtle interictal cognitive dysfunction in MwTA patients by using a visual oddball paradigm to elicit the P300 component [72]. Moreover, it was suggested that the visual oddball paradigm, particularly rare stimuli, could serve as a potential new tool for deep profiling of different clinical complexities, such as the presence of somatosensory and/or dysphasic symptoms during aura, among MwA patients [72]. Further confirmation of subtle interictal cognitive dysfunction, as well as dysfunction of semantic function, in MwTA patients, was provided in another study by using a picture–word priming paradigm to elicit the N400 component [73].

In addition, magnetoencephalography is considered to be superior to scalp electroencephalography because the skull, skin, and other tissues can distort electric signals, whereas magnetic signals can pass through these tissues without significant distortion [74]. Thus, studies using magnetoencephalography, combined with graph theory, may reveal the features of the intrinsic functional network of the brain in MwA patients [75]. Wu and colleagues reported that both conditions, migraine with and without aura, are characterized by distinctive topographic patterns of the neural network, showing that the migraine patients had significantly increased functional connectivity in the slow wave (0.1–1 Hz) band in the frontal area compared to HCs. Additionally, MwA patients had significantly increased functional connectivity in the theta (4–8 Hz) band in the occipital area compared to those who have migraine without aura [75]. These results imply that MwA is associated with functional brain reorganization.

6.2.2 *Neuroimaging Studies of Migraine with Typical Aura During the Ictal Phase*

The main goal of neuroimaging studies that investigate MwA during the ictal phase is to try to capture the changes in the brain that accurately reflect the occurrence of aura symptoms [76]. The first attempts to capture MwA attack were performed by using intra-arterial Xenon techniques [77, 78]. Those studies showed alterations in regional cerebral blood flow, indicating oligemia, during triggered migraine aura attacks occurring posteriorly and propagating forward at a rate compatible with cortical spreading depression. These studies provided neuroimaging evidence that cortical spreading depression likely mediates aura in human subjects who suffer from MwTA. In addition, another study demonstrated that during aura, relative cerebral blood flow was significantly decreased in the occipital cortex contralateral to the affected hemifield [79]. Also, relative cerebral blood volume was decreased and mean transit time increased, persisting up to 2.5 h into the headache phase. Moreover, in one patient who experienced both migraine with and without aura, perfusion deficits were observed only during MwA [79]. Subsequently, the functional MRI study case, on a patient who can provoke migraine with aura attack by physical activity, demonstrated BOLD signal changes that contained at least eight characteristics in common between the observed events and animal cortical spreading depression studies [16]. Those characteristics were as follows:

1. The BOLD signal in the occipital cortex was time-locked to the onset of the visual aura.
2. The quality of the aura was consistent with the function of the area where it started (area V3A).
3. Aura propagation was congruent with the retinotopy of the visual percept.
4. The initial focal BOLD signal increase possibly reflected vasodilation.
5. BOLD signal progressed contiguously and slowly over the occipital cortex to affect adjacent voxels, mirroring the 2–3 mm/min pace of cortical spreading depression and not respecting the supply territories of large arteries.
6. After this initial increase, the BOLD signal diminished (possibly reflecting vasoconstriction following the initial vasodilation).
7. BOLD signal was suppressed transiently.
8. During periods with no visual stimulation (periods of 32 s of flickering radial checkerboard) other than a fixation cross, but during which the subject was experiencing scintillations, the BOLD signal change followed the retinotopic progression of the visual percept.

This study, despite the limitation of collecting neuroimaging data on only three male patients, strongly suggested that a propagating event akin to cortical spreading depression generates the migraine visual aura in the human visual cortex.

In addition, another study investigated five migraine patients during various forms of aura symptoms induced by hypoxia, sham hypoxia, or physical exercise with concurrent photostimulation [80]. The study used BOLD signal response to visual stimulation measured in retinotopic mapping-defined visual cortex areas V1 to V4. Findings from this study demonstrated reduced BOLD response in patients reporting scotoma and increased response in patients who only experienced positive symptoms. Furthermore, patients with bilateral visual symptoms had corresponding bi-hemispherical changes in BOLD response. These findings suggest that different aura symptoms reflect different types of cerebral dysfunction, which corresponds with a theory of possible simultaneous multiple origins of cortical spreading depressions in the brains of MwA patients [17]. Furthermore, Hougaard and colleagues imaged patients who have migraine with visual aura and demonstrated increased ictal connectivity between the left pons and somatosensory cortex, as well as between V5/MT and the middle frontal gyrus, providing possible links between brain areas involved in the aura and those involved in headache [6]. Moreover, complex direct current magnetoencephalographic shifts were observed in spontaneous and visually induced MwA, but not in controls [81]. Two-dimensional inverse imaging showed multiple cortical areas activated in spontaneous and visually induced migraine aura [81]. These findings support the theory that spreading cortical depression can arise spontaneously or be visually triggered in widespread regions of the hyperexcitable occipital cortex. Interestingly, the pattern of ictal perfusion change can help distinguish migraine aura from stroke in terms of the number of vascular territories involved, and ictal abnormalities on magnetic resonance angiography can occur in migraine aura, such as vasoconstriction or mild dilation [82]. Moreover, in another study where 98 patients underwent contrast perfusion MRI within 24 h of aura onset, 22% of them had hemispheric cortical hypoperfusion [83].

Furthermore, a combined PET/MR study that used [11C]PBR28, a radioligand that binds to the 18 kDa translocator protein, a marker of glial activation, in MwA patients revealed increased signal interictally in areas previously shown to be involved in cortical spreading depression generation (primary visual cortex, visual areas V3A and MT, and Broca's area), as well as with areas involved in pain processing (thalamus and primary/secondary somatosensory and insular cortices) [84]. Increase of the signal was also positively associated with the frequency of migraine attacks. A subsequent study also suggested increased uptake of [11C]PBR28 in the meninges, possibly reflecting activation of dural macrophages following MwA attack [12, 85]. In addition, the study included control groups of HCs and patients with chronic lower back pain. The study found increased uptake in the parameningeal tissue overlying the occipital cortex, when compared to HCs and patients with chronic lower back pain [85]. Although a study suggested that there is no blood–brain barrier disruption during MwA attacks [86], one has to keep in mind that gadolinium (the tracer used in that study) only extravasates when there is a substantial breakdown of the blood–brain barrier. New quantitative MRI data suggest indeed that extravasation and cerebral edema observed in the animal model are also present in MwA patients [87].

Altogether, converging perfusion MRI evidence has demonstrated that abnormal cerebral blood flow, exceeding the boundaries of a single vascular territory, with a trend dominated by an initial brief hyperperfusion, followed by hypoperfusion (during the aura phenomenon but also in the first part of the headache phase) and then hyperperfusion, characterizes migraine with aura attack [88]. Furthermore, perfusion MRI findings tend to support the presence of perfusion abnormalities in areas involved in multisensory processing, in both patients with MwA and migraine without aura [88]. However, the generalizability of results is currently limited by heterogeneities regarding study design and documentation of clinical variables (e.g., relation of attacks to scanning timepoint, migraine subtypes) [89].

6.3 Neuroimaging Studies of Vestibular Migraine and Hemiplegic Migraine

Vestibular migraine (VM), listed in the appendix of the third edition of the International Classification of Headache Disorders (ICHD-3) [1], is a subtype of migraine characterized by pronounced vestibular symptoms and is regarded to be the most prevalent neurological cause of episodic vertigo [90]. The possible pathophysiological mechanisms of VM include dysfunction of the trigeminovascular and vestibular systems, including aberrant multisensory modulation or integration within the thalamo-cortical network [91].

Neuroimaging studies that investigated brain structural and functional changes in VM patients have significantly improved our understanding of this complex subtype of migraine, which is highly linked with pathophysiological mechanisms in MwA. Structural neuroimaging studies, such as voxel-based morphometry studies, revealed that VM patients have altered gray matter volume in multisensory vestibular cortices, including the prefrontal cortex; bilateral parietoinsular vestibular cortex; inferior parietal gyrus; precuneus; superior, inferior, and middle (MT/V5) temporal gyrus; supramarginal gyrus; and cerebellum [92–96]. However, the results of those studies vary significantly from one to another [97]. In addition, compared to MwTA patients and those without aura, VM had increased gray matter volume of the left thalamus [93]. Diffusion tensor imaging studies did not reveal any significant microstructural changes in VM patients [98].

Relative to HCs, VM patients demonstrated reduced resting-state activity in the left superior temporal gyrus and left midcingulate/paracingulate gyri and increased activity in the precuneus, right superior parietal gyrus, and right middle frontal gyrus [99]. Furthermore, as revealed by meta-regression analysis, the Dizziness Handicap Inventory scores were positively correlated with the activity in the precuneus, and higher Dizziness Handicap Inventory scores and Headache Impact Test-6 were associated with lower activity within the left midcingulate/paracingulate gyri [99]. Furthermore, increased functional connectivity was observed between the left primary somatosensory cortex and the left parietoinsular vestibular cortex in VM patients [96]. Also, VM patients exhibited increased functional connectivity between the right precentral gyrus and areas of the left postcentral gyrus, left cuneus, and right lingual gyrus, as well as decreased functional connectivity between the left insular cortex and regions of the left thalamus and right anterior cingulate cortex [97]. In addition, altered thalamo-cortical functional connectivity and aberrant dynamic functional network connectivity between sensory networks and networks related to cognitive, emotional, and attention implementation were noted [100, 101], as well as decreased intra-network functional connectivity in the executive control network, and weakened functional connectivity between the right frontoparietal network and the auditory network [102]. Also, a dynamic amplitude of low-frequency fluctuation and regional homogeneity study revealed altered temporal dynamics and concordance of regional intrinsic brain activity in the motor cortex, cerebellum, and occipital and temporoparietal cortex in VM patients relative to HCs

[103]. Moreover, when compared to patients who have migraine without aura, VM patients demonstrated decreased functional network connectivity between the dorsal attention network and posterior medial visual network, between the sensorimotor network and posterior medial visual network, and between the sensorimotor network and lateral visual network [104]. Additionally, a caloric vestibular stimulation task-state functional MRI study in VM patients suggested aberrant brain activation in the thalamus, in particular, a significantly increased thalamic activation in comparison with both patients with migraine without aura and HCs [105]. Moreover, compared with HCs, VM patients showed higher normalized cerebral blood flow in the right precentral gyrus, left postcentral gyrus, left superior frontal gyrus, and bilateral insular cortex. Furthermore, these variations in brain perfusion significantly correlated with the frequency of migraine and vestibular symptoms, as well as with disease duration [93]. Ultimately, a positron emission tomography study showed increased metabolism in the vestibulo-thalamo-cortical pathway and decreased metabolism in the visual pathway during a VM attack [106].

HM is a rare subtype of migraine with aura, characterized by sometimes prolonged hemiparesis during the aura phase [1], and is associated with mutations in specific genes such as CACNA1A, ATP1A2, and SCN1A, which affect ion channels in nerve cells, leading to abnormal neuronal activity. Conventional neuroimaging in acute HM attacks is often normal. However, imaging may reveal cerebral cortical hyperintensity and edema contralateral to the hemiparesis [107, 108]. These neuroimaging abnormalities, as well as the neurological deficit, often resolve within days to weeks after an attack. However, the occurrence of white matter hyperintensities in patients with sporadic HM is significantly higher in the parietal lobe when compared to those with other subtypes of migraine headaches [109].

Advanced neuroimaging findings in HM patients are limited because of the difficulty of designing a neuroimaging study with a large cohort of HM patients [110, 111]. However, MRI studies showed cerebellar and cerebral atrophy signs in HM patients [112–114], which is also accompanied by a significant increase in the apparent diffusion coefficient median values in the vermis and cerebellar hemispheres [115]. Furthermore, a single-voxel 7 Tesla 1H-MRS study showed that HM patients showed a significantly lower total N-acetyl aspartate/total creatine ratio in the cerebellum compared to HCs, suggesting cerebellar neuronal loss or dysfunction in HM [116]. In addition, patients with a CACNA1A mutation show the lowest total N-acetyl aspartate/total creatine ratio [116].

Moreover, cerebral blood flow changes during an HM attack beginning with multifocal hypoperfusion in the early phase followed by persistent hyperperfusion for several days in a prolonged aura attack [117]. Additionally, positron emission tomography revealed increased cerebral glucose metabolism in the regions corresponding to hyperperfusion when hemiparesis still persisted, while electroencephalography showed attenuated alpha activity without paroxysmal discharge in familial HM type 2 [117]. In addition, data from one study indicated increased habituation of visual-evoked potentials and nociception-specific blink reflexes in patients with familial HM types 1 and 2, whereas patients with MwA have deficient habituation, suggesting differences in central neuronal processing [118]. Furthermore, another study showed that the activation amplitude and the cluster extension of the activation area in the primary motor area determined by a specifically designed motor task functional MRI were smaller on the affected side in HM patients [119].

Understanding the neuroimaging findings in HM is crucial for accurate diagnosis and management. However, larger cohorts and longitudinal neuroimaging studies are needed to better understand the underlying HM mechanisms, which potentially could lead to more targeted and effective treatments.

6.4 Key Findings and Current Gaps in Neuroimaging Studies of Migraine with Aura

In summary, atypical brain responses to sensory stimuli and altered functional connectivity in multisensory processing regions and default mode network are consistent findings in MwA patients [120]. In addition, the interictal brain of MwA patients also presents microstructural, morphological, and metabolic differences, some of which may predispose individuals to specific MwA phenotypes, compared to HCs. However, it is still unclear whether these neuroimaging alterations are exclusive to MwA, as there are insufficient numbers of studies that investigate differences between MwA patients and those with other recurrent or chronic pain conditions. Moreover, the overall sample of patients included in the majority of studies is small; hence, the statistical potency of the results is limited if we consider that the results must be extrapolated to the 4.5% of people who have MwA worldwide. In addition to these gaps in neuroimaging MwA studies, most of the studies did not address the question of patient brain dominance; both genders were included in the study; the predominant laterality of MwA attacks was ignored; subtypes of MwA were neglected; heterogeneous post-processing neuroimaging techniques and statistical analysis were applied, etc. Further neuroimaging research should focus on distinguishing between migraine subtypes to discover specific biomarkers and accurate predictive models, allowing therapeutic strategies tailored to each subtype. This approach may enhance the precision of migraine classification and treatment.

References

1. Headache Classification Committee of the International Headache Society (IHS). The international classification of headache disorders, 3rd ed. Cephalalgia. 2018;38:1–211.
2. Petrušić I, Goadsby PJ, Tassorelli C, et al. Editorial: subtypes of typical migraine with aura: exploring markers for subtype classification and treatment response. Front Hum Neurosci. 2023;17:1301809.
3. Mitrovic K, Petrusic I, Dakovic M, et al. Migraine with aura detection and subtype classification using machine learning algorithms and morphometric magnetic resonance imaging data. Front Neurol. 2023;14:1106612.

4. Bridge H, Stagg CJ, Near J, et al. Altered neurochemical coupling in the occipital cortex in migraine with visual aura. Cephalalgia. 2015;35:1025–30.
5. Tedeschi G, Russo A, Conte F, et al. Increased interictal visual network connectivity in patients with migraine with aura. Cephalalgia. 2016;36:139–47.
6. Hougaard A, Amin F, Larsson HBW, et al. Increased intrinsic brain connectivity between pons and somatosensory cortex during attacks of migraine with aura. Hum Brain Mapp. 2017;38:2635–42.
7. Gaist D, Hougaard A, Garde E, et al. Migraine with visual aura associated with thicker visual cortex. Brain. 2018;141:776–85.
8. Faragó P, Tóth E, Kocsis K, et al. Altered resting state functional activity and microstructure of the white matter in migraine with aura. Front Neurol. 2019;10:1039.
9. Petrusic I, Viana M, Dakovic M, et al. Application of the migraine aura complexity score (MACS): clinical and neuroimaging study. Front Neurol. 2019;10:1112.
10. Coppola G, Di Renzo A, Tinelli E, et al. Thalamo-cortical networks in subtypes of migraine with aura patients. J Headache Pain. 2021;22:58.
11. Coppola G, Corbelli I, Di Renzo A, et al. Visual stimulation and frequency of focal neurological symptoms engage distinctive neurocognitive resources in migraine with aura patients: a study of resting-state functional networks. J Headache Pain. 2022;23:80.
12. Christensen RH, Gollion C, Amin FM, et al. Imaging the inflammatory phenotype in migraine. J Headache Pain. 2022;23:60.
13. Fu T, Liu L, Huang X, et al. Cerebral blood flow alterations in migraine patients with and without aura: an arterial spin labeling study. J Headache Pain. 2022;23:131.
14. Silvestro M, Tessitore A, Nardo FD, et al. Functional connectivity changes in complex migraine aura: beyond the visual network. Eur J Neurol. 2022;29:295–304.
15. Karsan N, Silva E, Goadsby PJ. Evaluating migraine with typical aura with neuroimaging. Front Hum Neurosci. 2023;17:1112790.
16. Hadjikhani N, Sanchez Del Rio M, Wu O, et al. Mechanisms of migraine aura revealed by functional MRI in human visual cortex. Proc Natl Acad Sci USA. 2001;98:4687–92.
17. Petrusic I, Zidverc-Trajkovic J. Cortical spreading depression: origins and paths as inferred from the sequence of events during migraine aura. Funct Neurol. 2014;29:207–12.
18. Fischl B, Dale AM. Measuring the thickness of the human cerebral cortex from magnetic resonance images. Proc Natl Acad Sci USA. 2000;97:11050–5.
19. Desikan RS, Ségonne F, Fischl B, et al. An automated labeling system for subdividing the human cerebral cortex on MRI scans into Gyral based regions of interest. NeuroImage. 2006;31:968–80.
20. Fischl B. FreeSurfer. NeuroImage. 2012;62:774–81.
21. Niddam DM, Lai K-L, Hsiao Y-T, et al. Grey matter structure within the visual networks in migraine with aura: multivariate and univariate analyses. Cephalalgia. 2024;44:3331024231222637.
22. Petrusic I, Viana M, Dakovic M, et al. Proposal for a migraine aura complexity score. Cephalalgia. 2018;39:732–41.
23. Granziera C, DaSilva A, Snyder J, et al. Anatomical alterations of the visual motion processing network in migraine with and without aura. PLoS Med. 2006;3:e402.
24. DaSilva A, Granziera C, Snyder J, et al. Thickening in the somatosensory cortex of patients with migraine. Neurology. 2007;69:1990–5.
25. Abagnale C, Renzo AD, Sebastianelli G, et al. Whole brain surface-based morphometry and tract-based spatial statistics in migraine with aura patients: difference between pure visual and complex auras. Front Hum Neurosci. 2023;17:1146302.
26. Hougaard A, Amin FM, Arngrim N, et al. Sensory migraine aura is not associated with structural grey matter abnormalities. Neuroimage Clin. 2016;11:322–7.
27. Messina R, Rocca M, Colombo B, et al. Cortical abnormalities in patients with migraine: a surface-based analysis. Radiology. 2013;268:170–80.

28. Petrusic I, Dakovic M, Kacar K, et al. Migraine with aura: surface-based analysis of the cerebral cortex with magnetic resonance imaging. Korean J Radiol. 2018;19:767–76.
29. Sheng LQ, Ma HR, Shi YY, et al. Cortical thickness in migraine: a coordinate-based meta-analysis. Front Neurosci. 2021;14:600423.
30. Coppola G, Renzo AD, Parisi V, et al. Comment on "lack of reproducibility of resting-state functional MRI findings in migraine with aura". Cephalalgia. 2024;44:3331024231225186.
31. Mitrović K, Savić AM, Radojičić A, et al. Machine learning approach for migraine aura complexity score prediction based on magnetic resonance imaging data. J Headache Pain. 2023;24:169.
32. Petrusic I, Dakovic M, Zidverc-Trajkovic J. Subcortical volume changes in migraine with aura. J Clin Neurol. 2019;15:448–53.
33. Petrusic I, Dakovic M, Zidverc-Trajkovic J. Volume alterations of brainstem subregions in migraine with aura. NeuroImage Clin. 2019;22:101714.
34. Kruit M, van Buchem M, Launer L, et al. Migraine is associated with an increased risk of deep white matter lesions, subclinical posterior circulation infarcts and brain iron accumulation: the population-based MRI CAMERA study. Cephalalgia. 2010;30:129–36.
35. Palm-Meinders I, Koppen H, Terwindt G, et al. Structural brain changes in migraine. JAMA. 2012;308:1889–97.
36. Bashir A, Lipton R, Ashina S, et al. Migraine and structural changes in the brain: a systematic review and meta-analysis. Neurology. 2013;81:1260–8.
37. Gaist D, Garde E, Blaabjerg M, et al. Migraine with aura and risk of silent brain infarcts and white matter hyperintensities: an MRI study. Brain. 2016;139:2015–23.
38. Dobrynina LA, Suslina AD, Gubanova MV, et al. White matter hyperintensity in different migraine subtypes. Sci Rep. 2021;11:10881.
39. DaSilva A, Granziera C, Tuch D, et al. Interictal alterations of the trigeminal somatosensory pathway and periaqueductal gray matter in migraine. Neuroreport. 2007;18:301–5.
40. Szabó N, Faragó P, Király A, et al. Evidence for plastic processes in migraine with aura: a diffusion weighted MRI study. Front Neuroanat. 2018;11:138.
41. Granziera C, Daducci A, Romascano D, et al. Structural abnormalities in the thalamus of migraineurs with aura: a multiparametric study at 3 T. Hum Brain Mapp. 2014;35:1461–8.
42. Petrušić I, Daković M, Kačar K, et al. Migraine with aura and white matter tract changes. Acta Neurol Belg. 2018;118:485–91.
43. Lo Buono V, Bonanno L, Corallo F, et al. Functional connectivity and cognitive impairment in migraine with and without aura. J Headache Pain. 2017;18:72.
44. Zielman R, Wijnen J, Webb A, et al. Cortical glutamate in migraine. Brain. 2017;140:1859–71.
45. Niddam D, Lai K, Fuh J, et al. Reduced functional connectivity between salience and visual networks in migraine with aura. Cephalalgia. 2016;36:53–66.
46. Datta R, Aguirre GK, Hu S, et al. Interictal cortical hyperresponsiveness in migraine is directly related to the presence of aura. Cephalalgia. 2013;33:365–74.
47. Hougaard A, Amin F, Hoffmann M, et al. Interhemispheric differences of fMRI responses to visual stimuli in patients with side-fixed migraine aura. Hum Brain Mapp. 2014;35:2714–23.
48. Sarchielli P, Tarducci R, Presciutti O, et al. Functional 1H-MRS findings in migraine patients with and without aura assessed interictally. NeuroImage. 2005;24:1025–31.
49. Russo A, Tessitore A, Silvestro M, et al. Advanced visual network and cerebellar hyperresponsiveness to trigeminal nociception in migraine with aura. J Headache Pain. 2019;20:46.
50. Sándor PS, Dydak U, Schoenen J, et al. MR-spectroscopic imaging during visual stimulation in subgroups of migraine with aura. Cephalalgia. 2005;25:507–18.
51. Michels L, Villanueva J, O'Gorman R, et al. Interictal hyperperfusion in the higher visual cortex in patients with episodic migraine. Headache. 2019;59:1808–20.
52. Arkink E, Bleeker E, Schmitz N, et al. Cerebral perfusion changes in migraineurs: a voxelwise comparison of interictal dynamic susceptibility contrast MRI measurements. Cephalalgia. 2012;32:279–88.

53. Tessitore A, Russo A, Conte F, et al. Abnormal connectivity within executive resting-state network in migraine with aura. Headache. 2015;55:794–805.
54. Hadjikhani N, Ward N, Boshyan J, et al. The missing link: enhanced functional connectivity between amygdala and visceroceptive cortex in migraine. Cephalalgia. 2013;33:1264–8.
55. Faragó P, Tuka B, Tóth E, et al. Interictal brain activity differs in migraine with and without aura: resting state fMRI study. J Headache Pain. 2017;18:8.
56. Veréb D, Szabó N, Tuka B, et al. Temporal instability of salience network activity in migraine with aura. Pain. 2020;161:856–64.
57. Hougaard A, Amin F, Magon S, et al. No abnormalities of intrinsic brain connectivity in the interictal phase of migraine with aura. Eur J Neurol. 2015;22:702–e46.
58. Hougaard A, Gaist D, Garde E, et al. Lack of reproducibility of resting-state functional MRI findings in migraine with aura. Cephalalgia. 2023;43:3331024231212574.
59. Vernieri F, Tibuzzi F, Pasqualetti P, et al. Increased cerebral vasomotor reactivity in migraine with aura: an autoregulation disorder? A transcranial Doppler and near-infrared spectroscopy study. Cephalalgia. 2008;28:689–95.
60. Podgorac A, Petrusic I, Radojicic A, et al. Breath holding index in episodic primary headaches. Vojnosanit Pregl. 2018;75:347–51.
61. Gollion C, Nasr N, Fabre N, et al. Cerebral autoregulation in migraine with aura: a case control study. Cephalalgia. 2019;39:635–40.
62. Dzator JS, Howe PR, Wong RH. Profiling cerebrovascular function in migraine: a systematic review and meta-analysis. J Cereb Blood Flow Metab. 2021;41:919–44.
63. Ornello R, Frattale I, Caponnetto V, et al. Cerebral vascular reactivity and the migraine-stroke relationship: a narrative review. J Neurol Sci. 2020;414:116887.
64. Reinhard M, Schork J, Allignol A, et al. Cerebellar and cerebral autoregulation in migraine. Stroke. 2012;43:987–93.
65. Petrušić I, Podgorac A, Radojičić A, et al. Transcranial Doppler evaluation of the cerebral vasculature in women patients who have migraine with aura. Pain Med. 2020;21:3012–7.
66. Mattle H, Evers S, Hildick-Smith D, et al. Percutaneous closure of patent foramen ovale in migraine with aura, a randomized controlled trial. Eur Heart J. 2016;37:2029–36.
67. Altamura C, Paolucci M, Costa CM, et al. Right-to-left shunt and the clinical features of migraine with aura: earlier but not more. Cerebrovasc Dis. 2019;47:268–74.
68. Shin DH, Lim TS, Yong SW, et al. Posterior circulation embolism as a potential mechanism for migraine with aura. Cephalalgia. 2012;32:497–9.
69. Petrusic I, Podgorac A, Zidverc-Trajkovic J, et al. Do interictal microembolic signals play a role in higher cortical dysfunction during migraine aura? Cephalalgia. 2016;36:561–7.
70. Schoenen J. Neurophysiological features of the migrainous brain. Neurol Sci. 2006;27:S77–81.
71. Ambrosini A, Coppola G. Neurophysiology of migraine with aura. In: Coppola G, Chen WT, editors. Neurophysiology of the migraine brain. Cham: Springer; 2021. p. 181–200.
72. Petrusic I, Jovanovic V, Kovic V, et al. P3 latency as a biomarker for the complexity of migraine with aura: event-related potential study. Cephalalgia. 2022;42:1022–30.
73. Petrusic I, Jovanovic V, Kovic V, et al. Characteristics of N400 component elicited in patients who have migraine with aura. J Headache Pain. 2021;22:157.
74. Barkley GL, Baumgartner C. MEG and EEG in epilepsy. J Clin Neurophysiol. 2003;20:163–78.
75. Wu D, Zhou Y, Xiang J, et al. Multi-frequency analysis of brain connectivity networks in migraineurs: a magnetoencephalography study. J Headache Pain. 2016;17:38.
76. Hadjikhani N, Vincent M. Neuroimaging clues of migraine aura. J Headache Pain. 2019;20:32.
77. Lauritzen M, Olsen TS, Lassen NA, et al. Changes in regional cerebral blood flow during the course of classic migraine attacks. Ann Neurol. 1983;13:633–41.
78. Olesen J, Friberg L, Olsen TS, et al. Timing and topography of cerebral blood flow, aura, and headache during migraine attacks. Ann Neurol. 1990;28:791–8.
79. Sanchez del Rio M, Bakker D, Wu O, et al. Perfusion weighted imaging during migraine: spontaneous visual aura and headache. Cephalalgia. 1999;19:701–7.

80. Arngrim N, Hougaard A, Ahmadi K, et al. Heterogenous migraine aura symptoms correlate with visual cortex functional magnetic resonance imaging responses. Ann Neurol. 2017;82:925–39.
81. Bowyer SM, Aurora KS, Moran JE, et al. Magnetoencephalographic fields from patients with spontaneous and induced migraine aura. Ann Neurol. 2001;50:582–7.
82. Förster A, Wenz H, Kerl H, et al. Perfusion patterns in migraine with aura. Cephalalgia. 2014;34:870–6.
83. Kellner-Weldon F, El-Koussy M, Jung S, et al. Cerebellar hypoperfusion in migraine attack: incidence and significance. AJNR Am J Neuroradiol. 2018;39:435–40.
84. Albrecht D, Mainero C, Ichijo E, et al. Imaging of neuroinflammation in migraine with aura—a [11C] PBR28 PET/MR study. Neurology. 2019;92:e2038–50.
85. Hadjikhani N, Albrecht DS, Mainero C, et al. Extra-axial inflammatory signal in parameninges in migraine with visual aura. Ann Neurol. 2020;87:939–49.
86. Hougaard A, Amin FM, Christensen CE, et al. Increased brainstem perfusion, but no blood-brain barrier disruption, during attacks of migraine with aura. Brain. 2017;140:1633–42.
87. Christensen RH, Ashina H, Al-Khazali HM, et al. Cortical inflammation in migraine measured with quantitative resonance imaging: a registry for migraine (REFORM) study. Manuscript in preparation
88. Russo A, Silvestro M, Tessitore A, et al. Arterial spin labeling MRI applied to migraine: current insights and future perspectives. J Headache Pain. 2023;24:71.
89. Schramm S, Börner C, Reichert M, et al. Perfusion imaging by arterial spin labeling in migraine: a literature review. J Cereb Blood Flow Metab. 2024; 271678X241237733
90. Smyth D, Britton Z, Murdin L, et al. Vestibular migraine treatment: a comprehensive practical review. Brain. 2022;145:3741–54.
91. Huang T-C, Wang S-J, Kheradmand A. Vestibular migraine: an update on current understanding and future directions. Cephalalgia. 2020;40:107–21.
92. Obermann M, Wurthmann S, Steinberg BS, et al. Central vestibular system modulation in vestibular migraine. Cephalalgia. 2014;34:1053–61.
93. Messina R, Rocca MA, Colombo B, et al. Structural brain abnormalities in patients with vestibular migraine. J Neurol. 2017;264:295–303.
94. Wang S, Wang H, Zhao D, et al. Grey matter changes in patients with vestibular migraine. Clin Radiol. 2019;74:898e1–5.
95. Zhe X, Gao J, Chen L, et al. Altered structure of the vestibular cortex in patients with vestibular migraine. Brain Behav. 2020;10:e01572.
96. Zhe X, Zhang X, Chen L, et al. Altered gray matter volume and functional connectivity in patients with vestibular migraine. Front Neurosci. 2021;15:683802.
97. Chen Z, Liu Y, Lin C, et al. Aberrant cerebral blood flow and functional connectivity in patients with vestibular migraine: a resting-state ASL and fMRI study. J Headache Pain. 2024;25:84.
98. Russo A, Marcuccio L, Conte F, et al. No evidence of microstructural changes in patients with vestibular migraine: a diffusion tensor tract based spatial statistic (TBSS) study. J Headache Pain. 2015;16:A161.
99. Du J, Liu Y, Zhu W. The altered functional status in vestibular migraine: a meta-analysis. Brain Behav. 2024;14:e3591.
100. Chen Z, Xiao L, Liu H, et al. Altered Thalamo–cortical functional connectivity in patients with vestibular migraine: a resting–state fMRI study. Neuroradiology. 2022;64:119–27.
101. Chen Z, Liu H, Wei XE, et al. Aberrant dynamic functional network connectivity in vestibular migraine patients without peripheral vestibular lesion. Eur Arch Otorrinolaringol. 2023;280:2993–3003.
102. Lin Han L, Jiajie LJ, Can Chen C, et al. Altered functional connectivity within and between resting-state networks in patients with vestibular migraine. Neuroradiology. 2023;65:591–8.
103. Xiong X, Dai L, Chen W, et al. Dynamics and concordance alterations of regional brain function indices in vestibular migraine: a resting-state fMRI study. J Headache Pain. 2024;25:1.

104. Zhang B, Wu D, Guo Y, et al. Altered large-scale internetwork functional connectivity in patients with vestibular migraine and migraine without aura. Neurosci Lett. 2023;800:137123.
105. Russo A, Marcelli V, Esposito F, et al. Abnormal thalamic function in patients with vestibular migraine. Neurology. 2014;82:2120–6.
106. Shin JH, Kim YK, Kim HJ, et al. Altered brain metabolism in vestibular migraine: comparison of interictal and ictal findings. Cephalalgia. 2014;34:58–67.
107. Dreier JP, Jurkat-Rott K, Petzold GC, et al. Opening of the blood-brain barrier preceding cortical edema in a severe attack of FHM type II. Neurology. 2005;64:2145–7.
108. Sugrue G, Bolster F, Crosbie I, et al. Hemiplegic migraine: neuroimaging findings during a hemiplegic migraine attack. Headache. 2014;54:716–8.
109. Nagarajan E, Bollu PC, Manjamalai S, et al. White matter hyperintensities in patients with sporadic hemiplegic migraine. J Neuroimaging. 2019;29:730–6.
110. Bosemani T, Burton VJ, Felling RJ, et al. Pediatric hemiplegic migraine: role of multiple MRI techniques in evaluation of reversible hypoperfusion. Cephalalgia. 2014;34:311–5.
111. Kim S, Kang M, Choi S. A case report of sporadic hemiplegic migraine associated cerebral hypoperfusion: comparison of arterial spin labeling and dynamic susceptibility contrast perfusion MR imaging. Eur J Pediatr. 2016;175:295–8.
112. Romaniello R, Zucca C, Tonelli S, et al. A wide spectrum of clinical, neurophysiological and neuroradiological abnormalities in a family with a novel CACNA1A mutation. J Neurol Neurosurg Psychiatry. 2010;81:840–3.
113. Pelzer N, Hoogeveen ES, Ferrari MD, et al. Brain atrophy following hemiplegic migraine attacks. Cephalalgia. 2018;38:1199–202.
114. Khaiboullina SF, Mendelevich EG, Shigapova LH, et al. Cerebellar atrophy and changes in cytokines associated with the CACNA1A R583Q mutation in a Russian familial hemiplegic migraine type 1 family. Front Cell Neurosci. 2017;11:263.
115. Grimaldi D, Tonon C, Cevoli S, et al. Clinical and neuroimaging evidence of interictal cerebellar dysfunction in FHM2. Cephalalgia. 2010;30:552–9.
116. Zielman R, Teeuwisse WM, Bakels F, et al. Biochemical changes in the brain of hemiplegic migraine patients measured with 7 tesla 1H-MRS. Cephalalgia. 2014;34:959–67.
117. Iizuka T, Tominaga N, Kaneko J, et al. Biphasic neurovascular changes in prolonged migraine aura in familial hemiplegic migraine type 2. J Neurol Neurosurg Psychiatry. 2015;86:344–53.
118. Hansen JM, Bolla M, Magis D, et al. Habituation of evoked responses is greater in patients with familial hemiplegic migraine than in controls: a contrast with the common forms of migraine. Eur J Neurol. 2011;18:478–85.
119. da Silva RVB, Sanchez TA, Gama TM, et al. The Digiti Quinti sign in hemiplegic migraine: an fMRI study. J Neuroimaging. 2022;32:690–6.
120. Raggi A, Leonardi M, Arruda M, et al. Hallmarks of primary headache: part 1—migraine. J Headache Pain. 2024;25:189.

Chapter 7
Neuroimaging Studies of Chronic Migraine and Medication Overuse Headache

Gianluca Coppola, Francesco Casillo, Yonggang Wang, and Yiheng Tu

7.1 Introduction

According to the Global Burden of Disease (GBD) study, which builds on epidemiological research, headache disorders are among the most prevalent and disabling conditions worldwide. The global prevalence estimate for migraine is 14.0%, and this figure has increased over the years [1]. However, headache centers frequently see patients with chronic migraine, defined as having headaches on 15 or more days per month for more than 3 months, with at least 8 of these days meeting the criteria for migraine, with or without aura, and/or responding to migraine-specific treatment [2]. Worldwide, up to 45% of patients presenting to headache clinics experience daily or near-daily headaches [3]. Therefore, chronic migraine (CM) should be recognized as a disabling, underdiagnosed, and undertreated disorder [4]. The prevalence of CM in the general population is estimated to be between 0.9% and 2.2% [5]. Although opinions vary, the most frequently cited modifiable factor contributing to the transformation of episodic migraine to CM is the overuse of symptomatic drugs. In fact, more than 70 % of CM patients overuse these medications, and limiting their use of withdrawal from them is always recommended in such cases [6].

G. Coppola (✉) · F. Casillo
Department of Medico-Surgical Sciences and Biotechnologies, Sapienza University of Rome Polo Pontino ICOT, Latina, Italy
e-mail: gianluca.coppola@uniroma1.it

Y. Wang
Department of Neurology, Headache Center, Beijing Tiantan Hospital, Capital Medical University, Beijing, China

Y. Tu
CAS Key Laboratory of Mental Health, Institute of Psychology, Chinese Academy of Sciences, Beijing, China

Department of Psychology, University of Chinese Academy of Sciences, Beijing, China

I. Petrušić, Y. Wang (eds.), *Neuroimaging of Headache Disorders*, Headache,
https://doi.org/10.1007/978-3-031-85402-6_7

Given the limited availability of prophylactic drugs indicated for the treatment of CM and medication overuse headache (MOH), it is common for patients to experience a rapid progression toward treatment refractoriness. Compounding the clinical picture and increasing the levels of disability are the numerous systemic and neurological comorbidities that can complicate CM.

It is precisely for these reasons that over the years, efforts have been made to investigate the pathophysiological aspects of chronicity and overuse of symptomatic drugs in greater depth. In this regard, help has come from the application of numerous and increasingly refined neuroimaging techniques. Virtually, all methods of analyzing MRI sequences have been used to study the brains of patients with CM and/or MOH, including diffusion tensor imaging (DTI), voxel-based morphometry (VBM), and task-related or resting-state functional MRI (rs-fMRI). The results of studies employing these MRI techniques are often conflicting, due to both their strictly experimental nature and the lack of standardization of acquisition parameters.

In this present chapter, we will summarize the results of structural and functional imaging studies on CM and MOH, demonstrating how functional neuroimaging has advanced our understanding of their pathophysiology. Moreover, we will provide insights for future investigations.

7.2 Structural Investigations in CM and in MOH

Structural MRI provides robust and high-resolution measures of brain morphometry and has superior test–retest reliability compared to functional MRI.

7.2.1 Voxel-based Morphometry in CM and in MOH

One established method to characterize the volume and density of gray matter in brain structures is voxel-based morphometry (VBM). The most widely used structural measures are volume- and surface-based analyses, which assess critical aspects of brain development, learning and memory processes, and normal aging [7, 8].

Using VBM to quantify the volume and density of gray matter, several neuroimaging studies have explored the macrostructural characteristics of the brain in patients with CM, yielding some inconsistent results. It should be noted that many of these studies had significant sources of bias, including the inclusion of patients with a history of MOH [9], concomitant use of preventive medications [9–12], mixed migraine (with and without aura) [10, 13, 14], and white matter (WM) abnormalities [13]. Despite these inconsistencies, a consistent finding is the significant abnormal gray matter (GM) volume in areas associated with pain processing [9–11, 13, 15, 16], multisensory integration [15, 17], and affective processing [18, 19] in patients with CM compared to healthy individuals. Other studies involving CM patients without a history of drug overuse and without prophylaxis found no statistically significant structural changes [18, 20, 21]. Due to these conflicting results, which are often (when significant) related to the choice of more liberal statistical thresholds, some authors conclude these findings may be epiphenomena of specific brain systems responding to the disease or its indirect cognitive consequences [22]. Focusing specifically on the volume of the hypothalamus, one study showed that hypothalamic volume was significantly decreased in CM patients compared with healthy controls. Receiver operating characteristics (ROC) curve analysis disclosed that the hypothalamic volume had good diagnostic accuracy for CM, with a sensitivity of 81.25% and specificity of 100% compared to episodic migraine and controls [23]. Additionally, examining the morphometry of the hippocampus, Aybakan et al. [19] found lower volumetric values for both episodic and chronic migraine compared to the healthy controls. In another study, CM sufferers exhibited a larger left thalamus and smaller frontal areas compared to those with episodic migraines [17].

Among patients with MOH, an increase in GM volume was observed in the periaqueductal gray matter, thalamus, and ventral striatum [24]. Conversely, there was a decrease in GM volume in the frontal regions, specifically the orbitofrontal cortex, anterior cingulate cortex, left and right insula, and precuneus. The authors noted that patients who experienced substantial clinical improvement after discontinuing analgesics had a reduced volume of GM in the midbrain. However, patients who did not experience recovery did not show any changes in midbrain volume. Additionally, individuals who did not respond to treatment exhibited reduced GM volume in the orbitofrontal cortex [24].

To analyze the brain areas associated with medication overuse, some authors processed MRI images through VBM in groups of CM patients with or without MOH [15]. They found that patients with MOH showed a significant reduction in GM volume in the orbitofrontal cortex and left middle occipital gyrus, along with an increase in the volume of the temporal pole and left parahippocampus. The volume of the orbitofrontal cortex increased only in those who responded well to treatment. Mehnert et al. discovered MOH-related GM volume decreases in the medial orbital gyrus, hippocampus, inferior frontal gyrus, and precuneus [25]. Other VBM studies found no significant differences between patients with MOH and healthy subjects [26–28], even when comparing before and after withdrawal from symptomatic drugs [27].

7.2.2 *Surface-based Morphometry (SBM) in CM and in MOH*

Unlike VBM, which only measures GM volume, SBM can assess other cortical characteristics such as cortical thickness, sulcal depth, gyrification index, and surface area [29]. The study conducted by Lai and colleagues found no major differences in terms of brain volume between a cohort of 30 individuals with CM and 30 healthy controls, as determined by VBM [21]. However, using SBM, they identified reduced thickness in the bilateral insular cortex, caudal middle frontal gyrus, precentral gyrus, and parietal lobes in chronic migraine patients compared to the control group [21].

A study examining alterations in the shape of cortical fissures found that patients with CM had a lower average depth compared to both the healthy control (HC) and episodic migraine (EM) groups [30]. Additionally, the CM group exhibited a greater average depth in the left anterior callosomarginal fissure compared to the HC group. Patients with CM showed increased cortical thickness in the left and right superior postcentral sulcus, as well as the left median frontal sulcus, when compared to both HCs and individuals with EM. Furthermore, patients with CM had greater cortical thickness in the right median frontal sulcus and left superior parietal sulcus compared to individuals in the EM groups. Both individuals with CM and EM exhibited a significant increase in the opening width of the left and right insula compared to the HC group [30].

Another fascinating application is that disparities in baseline cortical thickness (CT) measurements may independently forecast responses to specific therapies. Hubbard investigated this phenomenon in a sample of 23 individuals suffering from CM [31]. Prior to administering Botox as a preventive medication, all participants underwent MRI scans. During the pre-treatment MRI, patients who subsequently responded to the treatment showed higher CT in specific brain regions, including the right primary somatosensory cortex, anterior insula, left superior temporal gyrus, and inferior parietal gyrus (pars opercularis), compared to those who did not respond. Although this study is preliminary, the results warrant further investigation into changes in CT that could potentially indicate a response to treatment.

7.2.3 Diffusion Tensor Imaging (DTI) in CM and in MOH

Among the various techniques used to acquire MRI data, DTI is the most sensitive to microstructural changes, as it estimates the diffusivity of water molecules along the fiber bundles of white matter (WM) in the three main orthogonal directions of diffusion. DTI metrics include fractional anisotropy (FA), mean diffusivity (MD), axial diffusivity (AD), and radial diffusivity (RD). FA measures the magnitude of anisotropy and closely reflects the integrity of the membranes of WM axons as well as the directionality of water molecule movement [32]. MD, which comprises radial and axial diffusivity and typically changes inversely to FA, reflects the overall magnitude of water diffusion by indicating both cellular swelling and density [32]. AD and RD serve as in vivo surrogate markers of myelin and axonal damage, respectively. These metrics are closely associated with brain microstructural maturation processes and higher levels of cognitive function.

7.2.3.1 Tract-based Spatial Statistics (TBSS) in CM and in MOH

TBSS is a tool that employs a tensor-fitting technique to produce various diffusion metrics. The method is fully automated and user-friendly, allowing for the reconstruction and examination of the WM structure of the entire brain without the need for prior specification or localization of regions or features of interest. After generating these measurements, they can be extracted using region of interest (ROI) methods, similar to the approach used with functional magnetic resonance imaging (fMRI) data [33].

Previous investigations have been unsuccessful in detecting notable disparities in DTI measurements between individuals with CM and HCs [34–36]. The inclusion of patients who were taking preventative measures or frequently using medication may have influenced the natural progression of the disease and, consequently, affected the accuracy of the results [34, 35]. However, in one specific study, although no significant abnormalities were found in the CM population, DTI measurements of patients with CM showed significant differences compared to those with CM in various brain regions [35]. These differences included regions whose microstructures were also found to differ significantly between patients with CM and HCs in another study [20]. This study identified significant changes in the subcallosal region, paracingulate region, posterior limb of the internal capsule, genu and splenium of the corpus callosum, and superior longitudinal fasciculus [20]. The differences were particularly noticeable when examining RD and MD measurements. In addition, a comparison of the related FA and MD values revealed slight differences in the WM fiber tracts between patients with CM and those with medication overuse (MO), although they were roughly similar [20]. In summary, the majority of the tracts identified in this investigation showed aberrant diffusivity metrics in the WM of the brain. These tracts are part of a widely distributed system of fiber bundles that transmit information related to the perception of somatosensory, cognitive, and affective aspects of orofacial pain discrimination, internal pain regulation processes, and the integration of various sensory inputs [37, 38].

In a prospective study involving 27 patients diagnosed with MOH, Beckmann et al. conducted DTI scans using TBSS before and 6 months after drug withdrawal. The results did not reveal any structural changes between the patients and the control group, both at the initial phase of the clinical study and after the patients stopped taking medication [27].

Multi-compartmental diffusion models of WM microstructure have been developed to better define the diffusion signal in the presence of multiple tissue compartments or contexts. Among these techniques, neurite orientation dispersion and density imaging (NODDI) has been suggested as a clinically viable protocol. NODDI can provide more precise measurements of specific tissue properties, such as the apparent volume fraction of neurites and the index of orientation dispersion [39]. Shibata and Ishiyama discovered that individuals suffering from MOH exhibited decreased orientation dispersion compared to those with pure CM who did not overuse medication, using the NODDI MRI analysis technique. Furthermore, a significant negative correlation was observed between orientation dispersion in the corpus callosum and the frequency of migraine attacks [40].

7.2.3.2 DTI Techniques to Study the Glymphatic System in CM

The glymphatic system was found to remove solutes from brain interstitial fluid through perivascular clearance in 2012. In 2017, Taoka et al. proposed DTI along the perivascular space (DTI-ALPS) index to measure the glymphatic function non-invasively [41]. The cerebral WM region of interest is typically located on the left side, at the same level as the upper lateral ventricles. The deep medullary veins flow horizontally and are usually parallel to the image slice. This technique isolates and quantifies water diffusivity in perivascular areas aligned with these veins [42].

Yuan et al. [43] examined the association between increased perivascular spaces, which serve as an indicator of glymphatic system malfunction, and episodic and chronic migraines compared to controls. They found that an increase in perivascular spaces (PVS) width, particularly in the centrum semiovale and midbrain areas, predicts migraine in general but not chronic migraine [43].

Zhang et al. [44] investigated GS activity variations during chronic migraine. Chronic migraineurs had a higher DTI-ALPS score than episodic migraineurs and healthy individuals, most notably in the right hemisphere.

Wu et al. [45] assessed DTI-ALPS alongside dynamic contrast-enhanced MRI (DCE-MRI), which quantifies microvascular characteristics such as perfusion, vessel permeability, and fluid volume fractions. In contrast to the results of Zhang et al. [44], CM patients had impaired glymphatic and meningeal lymphatic activity, according to multimodal MRI. Chronic migraine with medication overuse headache patients had higher glymphatic system impairment. The DTI-ALPS index correlates negatively with numerous clinical indications, including headache intensity, migraine-related disability, body pain, and sleep quality, in all migraine patients [45].

7.3 Functional Magnetic Resonance Imaging (fMRI) in CM and in MOH

Functional magnetic resonance imaging measures the brain activity by detecting hemodynamic changes associated with blood flow, specifically the blood–oxygen-level dependent (BOLD) signal. fMRI can be utilized to identify BOLD responses resulting from tasks or stimuli, as well as to assess resting-state or negative-task states, which represent the participants' baseline BOLD variability. fMRI is based on the principle that an increase in BOLD corresponds to an increase in cerebral metabolic activity, although it is not possible to say whether this activity is inhibitory or excitatory.

After renewed interest in the hypothalamus as a potential generator of migraine [46], some authors have attempted to verify its role in chronic migraine. To do this, they recorded the BOLD signal in response to an intranasal pain stimulus. They found a hypothalamic activation as a function of noxious trigeminal stimulations in patients with CM, especially when scanning during the pain phase compared with controls and migraine patients not experiencing pain at the time of scanning [47]. In patients with CM, compared to patients with episodic migraine, some authors used task-free fMRI and ROI-to-ROI analysis and found increased connectivity between the hypothalamus and the trigeminal spinal nucleus, as well as with some brain areas that are part of the salience network, such as the insula, caudate nucleus, dorsolateral prefrontal cortex, anterior cingulate cortex, thalamus, superior/middle temporal gyrus, right hippocampus, left cerebellar vermis, and precuneus [48–50]. Another study showed a significant increase in degree centrality of the salience network/pain neuromatrix in CM patients versus episodic migraine in correlation with the dorsal raphe nucleus [48]. A major weakness of most of these studies was the lack of control group or the small number of enrolled patients; hence, it is unclear how the presence of CM could have impacted the neuroimaging findings.

Using a hypothesis-driven seed-based approach for the analysis of resting-state MRI in CM patients, some authors found that, aside from the hypothalamus, certain brain areas were involved in pain modulation and migraine chronification. Compared with HC, these authors [51] found that CM patients had a decreased functional connectivity between the marginal division (seed), located at the caudal extent of the neostriatum, and the right cuneus and left middle cingulum cortex (MCC), and increased functional connectivity with the bilateral middle frontal gyrus, left hippocampus, and middle temporal gyrus. Using bilateral caudate nuclei as the ROIs to explore the FC across the whole brain, the authors revealed that, compared with controls, CM patients had higher FC values across a broad range of brain regions, including the bilateral calcarine cortex, bilateral lingual gyrus, bilateral anterior cingulate cortex (ACC), right superior parietal cortex, right inferior parietal cortex, right precuneus, right temporal lobe, right insula, right orbital part of the inferior frontal gyrus, and right temporal pole of the superior temporal gyrus [52]. FC values between the bilateral precuneus, left ACC, right MCC, and right CN were remarkably higher in the CM group than that in the EM group [52]. Other authors found an increase in FC of the superior parietal gyrus with the medial occipital gyrus of the left hemisphere [18]. In a study assessing ROI-based intrinsic resting functional connectivity of the default-mode network (DMN), the salience network (SN), and the executive control network (ECN) in a group of 13 women with CM, some researchers [53] reported widespread disruptions between cortical and limbic areas in patients compared to HC, largely attributed to the consequence of medication overuse. In a group of CM patients, functional connectivity in the brainstem trigeminal nucleus was significantly enhanced during visual stimulation compared to HC and episodic migraineurs [54]. Major sources of bias in these studies included the inclusion of patients with previous or ongoing acute medication overuse and the concomitant use of preventive medications, which may have influenced the resting connectivity patterns [55, 56]. Indeed, a study comparing individuals who responded to medication overuse withdrawal therapy with those who did not respond found that successful withdrawal led to a decrease in functional connectivity (FC) with the visual cortex in the responders. Notably, individuals who responded to the treatment already exhibited distinct functional connectivity in the visual cortex compared to those who did not respond [57].

In a resting-state fMRI study carried out in pure CM, applying an analysis of independent components, researchers found abnormalities in terms of functional connectivity between large-scale neurocognitive networks, specifically between the DMN, dorsal attention system (DAS), and ECN, in patients with CM compared to controls [36, 58]. In this study studying patients compared with HCs, it has been found that functional connectivity between the DMN and the ECN is disrupted and that between the ECN and DAS is weaker, while that between the DMN and the left DAS is stronger [58]. Moreover, in a study investigating Higuchi's fractal dimension as a measure of multi-scale signal complexity, Porcaro et al. demonstrated that this kind of large-scale network involvement in CM is sustained by a loss or gain in nonlinear complexity in brain activity, especially in the DAS and DMN [36].

In an ROI-to-ROI analysis using the hypothalamus as the seed, the same group of researchers demonstrated that patients with CM have greater connectivity of the hypothalamus only with the DMN areas and the left dorsal visual network compared to controls. Within the brain areas that are included in the DMN, the MPFC and LP were the most connected. The authors argued that these areas seem to play a relevant role in the integrative processing of emotional and cognitive processes by combining emotional biasing signals or markers with decision-making processes [59]. Moreover, they observed that the greater the perceived migraine pain intensity, the lower the strength of the functional connectivity between the hypothalamus and the MPFC. As the MPFC is also considered to mediate attenuation of pain via cognitive-control mechanisms [60], a negative correlation between the perceived pain intensity and the MPFC-to-hypothalamus connectivity in CM could reflect a lack of physiological mechanisms to cognitively attenuate pain perception. Remarkably, the correlation between the MPFC and severity of pain has been found in other chronic painful conditions, such as chronic low back pain [61] and fibromyalgia [62], indicating that it is non-specific to migraine. Another finding in this study was that the resting-state intrinsic network functional activities are correlated with headache severity [58]. In CM, subjective perception of headache intensity, as assessed on a visual analogue scale, correlated positively with the Zmax scores of the DAS intrinsic functional connectivity, but negatively with the Zmax scores of the ECN intrinsic functional connectivity. In humans, the visual areas devoted to the attentional systems, of which the DAS is composed, are functionally and anatomically connected with the trigeminal system [63], playing a crucial role in pain perception and, under certain experimental conditions, in analgesia [64].

7.4 Arterial Spin Labelling (ASL) in CM and in MOH

ASL is an MRI technique used to quantify cerebral blood perfusion by labelling blood water as it flows throughout the brain, without the need for gadolinium contrast. However, the ASL signal-to-noise ratio (SNR) and temporal resolution are inherently low, resulting in a low contrast-to-noise ratio. Despite these limitations, four studies to date have used ASL to assess the mechanisms of migraine chronification [65].

In an MR 3D pseudo-continuous arterial spin labelling (3D PCASL) imaging study, Liu et al. disclosed significantly lower cerebral blood flow (CBF) in 13 CM patients compared to 15 controls in the nucleus accumbens. A negative correlation between the CBF value of the left nucleus accumbens and VAS was also noted [66]. The same patients analyzed in another study showed a plethora of brain and white matter fibers with decreased perfusion [67]. Brain regions with decreased perfusion included the left postcentral gyrus, bilateral middle frontal gyrus, left middle occipital gyrus, left superior parietal lobule, left medial segment of superior frontal gyrus, and right orbital part of the inferior frontal gyrus. Decreased perfusion in white matter fibers was observed in bilateral superior longitudinal tracts, superior corona radiata, external capsules, anterior and posterior limbs of the internal capsule, anterior corona radiata, inferior longitudinal fasciculus, and right corticospinal tract [67].

Compared with controls, patients with CM (both with and without MOH) were found to have increased arrival-time-corrected CBF and arterial cerebral blood volume values in the bilateral amygdalae, which were positively correlated with the MIDAS score [68].

7.5 Conclusions

The literature review shows that MRI data analysis techniques have been used that explore both the micro- and macrostructures of the brain of chronic migraine patients, with or without medication overuse, as well as their function through the analysis of cerebral hemodynamics at rest.

Although some studies detect variations from normality in CM patients, a common thread in many of these studies is the inconsistency of results or the complete absence of statistical significance. Several limitations found in a large proportion of the studies may help explain this inconsistency. First, the often low sample sizes (sometimes fewer than ten patients) limit the replicability and immediate generalizability of study results. Second, comparisons are frequently made between chronic migraine patients and those suffering from episodic forms, without including a control group. This makes it impossible to determine whether the changes found in one group exceed or fall within normal limits. Third, the inclusion of patients on prophylactic therapy may alter cortical excitability, which makes it predictable that inducing a change in function could also induce a change in structure. Further inconsistencies arise from the methodological heterogeneities inherent in different MRI acquisitions, such as the use of varying scanners, inconsistent sequence parameters, and completely different analysis pipelines and statistical approaches.

Despite these obvious limitations, the following data emerge from the review of studies using neuroimaging to investigate the brains of patients with chronic migraine:

1	A remodeling of brain macrostructure in the form of a significant abnormality of gray matter (GM) volume in areas attributable to pain processing, multisensory integration, and pain-related affective processing
2	Reduction in the volume of cortical areas, often associated with altered gray matter thickness as well as altered fissure shape and depth of brain sulcus
3	A reduction in the volume of the orbitofrontal cortex is common in studies of MOH patients, a finding that normalizes after withdrawal from symptomatic drugs
4	TBSS analysis revealed extensive alteration of the microstructure of the white matter fiber bundles. These bundles are part of a widely distributed system of fibers that transmit information related to the perception of somatosensory, cognitive, and affective aspects of orofacial pain discrimination, internal pain regulation processes, and the integration of multisensory inputs
5	Conflicting results were obtained from the study of the glymphatic system in chronic migraine: a reduction, an increase, or normality of this system was observed
6	An altered functional connectivity of the hypothalamus with the brainstem and other cortical areas/networks
7	From ROI-to-ROI fMRI analyses, alterations in functional connectivity of different and scattered cortical areas and subcortical structures have emerged in various studies, in most cases not replicated
8	In support of this widespread pattern of altered connectivity, resting-state fMRI studies applying independent component analysis reveal functional connectivity abnormalities between large-scale neurocognitive networks. The networks most affected are the DMN, DAS, SN, and ECN, especially in relation to the severity of pain perceived by patients
9	Data obtained using the arterial spin labelling technique show extensive hypoflow of blood into cortical structures and white fiber bundles

The lack of longitudinal studies makes it difficult to speculate on the true nature of these anatomic–functional abnormalities: are they the probably genetically determined cause of chronic migraine, or are they consequences of recurrent migraine pain and/or overuse of symptomatic treatments?

Furthermore, it is not clear how many of these abnormalities are specific to chronic migraine or are products of chronicity, regardless of the underlying pathology, such as migraine, chronic low back pain, fibromyalgia, etc.

To address this question, it will be crucial to improve the comparability of results between studies and enhance the replicability by adopting standardized acquisition parameters and analysis pipelines. This will contribute to a better understanding of the pathophysiology of migraine as investigated through various neuroimaging techniques.

References

1. Steiner TJ, Stovner LJ, Jensen R, et al. Migraine remains second among the world's causes of disability, and first among young women: findings from GBD2019. J Headache Pain. 2020;21:137.
2. Headache Classification Committee of the International Headache Society (IHS). The international classification of headache disorders, 3rd edition. Cephalalgia. 2018;38:1–211.
3. Diener HC, Solbach K, Holle D, et al. Integrated care for chronic migraine patients: epidemiology, burden, diagnosis and treatment options. Clin Med (Northfield Il). 2015;15:344–50.
4. Bigal ME, Serrano D, Reed M, et al. Chronic migraine in the population: burden, diagnosis, and satisfaction with treatment. Neurology. 2008;71:559–66.
5. Buse DC, Manack AN, Fanning KM, et al. Chronic migraine prevalence, disability, and sociodemographic factors: results from the American migraine prevalence and prevention study. Headache. 2012;52:1456–70.
6. Ashina S, Terwindt GM, Steiner TJ, et al. Medication overuse headache. Nat Rev Dis Prim. 2023;9:5.
7. Ashburner J, Friston KJ. Voxel-based morphometry – the methods. Neuroimage. 2000;11:805–21.
8. Good CD, Johnsrude IS, Ashburner J, et al. A voxel-based morphometric study of ageing in 465 normal adult human brains. Neuroimage. 2001;14:21–36.
9. Neeb L, Bastian K, Villringer K, et al. Structural gray matter alterations in chronic migraine: implications for a progressive disease? Headache. 2017;57:400–16.
10. Valfrè W, Rainero I, Bergui M, et al. Voxel-based morphometry reveals gray matter abnormalities in migraine. Headache. 2008;48:109–17.
11. Schmidt-Wilcke T, Gänssbauer S, Neuner T, et al. Subtle grey matter changes between migraine patients and healthy controls. Cephalalgia. 2008;28:1–4.
12. Hubbard CS, Khan SA, Keaser ML, et al. Altered brain structure and function correlate with disease severity and pain catastrophizing in migraine patients. eNeuro. 2014;1:e20.14.
13. Bilgic B, Kocaman G, Arslan AB, et al. Volumetric differences suggest involvement of cerebellum and brainstem in chronic migraine. Cephalalgia. 2016;36:301–8.
14. Liu HY, Lee PL, Chou KH, et al. The cerebellum is associated with 2-year prognosis in patients with high-frequency migraine. J Headache Pain. 2020;21:29.
15. Lai T-H, Chou K-H, Fuh J-L, et al. Gray matter changes related to medication overuse in patients with chronic migraine. Cephalalgia. 2016;36:1324–33.
16. Christensen RH, Ashina H, Al-Khazali HM, et al. Differences in cortical morphology in people with and without migraine: a registry for migraine (REFORM) MRI study. Neurology. 2024;102:e209305.
17. Chen XY, Chen ZY, Dong Z, et al. Regional volume changes of the brain in migraine chronification. Neural Regen Res. 2020;15:1701–8.
18. Dong L, Fan X, Fan Y, et al. Impairments to the multisensory integration brain regions during migraine chronification: correlation with the vestibular dysfunction. Front Mol Neurosci. 2023;16:1153641.
19. Aybakan MN, Gürsoy G, Pazarci N. Changes in the hippocampal volume in chronic migraine, episodic migraine, and medication overuse headache patients. Ideggyogy Sz. 2023;76:373–8.
20. Coppola G, Di Renzo A, Tinelli E, et al. Patients with chronic migraine without history of medication overuse are characterized by a peculiar white matter fiber bundle profile. J Headache Pain. 2020;21:92.
21. Lai KL, Niddam DM, Fuh JL, et al. Cortical morphological changes in chronic migraine in a Taiwanese cohort: surface- and voxel-based analyses. Cephalalgia. 2020;40:575–85.
22. Mehnert J, Schulte L, May A. No grey matter alterations in longitudinal data of migraine patients. Brain. 2020;143:e93.
23. Chen Z, Chen X, Liu M, et al. Volume of hypothalamus as a diagnostic biomarker of chronic migraine. Front Neurol. 2019;10:606.

24. Riederer F, Gantenbein AR, Marti M, et al. Decrease of gray matter volume in the midbrain is associated with treatment response in medication-overuse headache: possible influence of orbitofrontal cortex. J Neurosci. 2013;33:15343–9.
25. Mehnert J, Hebestreit J, May A. Cortical and subcortical alterations in medication overuse headache. Front Neurol. 2018;9:499.
26. Schmidt-Wilcke T, Leinisch E, Straube A, et al. Gray matter decrease in patients with chronic tension type headache. Neurology. 2005;65:1483–6.
27. Beckmann Y, Gökçe S, Zorlu N, et al. Longitudinal assessment of gray matter volumes and white matter integrity in patients with medication-overuse headache. Neuroradiol J. 2018;31:150–6.
28. Chanraud S, Di S, Dilharreguy B, et al. Brain functional connectivity and morphology changes in medication-overuse headache: clue for dependence-related processes? Cephalalgia. 2014;34:605–15.
29. Winkler AM, Kochunov P, Blangero J, et al. Cortical thickness or grey matter volume? The importance of selecting the phenotype for imaging genetics studies. Neuroimage. 2010;53:1135–46.
30. Liu S, Hou X, Shi M, et al. Cortical sulcal abnormalities revealed by sulcal morphometry in patients with chronic and episodic migraine. J Pain Res. 2024;17:477.
31. Hubbard CS, Becerra L, Smith JH, et al. Brain changes in responders vs. non-responders in chronic migraine: markers of disease reversal. Front Hum Neurosci. 2016;10:497.
32. Beaulieu C. The basis of anisotropic water diffusion in the nervous system – a technical review. NMR Biomed. 2002;15:435–55.
33. Smith SM, Jenkinson M, Johansen-Berg H, et al. Tract-based spatial statistics: voxelwise analysis of multi-subject diffusion data. Neuroimage. 2006;31:1487–505.
34. Neeb L, Bastian K, Villringer K, et al. No microstructural white matter alterations in chronic and episodic migraineurs: a case-control diffusion tensor magnetic resonance imaging study. Headache. 2015;55:241–51.
35. Planchuelo-Gómez Á, García-Azorín D, Guerrero ÁL, et al. White matter changes in chronic and episodic migraine: a diffusion tensor imaging study. J Headache Pain. 2020;21:1.
36. Porcaro C, Di Renzo A, Tinelli E, et al. Haemodynamic activity characterization of resting state networks by fractal analysis and thalamocortical morphofunctional integrity in chronic migraine. J Headache Pain. 2020;21:112.
37. Morecraft RJ, Binneboese A, Stilwell-Morecraft KS, et al. Localization of orofacial representation in the corona radiata, internal capsule and cerebral peduncle in Macaca mulatta. J Comp Neurol. 2017;525:3429–57.
38. Millan MJ. Descending control of pain. Prog Neurobiol. 2002;66:355–474.
39. Zhang H, Schneider T, Wheeler-Kingshott CA, et al. NODDI: practical in vivo neurite orientation dispersion and density imaging of the human brain. Neuroimage. 2012;61:1000–16.
40. Shibata Y, Ishiyama S. Neurite damage in patients with migraine. Neurol Int. 2024;16:299–311.
41. Taoka T, Masutani Y, Kawai H, et al. Evaluation of glymphatic system activity with the diffusion MR technique: diffusion tensor image analysis along the perivascular space (DTI-ALPS) in Alzheimer's disease cases. Jpn J Radiol. 2017;35:172–8.
42. Ringstad G. Glymphatic imaging: a critical look at the DTI-ALPS index. Neuroradiology. 2024;66:157–60.
43. Yuan Z, Li W, Tang H, et al. Enlarged perivascular spaces in patients with migraine: a case-control study based on 3T MRI. Ann Clin Transl Neurol. 2023;10:1160–9.
44. Zhang X, Wang W, Bai X, et al. Increased glymphatic system activity in migraine chronification by diffusion tensor image analysis along the perivascular space. J Headache Pain. 2023;24:147.
45. Wu CH, Chang FC, Wang YF, et al. Impaired glymphatic and meningeal lymphatic functions in patients with chronic migraine. Ann Neurol. 2024;95:583–95.
46. Schulte LH, May A. The migraine generator revisited: continuous scanning of the migraine cycle over 30 days and three spontaneous attacks. Brain. 2016;139:1987–93.

47. Schulte LH, Allers A, May A. Hypothalamus as a mediator of chronic migraine. Neurology. 2017;88:2011–6.
48. Lee MJ, Park BY, Cho S, et al. Increased connectivity of pain matrix in chronic migraine: a resting-state functional MRI study. J Headache Pain. 2019;20:29.
49. Lerebours F, Boulanouar K, Barège M, et al. Functional connectivity of hypothalamus in chronic migraine with medication overuse. Cephalalgia. 2019;39:892–9.
50. Lim M, Jassar H, Kim DJ, et al. Differential alteration of fMRI signal variability in the ascending trigeminal somatosensory and pain modulatory pathways in migraine. J Headache Pain. 2021;22:4.
51. Chen Z, Chen X, Liu M, et al. Altered functional connectivity of the marginal division in migraine: a resting-state fMRI study. J Headache Pain. 2016;17:89.
52. Yuan Z, Wang W, Zhang X, et al. Altered functional connectivity of the right caudate nucleus in chronic migraine: a resting-state fMRI study. J Headache Pain. 2022;23:154.
53. Androulakis XM, Krebs K, Peterlin BL, et al. Modulation of intrinsic resting-state fMRI networks in women with chronic migraine. Neurology. 2017;89:163–9.
54. Schulte LH, Allers A, May A. Visual stimulation leads to activation of the nociceptive trigeminal nucleus in chronic migraine. Neurology. 2018;90:e1973–8.
55. Hebestreit JM, May A. Topiramate modulates trigeminal pain processing in thalamo-cortical networks in humans after single dose administration. PLoS One. 2017;12:e0184406.
56. Hebestreit JM, May A. The enigma of site of action of migraine preventives: no effect of metoprolol on trigeminal pain processing in patients and healthy controls. J Headache Pain. 2017;18:116.
57. Mäki-Marttunen V, Kies DA, Pijpers JA, et al. Functional connectivity of the visual cortex in chronic migraine before and after medication withdrawal therapy. NeuroImage Clin. 2023;40:103543.
58. Coppola G, Di Renzo A, Petolicchio B, et al. Aberrant interactions of cortical networks in chronic migraine. Neurology. 2019;92:e2550–8.
59. Raichle M, MacLeod AM, Snyder AZ, et al. A default mode of brain function. Proc Natl Acad Sci USA. 2001;98:676–82.
60. Wiech K, Ploner M, Tracey I. Neurocognitive aspects of pain perception. Trends Cogn Sci. 2008;12:306–13.
61. Tu Y, Jung M, Gollub RL, et al. Abnormal medial prefrontal cortex functional connectivity and its association with clinical symptoms in chronic low back pain. Pain. 2019;160:1308–18.
62. Schreiber KL, Loggia ML, Kim J, et al. Painful after-sensations in fibromyalgia are linked to catastrophizing and differences in brain response in the medial temporal lobe. J Pain. 2017;18:855–67.
63. Sava SL, de Pasqua V, Magis D, et al. Effects of visual cortex activation on the nociceptive blink reflex in healthy subjects. PLoS One. 2014;9:e100198.
64. Martini M. Real, rubber or virtual: The vision of "one's own" body as a means for pain modulation. A narrative review. Conscious Cogn. 2016;43:143–51.
65. Petcharunpaisan S, Ramalho J, Castillo M. Arterial spin labeling in neuroimaging. World J Radiol. 2010;2:384.
66. Liu M, Sun Y, Li X, et al. Hypoperfusion in nucleus accumbens in chronic migraine using 3D pseudo-continuous arterial spin labeling imaging MRI. J Headache Pain. 2022;23:72.
67. Li X, Liu M, Zhao S, et al. Decreased cerebral perfusion in chronic migraine: a voxel-based cerebral blood flow analysis using 3D pseudo-continuous arterial spin labeling. Curr Med Imaging. 2024;20:e15734056219963.
68. Bai X, Wang W, Zhang X, et al. Hyperperfusion of bilateral amygdala in patients with chronic migraine: an arterial spin-labeled magnetic resonance imaging study. J Headache Pain. 2023;24:1–12.

Chapter 8
Neuroimaging Studies in Cluster Headache and Other Trigeminal Autonomic Cephalalgias

Diana Y. Wei and Peter J. Goadsby

8.1 Introduction

Trigeminal autonomic cephalalgias (TACs) are primary headache disorders with unique features that separate them from migraine. TACs are strictly unilateral headache disorders that present with ipsilateral cranial autonomic symptoms, such as lacrimation, conjunctival injection and nasal congestion or rhinorrhoea. TACs encompass four distinct headache disorders, i.e. hemicrania continua, cluster headache, paroxysmal hemicrania and short-lasting unilateral neuralgiform headache attacks (SUNHA), each differing in duration and individual characteristic features [1].

Cluster headache is the most common TAC with a prevalence of approximately 0.1% [2, 3]. Cluster headache is an extremely debilitating disorder, whereby patients experience attacks of severe pain typically in the first two trigeminal regions lasting between 15 min and 3 h, which can recur up to eight times a day and often waking them from their sleep. Patients describe the pain to be the worst pain imaginable and

D. Y. Wei
Department of Neurology, King's College Hospital, London, UK

Wolfson Sensory, Pain and Regeneration Centre, London, UK
e-mail: Diana.Wei@kcl.ac.uk

P. J. Goadsby (✉)
Department of Neurology, King's College Hospital, London, UK

Wolfson Sensory, Pain and Regeneration Centre, London, UK

NIHR King's Clinical Research Facility, Institute of Psychiatry, Psychology & Neuroscience, King's College, London, UK
e-mail: Peter.Goadsby@kcl.ac.uk

I. Petrušić, Y. Wang (eds.), *Neuroimaging of Headache Disorders*, Headache,
https://doi.org/10.1007/978-3-031-85402-6_8

comparable to the pain from gunshot wounds and childbirth [4]. A sense of agitation and restlessness accompanies the attacks; patients are unable to lie still as they would do if they had a migraine attack. The attacks can come in a particular time of the year, lasting for a few weeks to months; these are called bouts. Patients can have episodic cluster headache (ECH), whereby they have bouts with breaks between them of at least 3 months; if they have attacks with less than the 3-month break between them, then they are classified as having chronic cluster headache (CCH) [1].

Hemicrania continua [5] and paroxysmal hemicrania [6] are indomethacin-sensitive headache disorders. This means that as part of their diagnostic workup, the patient will receive indomethacin and will have a significant, if not absolute, response to it. Hemicrania continua is a continuous unilateral headache disorder with a baseline level of pain with exacerbations. Patients with paroxysmal hemicrania will have attacks of unilateral headache lasting between 2 and 30 min.

There are two types of SUNHA disorders: short-lasting unilateral neuralgiform headache attacks with conjunctival injection and tearing (SUNCT) and short-lasting unilateral neuralgiform headache attacks with cranial autonomic symptoms (SUNA). These are extremely short attacks of unilateral pain lasting 1–600 s, which can occur as a single stab, series of stabs or in a saw-tooth pattern [7].

Neuroimaging has allowed us to deepen our knowledge on TACs, particularly cluster headache, with an understanding that the hypothalamus is pivotal in TAC pathophysiology. However, there are several challenges given the conditions' rarity and the unilateral aspect of the attacks. We present the key findings of the acute cluster headache attack phase, and comparing in and out of bout phases provides different aspects to the pathophysiology along with the key imaging findings of hemicrania continua, paroxysmal hemicrania and SUNHA.

8.2 Neuroimaging Studies of Cluster Headache

8.2.1 Studies Investigating Acute Attacks

There are several challenges to imaging cluster headache attacks; indeed, the most significant challenge remains the logistics of capturing enough spontaneous attacks in the scanner. Therefore, using nitroglycerin (NTG) to trigger cluster headache attacks, we can study cluster headache in a controlled experimental environment. Studies using PET and functional MRI (fMRI) have highlighted the cerebral blood flow (CBF) changes during headache, whereby regional CBF can be used as a surrogate of cerebral neuronal activity.

The first PET study with NTG-triggered cluster headache attacks consisted of four ECH patients, two with right-sided attacks and two with left-sided attacks [8].

In this study, the authors found significant increases in CBF in the right caudal anterior cingulate cortex (ACC), rostrocaudal ACC, temporopolar region, supplementary motor area bilaterally, primary motor area (foci corresponding to face, upper and lower extremities), premotor areas, opercular region, insula and lateral inferior frontal cortex. Meanwhile, there were reductions in the CBF in bilateral posterior parietal cortex, occipito-temporal region and prefrontal cortex. These early findings demonstrated that centralised pain processing regions were involved during the cluster headache attacks. The small sample size limited the conclusions that could be made from the study; therefore, they were unable to analyse the data based on the laterality of attacks. The authors suggested that the right-sided cerebral blood flow increases were due to pain sensitivity lateralising to the non-dominant hemisphere.

The subsequent PET study was pivotal, as it acknowledged the laterality of the condition and flipped the images of right-sided cluster headache attacks to analyse all the attacks to be left-sided [9]. The study involved NTG-triggered attacks in nine CCH patients. The authors found significant increases in the CBF in several regions, including the bilateral ACC, contralateral posterior thalamus, ipsilateral basal ganglia, bilateral insulae and cerebellar hemispheres. Beyond this, a regional CBF increase was observed in the posterior hypothalamic grey region ipsilateral to the attack side. This finding is particularly relevant, not only because of the circannual and circadian pattern seen in cluster headache, but there are also changes in neuroendocrine levels in cluster headache patients that implicate the hypothalamus in the pathophysiology.

More than a decade following the pivotal PET study, MRI with arterial spin labelling was used to study the CBF changes during NTG-triggered attacks in 18 cluster headache patients when compared with placebo [10]. In the whole-brain analysis during the cluster headache attack, there were regions of significantly elevated CBF in the medial frontal gyrus, superior frontal gyrus, inferior frontal gyrus and cingulate gyrus, ipsilateral to the attack side when compared with placebo. There was also a significant decrease in CBF in the precuneus, cuneus, superior parietal lobe and occipital lobe contralateral to the attack side. When using region of interest (ROI) analysis, both the hypothalamus and ipsilateral ventral pons showed higher CBF.

Five studies have managed to image spontaneous attacks despite the challenges of capturing them in the scanner environment [11–15]. However, these studies have several limitations; the main drawback is the small sample size. Despite this, the spontaneous attacks captured by Morelli showed ipsilateral hypothalamic grey matter activation using BOLD with single-subject and multi-subject general linear model analysis, supporting the findings from the seminal PET study by May and colleagues [13, 15]. Sprenger and colleagues observed activation in the ipsilateral inferior hypothalamic grey matter, medial thalamus and contralateral perigenual ACC using a priori ROI small-volume correction analysis of PET images of a spontaneous attack in a 30-year-old CCH patient. This patient had deep brain stimulation of the left posterior hypothalamus inserted 2 months earlier for treatment for his CCH [12].

The largest study capturing spontaneous attacks involved 12 ECH patients with right-sided spontaneous attacks and 12 healthy controls [14]. They used resting-state functional MRI (rs-fMRI) to image during an attack ('in attack') and at least 4 h after the previous attack ('out of attack'). The study identified increases in regional homogeneity (ReHo) in the bilateral posterior cingulate cortex (PCC) and ventromedial prefrontal cortex during 'in attack' compared with 'out of attack'. ReHo analysis is a voxel-based measure of the similarity between the time series of a given voxel and its nearest neighbours. When comparing 'out of attack' with 'in attack', ReHo increases in the right middle frontal gyrus and parahippocampal gyrus were observed. They did not find changes in ReHo in the hypothalamus; the reason for this could be the time elapsed between the fMRI and the cluster headache attack. They did find changes in the occipital cortex when comparing 'out of attack' with 'in attack'. The occipital changes were an unexpected finding in cluster headache. In migraine imaging studies, changes in the occipital cortex are found in migraine with aura patients, hypoperfusion in the occipital cortex in spontaneous migraine attacks [16–20], carotid–artery puncture-induced migraine attacks [21] and occipital activation in NTG-induced migraine with aura attacks [22]. The authors hypothesised that these occipital changes may reflect the phenomenon of cortical spreading depression (CSD) of Leão observed in aura [23, 24]. Aura can occur in cluster headache with a reported incidence that ranges from 1% to 23% [25–31]; however, whether cortical spreading depression is involved in cluster headache is yet to be found. Although there could be a hypothetical involvement of CSD in cluster headache, as CSD leads to nitric oxide production [32], it is still unclear what leads to the occipital changes observed (Table 8.1).

Table 8.1 Imaging studies of cluster headache during acute attacks, either spontaneous or triggered with nitroglycerin (NTG)—significant findings

References	Number of patients (ECH or CCH)	Side of attacks	Controls	Nitroglycerin or spontaneous	Imaging modality	Mirroring of images on y-axis	Results
Hsieh et al. [33]	7 ECH enrolled, 4 in bout scanned	2 right, 2 left	No	1 mg sublingual NTG	PET with [^{15}O]butanol tracer	No	In CH attacks: Significant increase in rCBF in right caudal ACC, rostrocaudal ACC, temporopolar region, supplementary motor area bilaterally, primary motor area (foci corresponding to face, upper and lower extremities), premotor areas, opercular region, insula, lateral inferior frontal cortex Reduction in bilateral posterior parietal cortex, occipito-temporal region and prefrontal cortex
May et al. [9]	9 CCH	5 right, 4 left	8 ECH out of bout	1.0–1.2 mg NTG inhalation	PET with $H_2{}^{15}O$	Yes, all attacks on left	Acute attack: Ipsilateral hypothalamic grey (MNI [−2, −18, −8), bilateral ACC, contralateral posterior thalamus, ipsilateral basal ganglia, bilateral insulae and cerebellar hemispheres
May et al. [11]	18 CH, 9 CCH, 8 out of bout ECH, 1 spontaneous attack	5 right, 4 left	4 volunteers for MRA study	9 induced attacks with NTG and 1 spontaneous attack 1.0–1.2 mg NTG inhalation	PET with $H_2{}^{15}O$ and MRA	Yes, all attacks on the left	Acute attack reported in the 1998 *the lancet* paper NTG headache compared to rest: Bilateral anterior cingulate, right posterior thalamus, left basal ganglia, both frontal lobes, bilateral insulae and left temporal lobe, no hypothalamic activation MRA findings: Significant activation in large intracranial vessels (internal carotid arteries) after NTG spray in both CH and out of bout group, persisted during CH attacks but not in those with NTG headache Comparison of CH attack vs. post-NTG spray: Greater activations for CH attack in the left insula, right inferior frontal cortex and left hypothalamic grey area

(continued)

Table 8.1 (continued)

References	Number of patients (ECH or CCH)	Side of attacks	Controls	Nitroglycerin or spontaneous	Imaging modality	Mirroring of images on y-axis	Results
Wei et al. [10]	18 paired headache and placebo scans CH (9 ECH and 9 CCH)	9 left 9 right	No	IV NTG infusion 0.5 μg/kg/min over 20 min	3 T MRI arterial spin labelling		In the whole-brain analysis during the cluster headache attack, there were regions of significantly elevated CBF in the medial frontal gyrus, superior frontal gyrus, inferior frontal gyrus and cingulate gyrus, ipsilateral to attack side when compared with placebo. There was also a significant decrease in CBF in the precuneus, cuneus, superior parietal lobe and occipital lobe contralateral to the attack side. When using region of interest analysis, both the hypothalamus and ipsilateral ventral pons showed higher CBF
Sprenger et al. [12]	1 CCH, with left posterior hypothalamus electrode for deep brain stimulation	Left	No	Spontaneous	$H_2{}^{15}O$ -PET	N/A	Activation in ipsilateral hypothalamus (cluster size 14 voxels, Talairach −4, −14, −6: z-value 3.64), medial thalamus and contralateral perigenual ACC ($p < 0.001$, corrected for multiple comparisons using small volume correction) Statistical trend towards the activation in periaqueductal grey matter (cluster size 18 voxels, Talairach coordinates −2, −28, −10, Z value 4.69)
Morelli et al. [13]	4 ECH		No	Spontaneous	1.5 T MRI T2-weighted gradient echo-EPI (BOLD)		Each in-eCH patient showed significant activation in the ipsilateral hypothalamic area (Tal [−5, −8, −1]) in the comparison of the pain with the pain-free state. A trend of activation was also detected in the prefrontal cortex, cingulate cortex, insula, cerebellum, thalamus and basal ganglia

Qiu et al. [14]	12 ECH	12 Right	12 controls	Spontaneous	3.0 T scanner, echo planar imaging EPI	No	Attack vs. out of attack in CG had significant increases in bilateral posterior cingulate cortex (PCC) and ventromedial prefrontal cortex (VMPFC) Out of attack vs. in attack showed increases in right middle frontal gyrus (MFG) and parahippocampal gyrus, lingual gyrus, parahippocampal gyrus, superior frontal gyrus, postcentral gyrus, precuneus, middle occipital gyrus, postcentral gyrus ($p < 0.05$, corrected) Out of attack CH compared with controls, significant increases in bilateral ACC, rectal gyrus, orbital gyrus Increases in bilateral MPFC and right PCC and insular cortex and left dorsolateral prefrontal cortex in controls compared with CH out of attack
Morelli et al., 2013 [15]	1 CCH	Left-sided	No	Two consecutive spontaneous attacks	1.5 T MRI	No	Significant cerebral activation in ipsilateral to post-hypothalamic region (Talairach coordinates −3, −3, −8), ipsilateral trigeminal root entry zone, bilateral red nucleus (5/−5, −18, −4) and ventral pons (0, −16, −20)

8.3 Ligand PET Imaging Studies

The use of a non-selective opioid antagonist diprenorphine in a PET study demonstrated decreased opioidergic receptor binding in the pineal gland when comparing seven men with left-sided episodic cluster headache patients in bout when compared with eight healthy controls [34]. The pineal gland is responsible for melatonin synthesis, and melatonin plays a key role in cluster headache pathophysiology. Another key finding from this study was an inverse relationship between cluster headache duration and opioid receptor binding in the ipsilateral hypothalamus and the ACC. The authors noted that in rats, nocturnal melatonin supplementation decreased opiomelanocortinergic activity in the hypothalamus [35] and postulated that the melatonin deficiency seen in cluster headache patients could lead to an increased opioidergic function in the hypothalamus and, in turn, cause a reduced availability of opioid receptors.

In a study using ^{18}F-fluoro-2-deoxy-D-glucose (FDG) PET scans of 11 ECH patients and healthy controls [36], areas of hypometabolism in the orbitofrontal cortex, prefrontal cortex and dorsolateral prefrontal cortex were identified. When comparing ‘in bout’ scans with ‘out of bout’ scans, increased metabolism was noted in the perigenual ACC, posterior cingulate cortex (PCC) and orbitofrontal cortex including nucleus accumbens, ventrolateral prefrontal cortex, dorsolateral prefrontal cortex and temporal cortex (middle temporal gyrus), as well as decreases in the metabolism in the cerebellopontine area bilaterally. These findings suggest that first, there are changes in cellular activity in the pain processing system in cluster headache patients; secondly, there are dynamic changes between the in bout and out of bout phases in the central descending pain processing system.

8.4 Structural MRI

The first voxel-based morphometry (VBM) study using 2 T T1-weighted MRI scans involved 25 cluster headache patients and 29 healthy controls [37]. In this study, they found increased grey matter volume in the inferior posterior hypothalamus, both in bout and out of bout, when compared with healthy controls. This change was bilateral; when the attack side was taken into account and images flipped, there was slight lateralisation to the attack side. These changes in the hypothalamus were not seen in a subsequent VBM study [38]. In the study performed by Absinta and colleagues, there was reduced grey matter volume in the right thalamus, right posterior cingulate cortex, left inferior parietal lobule, head of the right caudate nucleus, bilateral middle frontal gyrus, right middle temporal gyrus, right precentral gyrus and left insula in cluster headache patients when compared with healthy controls. There was an increased grey matter volume of the right cuneus. In addition, they found a correlation between disease duration and the decreased left middle frontal gyrus volume. One reason that can account for the lack of changes in the hypothalamus is that in the study performed by Absinta and colleagues, all ECH patients were out of bout at the time of the scan, whereas in the study performed by May and colleagues, it included 14 cluster headache patients in active headache phase and 11 who were out of bout, bolstering the idea that the hypothalamus is involved in the acute cluster headache phase with a potentially dynamic process where the hypothalamus changes when patients are out of bout.

Cortical thickness can also be measured with a high-resolution MRI and can vary between individuals and between different regions of the brain. Before high-resolution MRI is allowed for in vivo studies, post-mortem studies demonstrated structural correlations between anatomical regions of the brain over a population; this is a phenomenon called structural covariance [39]. A common interpretation of structural covariance is that it reflects the underlying brain connectivity and has been used to study neurological conditions such as Alzheimer's disease and schizophrenia. Seifert and colleagues compared the cortical thickness in out of bout ECH patients with age- and sex-matched healthy controls and found a decrease in the cortical thickness in the angular gyrus and precentral gyrus contralateral to the attack side [40]. The angular gyrus (inferior parietal lobule) is involved in pain processing and medication overuse headache [41, 42]. In addition, Seifert and colleagues found a positive correlation in the postcentral gyrus thickness contralateral to the attack side with disease duration.

Comparing the in bout with out of bout phase in ECH patients in a longitudinal VBM study [43], the 'in bout' scans showed increases in the frontal structures, such as the left anterior cingulate, insula and fusiform gyrus. These regions are mainly involved in the modulation of cortical and subcortical nociceptive pathways and therefore suggest that the descending nociceptive modulation system is impaired when in bout due to a neuroplasticity response to the extreme pain. There were no hypothalamic volume changes found on small volume correction.

A large VBM study examined the 91 cluster headache patients, of which 23 had CCH, 46 were out of bout ECH patient and 22 in bout ECH patients, and 78 healthy controls [44]. There were grey matter changes in various brain regions, including the temporal lobe, hippocampus, insular cortex and cerebellum in cluster headache patients compared with controls. There were no changes identified in the hypothalamus in this study, including the sub-analysis of the ECH patients in bout; however, they did not perform small volume correction over the hypothalamus.

A recent structural study using 3 T MRI comparing 12 out of bout ECH patients with 13 healthy controls and 13 migraine patients without aura found decreases in the frontal cortex and increases in the cerebellum and occipital cortex, similar to the studies mentioned earlier [45].

Another analysis method is graph theory, which is a mathematical tool that reduces complex brain network structures to small-world architectures and allows studying the brain using nodes and edges [46]. Applying this method, Ha and colleagues found significant decreases in cortical structures in ECH patients when compared with healthy age- and sex-matched controls; the structures with reduced volumes were the left caudal anterior cingulate and postcentral gyrus [47]. These findings are consistent with previous VBM findings, showing reductions in volume in the cingulate gyrus.

An exploratory study of the telencephalic and cerebellar cortical thickness in 28 CCH patients compared with matched healthy individuals showed cortical thinning in the right middle cingulate cortex and the left posterior insula, and in the cerebellum, there was cortical thinning in the left anterior superior temporal sulcus and the left collateral/lingual sulcus [48].

8.5 Diffusor Tensor Imaging

Several small studies have used diffusor tensor imaging (DTI) to compare the white matter microstructural changes in cluster headache patients with healthy controls.

The first DTI study had seven ECH patients, of which one was in bout and six were out of bout and seven healthy controls [49]. The whole-brain analysis showed regional changes in pain processing networks as well as the brainstem, thalamus, internal capsule, superior and inferior temporal region, frontal lobe, occipital lobe and cerebellum. However, they did not include the hypothalamus in their analysis due to limitations of the DTI methodology.

In a small study comparing 13 cluster headache patients out of bout with healthy controls, they found more widespread white matter changes, in particular the frontal, parietal, temporal and occipital lobe, contralateral side to the pain [50]. However, in a more recent study with 12 ECH patients out of bout, they did not find any significant changes as none of the DTI measures survived statistical correction [45].

To investigate the white matter changes in cluster headache in bout and out of bout, Chou and colleagues scanned 17 ECH patients in bout and again when they were out of bout, comparing them with 17 age-, sex- and handedness-matched healthy controls [51]. They found white matter microstructural differences in the frontal and limbic areas in bout when compared with healthy controls; all changes, except for those seen in the cerebellum, persisted when patients were out of bout. There were also changes seen between anatomical connections to the ipsilateral hypothalamus when post-hoc probabilistic tractography was used.

8.6 Functional Connectivity

Studies used seed analysis at the hypothalamus to explore its functional connectivity (FC). In keeping up with previous studies involving acute attacks, resting-state fMRI (rs-fMRI) comparing spontaneous attack and out of bout showed altered resting-state FC of the hypothalamus ipsilateral to the pain side with regions in the pain matrix, regions involved in cognitive and emotional modulation of pain and occipital cortex [52]. Furthermore, when comparing out of bout ECH patients with healthy controls, FC increases from the hypothalamus and the ACC, bilateral secondary sensorimotor cortex, left V1, right middle occipital gyrus, right thalamus and right insula [53]. Another study found hypothalamic FC changes with frontal and occipital regions when comparing cluster headache patients with healthy controls [54]. Interestingly, this study found the annual bout frequency negatively correlated with the hypothalamic FC with the cerebellar region.

Moreover, a study with ECH patient in bout but outside of acute attacks showed reduced FC between the hypothalamus and the salience network compared with healthy controls [55]. The salience network refers to brain regions, including the ACC, ventral anterior insular cortices, amygdala, hypothalamus, ventral striatum, thalamus and specific brainstem nuclei [56]. Hence, the authors of the study suggest the changes identified reflect changes in pain processing, cognitive and emotional modulation of pain and autonomic dysfunction in cluster headache during the in bout phase [55].

A study combining rs-fMRI with network-sensitive independent component analysis (ICA) investigated the FC changes in resting-state networks outside traditional pain processing areas and between in bout and out of bout [57]. Changes were observed in resting-state networks when comparing ECH patients with controls; they were in the temporal, frontal, salience, default mode, somatosensory, dorsal attention and visual networks. Furthermore, when comparing ECH in and out of bout, there was reduced FC in the frontal and dorsal attention networks, and lower FC in the frontal network was associated with longer disease duration, suggesting that dynamic changes in the frontal pain modulation networks may play a role in shifting between bout periods and disease progression.

Dysfunctional connectivity within the attention network (the superior frontal gyrus and medial frontal cortex) ipsilateral to the headache side and the cerebellar network contralateral to the headache side was found in ECH patients out of bout [58]. When comparing out of bout ECH patients with migraine and healthy controls, they observed increased short-range FC in the working memory network (inferior frontal gyrus), executive control network (superior frontal gyrus) and default mode network (superior parietal lobule) [45]. In addition, there were changes to the long-range FC in the cerebellar and auditory language comprehension networks compared to migraine. Using graph theory to assess the FC in ECH patients compared to healthy controls, there were no global structural connectivity differences. However, there was a significant decrease in strength in the right frontopolar, left pericalcarine and left posterior cingulate gyrus in local structural connectivity, reflecting the changes in brain connectivity regions important for information processing [47].

In CCH patients, there were FC changes observed in the posterior hypothalamus ipsilateral to the headache side and diencephalic–mesencephalic regions, such as the ventral tegmental area, dorsal nuclei of raphe, bilateral substantia nigra, subthalamic nucleus and red nucleus. However, there were no changes in FC seen from the contralateral hypothalamus [59].

In a recent pilot study exploring the connectivity between the thalamus and salience network, comparing 21 CH patients in bout with age- and sex-matched healthy controls, the authors found decreased functional connectivity between the bilateral thalamus and the salience network in both right- and left-sided CH patients in the headache remission state during in bout periods [60].

A study used the fractional amplitude of low-frequency fluctuation (fALFF) in rs-fMRI, which can reflect the local spontaneous activity in brain areas, to compare

23 cluster headache patients with 23 age- and sex-matched healthy controls [61]. They divided the cluster headache cohort by their attack side and studied them separately and found that in the patients experiencing left-sided attack, there were ipsilateral decrease in fALDD in the left cerebellum, left lentiform nucleus, left frontal lobe, left anterior cingulate and right postcentral gyrus. In those experiencing right-sided attacks, there were ipsilateral decrease in fALDD in the right cerebellum, right cingulate gyrus, right superior parietal lobule, right inferior parietal lobule, right postcentral gyrus and left precuneus.

8.7 Exploring Localised Structures

To investigate the hypothalamus in detail, Arkink and colleagues used VBM with two methods to assess the structural hypothalamic changes, first with region-of-interest (ROI) analysis in whole-brain VBM and manual segmentation of the hypothalamus [62]. When using flipped ROI analysis, the anterior hypothalamus volume was increased ipsilateral to the headache side in CCH patients compared with controls. In addition, there was increased volume in the anterior hypothalamus contralateral to the headache side compared to typical CH with migraineurs. There were no changes seen in the unflipped analyses. When manual segmentation was used, bilateral hypothalamic volumes were larger in cluster headache patients when compared with healthy controls and migraineurs. This study highlights the structural hypothalamic changes in cluster headache that were not seen in migraineurs.

A retrospective study investigating both the structure volumes of the hypothalamus was performed in 18 ECH patients and compared with 18 age- and sex-matched healthy controls [63]. They did not find any significant differences in the structural volumes of the whole hypothalamus and the hypothalamic subunits.

In a larger study using the same algorithm for automatic segmentation of the hypothalamic subunits, they included a total of 105 cluster headache patients, of which 57 were CCH and 48 were ECH patients, and 59 self-reported healthy individuals was performed [64]. They found that there were volumetric differences in CCH and not ECH, where there was increased volumes of the ipsilateral anterosuperior subunit of the hypothalamus. Their findings align with the findings from that of Arkink and colleagues.

The sphenopalatine ganglion (SPG) is another structure of importance in cluster headache, as it plays a key role in the trigeminal autonomic reflex and gives rise to the cranial autonomic symptoms during an attack [65]. One neuroimaging study measured and compared the volume of the SPG in 80 ECH patients with 40 non-headache and healthy controls [66]. The volume was measured manually by two neuroimaging specialists, who calculated the sum of the cross-sectional area and multiplied by slice thickness. They found that the mean bilateral average SPG volume was larger in ECH patients than in controls; the SPG volume was larger ipsilateral to the pain side with the number of cranial autonomic symptoms noted by patients to be positively correlated with the SPG volume.

8.8 Comparison Between Migraine and Cluster Headache

There are only a few neuroimaging studies that have directly compared migraine with cluster headache [45, 62, 67]; the key findings were bilateral enlargement of the hypothalamus, reduced grey matter (GM) volume of frontal and occipital areas and increased functional activity of brain cognitive networks in cluster headache patients compared to migraine.

A recent key imaging study used a supervised machine learning approach to identify interictal MRI biomarkers to differentiate between 20 migraine patients, 20 cluster headache patients and 15 healthy controls. The study used multimodal imaging data, including brain volumetric maps, DTI, arterial spin labelling, and rsfMRI [68]. Bilateral hypothalamic and periaqueductal grey (PAG) functional networks were the most important MRI features in terms of classifying migraine and cluster headache patients from controls. When comparing cluster headache patients to migraine patients, it showed decreased functional interaction between the left thalamus and cortical areas mediating interoception and sensory integration. The presence of restlessness was the most important clinical feature in discriminating the two groups of patients.

8.9 Key Neuroimaging Findings and Structures in Cluster Headache

The neuroimaging findings in cluster headache so far can be summarised dependent on the different states of cluster headache.

There are dynamic changes in the frontal structures during in bout and out of bout states, which are involved in the nociceptive modulation. There is also decreased functional connectivity between the hypothalamus and thalamus with the salience network during the in bout state, which also contribute to alterations in pain processing and emotional modulation of pain. Lastly, the hypothalamus is likely to be involved during acute cluster headache attacks.

8.10 Neuroimaging Studies of Hemicrania Continua, Paroxysmal Hemicrania and SUNHA

8.10.1 Hemicrania Continua

There is one PET study involving seven right-handed HC patients comparing with healthy controls [69]. HC patients were scanned in two sessions, with six scans in each session. The patients were advised to stop taking indomethacin 24 to 36 hours before each scanning session. In one session, the patients were scanned for the pain and completely pain-free after being administered indomethacin 100 mg intramuscularly (IM). In the other session, the patients were scanned in the following two states: patients in pain and patients in pain after being administered placebo (normal saline) intramuscularly. In the pain state, involved were the contralateral posterior hypothalamus, ipsilateral dorsal rostral pons, ipsilateral ventrolateral midbrain region, pontomedullary junction, ipsilateral thalamus, bilateral insulae, ipsilateral cingulate gyrus, posterior cingulate cortex, bilateral frontal cortices including the contralateral precentral gyrus, contralateral postcentral gyrus, ipsilateral parietal cortex, bilateral temporal cortices, contralateral occipital cortex, ipsilateral cuneus, precuneus and the cerebellum ($P < 0.001$ uncorrected for multiple comparisons). Small volume corrections were applied to the regions identified according to their a priori hypotheses, which showed significant voxels ($P < 0.05$, corrected for multiple comparisons) at the dorsal rostral pons and at the right hypothalamus. The activity at the right posterior hypothalamus and dorsal rostral pons was significantly reduced when patients were pain-free following indomethacin administration, but remained unaltered by placebo.

8.10.2 Paroxysmal Hemicrania

Similar to hemicrania continua and given the rarity of the condition, only one neuroimaging study has been published in paroxysmal hemicrania. In this PET study, they compared seven patients with paroxysmal hemicrania, and PET imaging was obtained in the attack pain-state off indomethacin and pain-free state off indomethacin and then pain-free following administering IM indomethacin 100 mg [70]. There were no areas of significance when during the attack and out of attack. When comparing pain-state off indomethacin with pain-free state with IM indomethacin 100 mg, the contralateral posterior hypothalamus, contralateral ventral midbrain, ipsilateral lentiform nucleus, anterior and posterior cingulate cortices, bilateral insulae, bilateral frontal cortices, contralateral temporal cortex, contralateral postcentral gyrus, precuneus and contralateral cerebellum had significant activation. There was a significant regional cerebral blood flow in the contralateral hypothalamus during a paroxysmal hemicrania attack, compared with when rendered pain-free with IM indomethacin; however, not when the attack spontaneously resolved. This was explained as there would be persistent activation of the pain neuromatrix after a spontaneous attack.

8.10.3 SUNHA

There are two neuroimaging studies involving single patients with SUNHA. The first study captured spontaneous SUNCT attacks in a 71-year-old woman with left-sided attacks lasting 60 to 90 seconds with ipsilateral lacrimation, rhinorrhoea and conjunctival injection [71], using 2 T fMRI during one session. They captured six spontaneous attacks, and activation was seen in the ipsilateral inferior posterior hypothalamic grey with the BOLD contrast signal closely tracking the attacks. The second study captured spontaneous SUNA attacks in a 60-year-old male with left-sided attacks lasting 30–150 seconds with ipsilateral conjunctival injection, tearing, eyelid oedema, nasal congestion and rhinorrhoea [72]. Using 1 T fMRI, they captured the three attacks with a mean duration of 58.3 seconds where they found activation in the brainstem, right precentral, superior frontal, inferior frontal (opercular part) gyri, as well as in the superior frontal (medial part), middle frontal gyri, and supplementary motor areas bilaterally.

8.10.4 Key Neuroimaging Findings and Structures in Hemicrania Continua, Paroxysmal Hemicrania and SUNHA

From the limited neuroimaging studies available in hemicrania continua, paroxysmal hemicrania and SUNHA, beyond the pain areas involved, the hypothalamus seems to be implicated and appear to be a finding across the TACs and, perhaps similar to cluster headache, have a role in the acute attacks of pain. However, the challenge lies in the rarity of these conditions.

References

1. Headache Classification Committee of the International Headache Society (IHS). The international classification of headache disorders, 3rd edition. Cephalalgia. 2018;38:1–211.
2. Russell MB. Epidemiology and genetics of cluster headache. Lancet Neurol. 2004;3:279–83.
3. Crespi JGS, Salvesen Ø, Bratbak DF, et al. Epidemiology of diagnosed cluster headache in Norway. Cephalalgia Rep. 2022;5:1–15.
4. Burish MJ, Pearson SM, Shapiro RE, et al. Cluster headache is one of the most intensely painful human conditions: results from the international cluster headache questionnaire. Headache. 2021;61:117–24.
5. Cittadini E, Goadsby PJ. Hemicrania continua: a clinical study of 39 patients with diagnostic implications. Brain. 2010;133:1973–86.
6. Cittadini E, Matharu MS, Goadsby PJ. Paroxysmal hemicrania: a prospective clinical study of 31 cases. Brain. 2008;131:1142–55.
7. Cohen AS, Matharu MS, Goadsby PJ. Short-lasting unilateral neuralgiform headache attacks with conjunctival injection and tearing (SUNCT) or cranial autonomic features (SUNA) – a prospective clinical study of SUNCT and SUNA. Brain. 2006;129:2746–60.
8. Hsieh J-C, Hannerz J, Ingvar M. Right-lateralised central processing for pain of nitroglycerin-induced cluster headache. Pain. 1996;67:59–68.
9. May A, Bahra A, Büchel C, et al. Hypothalamic activation in cluster headache attacks. Lancet. 1998;352:275–8.
10. Wei DY, O'Daly O, Zelaya FO, Goadsby PJ. Areas of cerebral blood flow changes on arterial spin labelling with the use of symmetric template during nitroglycerin triggered cluster headache attacks. NeuroImage Clin. 2022;33:102920.

11. May A, Bahra A, Büchel C, et al. PET and MRA findings in cluster headache and MRA in experimental pain. Neurology. 2000;55:1328–35.
12. Sprenger T, Boecker H, Tolle TR, et al. Specific hypothalamic activation during a spontaneous cluster headache attack. Neurology. 2004;62:516–7.
13. Morelli N, Pesaresi I, Cafforio G, et al. Functional magnetic resonance imaging in episodic cluster headache. J Headache Pain. 2009;10:11–4.
14. Qiu EC, Yu SY, Liu RZ, et al. Altered regional homogeneity in spontaneous cluster headache attacks: a resting-state functional magnetic resonance imaging study. Chin Med J. 2012;125:705–9.
15. Morelli N, Rota E, Gori S, et al. Brainstem activation in cluster headache: an adaptive behavioural response? Cephalalgia. 2013;33:416–20.
16. Olesen J, Larsen B, Lauritzen M. Focal hyperemia followed by spreading oligemia and impaired activation of rCBF in classic migraine. Ann Neurol. 1981;9:344–52.
17. Woods RP, Iacoboni M, Mazziotta JC. Brief report: bilateral spreading cerebral hypoperfusion during spontaneous migraine headache. N Engl J Med. 1994;331:1689–92.
18. Cutrer FM, Sorensen AG, Weisskoff RM, et al. Perfusion-weighted imaging defects during spontaneous migrainous aura. Ann Neurol. 1998;43:25–31.
19. Sanchez del Rio M, Bakker D, Wu O, et al. Perfusion weighted imaging during migraine: spontaneous visual aura and headache. Cephalalgia. 1999;19:701–7.
20. Hadjikhani N, Sanchez Del Rio M, Wu O, et al. Mechanisms of migraine aura revealed by functional MRI in human visual cortex. Proc Natl Acad Sci USA. 2001;98:4687–92.
21. Lauritzen M, Olsen TS, Lassen NA, Paulson OB. Regulation of regional cerebral blood flow during and between migraine attacks. Ann Neurol. 1983;14:569–72.
22. Afridi S, Kaube H, Goadsby PJ. Occipital activation in glyceryl trinitrate induced migraine with visual aura. J Neurol Neurosurg Psychiatry. 2005;76:1158–60.
23. Leao AAP. Spreading depression of activity in the cerebral cortex. J Neurophysiol. 1944;7:359–90.
24. Leao AAP. Pial circulation and spreading of depression of activity in the cerebral cortex. J Neurophysiol. 1944;7:391–6.
25. Silberstein SD, Niknam R, Rozen TD, Young WB. Cluster headache with aura. Neurology. 2000;54:219–21.
26. Bahra A, May A, Goadsby PJ. Cluster headache: a prospective clinical study with diagnostic implications. Neurology. 2002;58:354–61.
27. Lin KH, Wang PJ, Fuh JL, et al. Cluster headache in the Taiwanese – a clinic-based study. Cephalalgia. 2004;24:631–8.
28. Schurks M, Kurth T, de Jesus J, et al. Cluster headache: clinical presentation, lifestyle features, and medical treatment. Headache. 2006;46:1246–54.
29. Donnet A, Lanteri-Minet M, Guegan-Massardier E, et al. Chronic cluster headache: a French clinical descriptive study. J Neurol Neurosurg Psychiatry. 2007;78:1354–8.
30. Rozen TD, Fishman RS. Cluster headache in The United States of America: demographics, clinical characteristics, triggers, suicidality, and personal burden. Headache. 2012;52:99–113.
31. de Coo IF, Wilbrink LA, Ie GD, et al. Aura in cluster headache: a cross-sectional study. Headache. 2018;58:1203–10.
32. Obrenovitch TP, Urenjak J, Wang M. Nitric oxide formation during cortical spreading depression is critical for rapid subsequent recovery of ionic homeostasis. J Cereb Blood Flow Metab. 2002;22:680–8.
33. Hsieh J-C, Hannerz J, Ingvar M. Right-lateralised central processing for pain of nitroglycer-induced cluster headache. Pain. 1996;67:59–68.
34. Sprenger T, Willoch F, Miederer M, et al. Opioidergic changes in the pineal gland and hypothalamus in cluster headache: a ligand PET study. Neurology. 2006;66:1108–10.
35. Rasmussen DD, Marck BT, Boldt BM, et al. Suppression of hypothalamic pro-opiomelanocortin (POMC) gene expression by daily melatonin supplementation in aging rats. J Pineal Res. 2003;34:127–33.

36. Sprenger T, Ruether KV, Boecker H, et al. Altered metabolism in frontal brain circuits in cluster headache. Cephalalgia. 2007;27:1033–42.
37. May A, Ashburner J, Buchel C, et al. Correlation between structural and functional changes in brain in an idiopathic headache syndrome. Nat Med. 1999;5:836–83.
38. Absinta M, Rocca MA, Colombo B, et al. Selective decreased grey matter volume of the pain-matrix network in cluster headache. Cephalalgia. 2012;32:109–15.
39. Alexander-Bloch A, Giedd JN, Bullmore E. Imaging structural co-variance between human brain regions. Nat Rev Neurosci. 2013;14:322–36.
40. Seifert CL, Magon S, Staehle K, et al. A case-control study on cortical thickness in episodic cluster headache. Headache. 2012;52:1362–8.
41. Ferraro S, Grazzi L, Mandelli ML, et al. Pain processing in medication overuse headache: a functional magnetic resonance imaging (fMRI) study. Pain Med. 2012;13:255–62.
42. Fumal A, Laureys S, Di Clemente L, et al. Orbitofrontal cortex involvement in chronic analgesic-overuse headache evolving from episodic migraine. Brain. 2006;129:543–50.
43. Yang FC, Chou KH, Fuh JL, et al. Altered gray matter volume in the frontal pain modulation network in patients with cluster headache. Pain. 2013;154:801–7.
44. Naegel S, Holle D, Desmarattes N, et al. Cortical plasticity in episodic and chronic cluster headache. NeuroImage Clin. 2014;6:415–23.
45. Giorgio A, Lupi C, Zhang J, et al. Changes in grey matter volume and functional connectivity in cluster headache versus migraine. Brain Imaging Behav. 2020;14:496–504.
46. Bullmore E, Sporns O. Complex brain networks: graph theoretical analysis of structural and functional systems. Nat Rev Neurosci. 2009;10:186–98.
47. Ha SY, Park KM. Alterations of structural connectivity in episodic cluster headache: a graph theoretical analysis. J Clin Neurosci. 2019;62:60–5.
48. Demichelis G, Pinardi C, Giani L, et al. Chronic cluster headache: a study of the telencephalic and cerebellar cortical thickness. Cephalalgia. 2022;42:444–54.
49. Teepker M, Menzler K, Belke M, et al. Diffusion tensor imaging in episodic cluster headache. Headache. 2012;52:274–82.
50. Szabo N, Kincses ZT, Pardutz A, et al. White matter disintegration in cluster headache. J Headache Pain. 2013;14:64.
51. Chou KH, Yang FC, Fuh JL, et al. Altered white matter microstructural connectivity in cluster headaches: a longitudinal diffusion tensor imaging study. Cephalalgia. 2014;34:1040–52.
52. Qiu E, Wang Y, Ma L, et al. Abnormal brain functional connectivity of the hypothalamus in cluster headaches. PLoS One. 2013;8:e57896.
53. Rocca MA, Valsasina P, Absinta M, et al. Central nervous system dysregulation extends beyond the pain-matrix network in cluster headache. Cephalalgia. 2010;30:1383–91.
54. Yang FC, Chou KH, Fuh JL, et al. Altered hypothalamic functional connectivity in cluster headache: a longitudinal resting-state functional MRI study. J Neurol Neurosurg Psychiatry. 2015;86:437–45.
55. Qiu E, Tian L, Wang Y, et al. Abnormal coactivation of the hypothalamus and salience network in patients with cluster headache. Neurology. 2015;84:1402–8.
56. Seeley WW. The salience network: a neural system for perceiving and responding to homeostatic demands. J Neurosci. 2019;39:9878.
57. Chou KH, Yang FC, Fuh JL, et al. Bout-associated intrinsic functional network changes in cluster headache: a longitudinal resting-state functional MRI study. Cephalalgia. 2017;37:1152–63.
58. Farago P, Szabo N, Toth E, et al. Ipsilateral alteration of resting state activity suggests that cortical dysfunction contributes to the pathogenesis of cluster headache. Brain Topogr. 2017;30:281–9.
59. Ferraro S, Nigri A, Bruzzone MG, et al. Defective functional connectivity between posterior hypothalamus and regions of the diencephalic-mesencephalic junction in chronic cluster headache. Cephalalgia. 2018;38:1910–8.
60. Qiu E, Xing X, Wang Y, Tian L. Altered functional connectivity of the thalamus and salience network in patients with cluster headache: a pilot study. Neurol Sci. 2024;45:269–76.

61. Chen Y, Xing X, Dai W, et al. Brain regions involved in fractional amplitude of low-frequency fluctuation in cluster headache patients: a resting-state functional MRI study. BMC Neurol. 2022;22:336.
62. Arkink EB, Schmitz N, Schoonman GG, et al. The anterior hypothalamus in cluster headache. Cephalalgia. 2017;37:1039–50.
63. Lee DA, Lee HJ, Kim HC, Park KM. Alterations of the structural covariance network in the hypothalamus of patients with cluster headache. J Neurol. 2022;269:316–22.
64. Ferraro S, Nigri A, Bruzzone MG, et al. Involvement of the ipsilateral-to-the-pain anterior-superior hypothalamic subunit in chronic cluster headache. J Headache Pain. 2024;25:7.
65. Wei DY, Goadsby PJ. Cluster headache pathophysiology – insights from current and emerging treatments. Nat Rev Neurol. 2021;17:308–24.
66. Wu JW, Chen ST, Wang YF, et al. Sphenopalatine ganglion volumetry in episodic cluster headache: from symptom laterality to cranial autonomic symptoms. J Headache Pain. 2023;24:2.
67. Chong CD, Aguilar M, Schwedt TJ. Altered hypothalamic region covariance in migraine and cluster headache: a structural MRI study. Headache. 2020;60:553–63.
68. Messina R, Sudre CH, Wei DY, et al. Biomarkers of migraine and cluster headache: differences and similarities. Ann Neurol. 2023;93:729–42.
69. Matharu MS, Cohen AS, McGonigle DJ, et al. Posterior hypothalamic and brainstem activation in hemicrania continua. Headache. 2004;44:747–61.
70. Matharu MS, Cohen AS, Frackowiak RS, Goadsby PJ. Posterior hypothalamic activation in paroxysmal hemicrania. Ann Neurol. 2006;59:535–45.
71. May A, Bahra A, Buchel C, et al. Functional magnetic resonance imaging in spontaneous attacks of SUNCT: short-lasting neuralgiform headache with conjunctival injection and tearing. Ann Neurol. 1999;46:791–4.
72. Auer T, Janszky J, Schwarcz A, et al. Attack-related brainstem activation in a patient with SUNCT syndrome: an ictal fMRI study. Headache. 2009;49:909–12.

Chapter 9
Neuroimaging Studies of Other Primary Headache Disorders

Wei Wang, Yonggang Wang, and Yiheng Tu

9.1 Introduction

Primary headache disorders represent a complex and diverse group of conditions that pose significant challenges in diagnosis and management. While migraines and tension-type headaches have been extensively studied, leading to substantial advances in understanding their pathophysiology, other primary headache disorders remain relatively underexplored. These include primary cough headache, primary exercise headache, primary headache associated with sexual activity, primary thunderclap headache, new daily persistent headache (NDPH), primary stabbing headache, cold-stimulus headache, external pressure headache, nummular headache, and hypnic headache [1]. Recent advancements in neuroimaging techniques offer new avenues to investigate these lesser-known disorders. Neuroimaging studies on other primary headaches are relatively scarce, with most of the existing evidence reported in patients with NDPH.

W. Wang (✉)
Department of Neurology, Sir Run Run Shaw Hospital, School of Medicine, Zhejiang University, Hangzhou, China

Y. Wang
Department of Neurology, Headache Center, Beijing Tiantan Hospital, Capital Medical University, Beijing, China

Y. Tu
CAS Key Laboratory of Mental Health, Institute of Psychology, Chinese Academy of Sciences, Beijing, China

Department of Psychology, University of Chinese Academy of Sciences, Beijing, China

I. Petrušić, Y. Wang (eds.), *Neuroimaging of Headache Disorders*, Headache,
https://doi.org/10.1007/978-3-031-85402-6_9

9.2 Neuroimaging on New Daily Persistent Headache

New daily persistent headache (NDPH) is a rare and complex primary headache disorder characterized by a sudden onset of unremitting headache that persists for more than 3 months [1]. Despite the lack of clarity on its pathogenesis, recent neuroimaging studies have shed light on potential structural, functional, and connectivity abnormalities associated with NDPH. Notably, some studies using voxel-based morphometry (VBM) and surface-based morphometry (SBM) failed to identify significant structural changes in the gray matter of NDPH patients, suggesting an absence of gross structural alterations [2]. However, contrasting evidence from diffusion tensor imaging (DTI) studies revealed widespread microstructural white matter abnormalities, including decreased fractional anisotropy (FA) and increased mean diffusivity (MD) and radial diffusivity (RD) across multiple white matter tracts, indicating potential disruptions in white matter integrity [3]. Further complicating the picture, functional imaging studies have demonstrated altered brain activity and connectivity patterns in NDPH. Resting-state functional MRI (rs-fMRI) analyses showed abnormal functional connectivity (FC) in regions involved in pain perception and regulation [4, 5]. For instance, Wang et al. identified aberrant FC in the brainstem nuclei, including regions such as the periaqueductal gray and ventral tegmental areas [5]. Additionally, abnormal functional connectivity was noted in other brain regions like the left inferior occipital gyrus and right thalamus, suggesting disruptions in networks related to pain and emotion regulation [4]. These findings are further supported by observations of increased amplitude of low-frequency fluctuations (ALFF) and regional homogeneity (ReHo) in the left middle occipital gyrus, indicating abnormal activation of the visual system [6].

Interestingly, studies employing magnetoencephalography (MEG) and structural MRI revealed that NDPH is associated with decreased cortical thickness in specific regions, such as the left rostral cortex of the middle frontal gyrus, along with increased gray matter volume in the left calcarine [7]. These structural changes are coupled with abnormal high-frequency cortical activity, suggesting that cortical hyperexcitability might contribute to the pain experience in NDPH. Despite these changes, investigations into glymphatic system function revealed normal findings, indicating that glymphatic dysfunction might not be a contributing factor to NDPH [8]. However, contrastingly, arterial spin-labeled MRI studies identified decreased cerebral blood flow (CBF) and arterial cerebral blood volume (aCBV) in multiple right hemisphere regions of NDPH patients, suggesting potential vascular dysregulation [9]. Further adding to the complexity, magnetic resonance spectroscopy (MRS) studies examining neurotransmitter levels, specifically gamma-aminobutyric acid (GABA) and glutamate/glutamine (Glx), found no significant differences between NDPH patients and healthy controls. However, moderate to severe NDPH patients exhibited lower Glx levels, suggesting that neurotransmitter imbalances, while not the primary cause, may still play a role in symptom severity [10]. Moreover, studies using graph theory and MEG analyses have identified altered functional network topology in NDPH, such as increased global efficiency and changes in the clustering coefficients of brain networks, which point to potential disruptions in how pain and sensory information are processed [11].

In summary, while NDPH does not appear to involve overt gray matter structural changes, there are evident microstructural abnormalities, altered functional connectivity, and disrupted brain activity patterns that collectively point to a complex and multifaceted pathophysiology. These findings highlight the importance of continued research using advanced neuroimaging techniques to unravel the mechanisms underlying NDPH and identify potential diagnostic markers and treatment targets.

9.3 Neuroimaging on Primary Cough Headache

Primary cough headache is characterized by sudden, short-lasting headaches precipitated by coughing, sneezing, or straining. The pathogenesis remains elusive, but neuroimaging studies have provided some clues. Initially, imaging focuses on excluding secondary causes like Chiari malformations [12]. Most research evidence indicates that MRI scans on patients and found no significant structural abnormalities, supporting a primary headache diagnosis [13]. However, some studies reported cases with cerebellar tonsillar ectopia, suggesting that minimal Chiari malformations could contribute to symptoms in some individuals [12]. Some evidence shows a significant incidence of venous stenosis diagnosed by magnetic resonance venography in primary cough headache patients compared to controls [13]. Functional imaging studies are scarce for primary cough headache due to the transient nature of attacks. Nevertheless, future research utilizing techniques like arterial spin labeling (ASL) MRI could assess cerebral blood flow changes during induced Valsalva maneuvers, potentially uncovering functional alterations associated with headache episodes. Moreover, MR venography might evaluate venous sinus compliance, as changes in intracranial venous pressure could play a role in pathophysiology.

9.4 Neuroimaging on Other Rare Types of Primary Headache

Primary exercise headache (PEH) is characterized by pulsatile headaches occurring during or after physical exertion without any underlying structural abnormalities [1]. While the exact pathophysiology remains unclear, vascular mechanisms have been proposed, and neuroimaging plays a crucial role in excluding secondary causes and exploring potential functional changes associated with PEH. Neuroimaging is essential in the diagnostic workup of PEH to rule out secondary causes such as subarachnoid hemorrhage, arterial dissection, or intracranial tumors [14]. Functional neuroimaging studies specific to PEH are limited, but existing research suggests possible transient vascular changes during episodes of exertion [15]. Additionally, cases of reversible cerebral vasoconstriction syndrome (RCVS) presenting as exercise-induced headaches have been reported [16, 17]. Although RCVS is considered a secondary headache disorder, this case highlights the potential role of transient vascular changes in exercise-related headaches. Because primary headache associated with sexual activity (PHASA), is diagnosed by excluding other conditions, the diagnostic approach focuses on ruling out secondary causes. The differential diagnosis should align with the specific presentation; for instance, a thunderclap headache warrants exclusion of a subarachnoid hemorrhage, which is precipitated by sexual intercourse in 5–12% of cases [18]. Other potential diagnoses include reversible cerebral vasoconstriction syndrome (RCVS), arterial dissection, cerebral aneurysm, venous abnormalities, intracranial masses, hemorrhages, cerebral venous sinus thrombosis, meningitis, and vasculitis. A comprehensive history and detailed neurological examination are crucial for all patients reporting headaches during sexual activity, as any focal neurological deficits may suggest a secondary etiology. For thunderclap headaches, at minimum, a non-contrast head CT scan and lumbar puncture are recommended. If no hemorrhage is detected, vascular imaging with CT or MR angiography (CTA/CTV or MRA/MRV) should be pursued [19]. There is limited neuroimaging evidence for cold stimulus headache. Wolf and Hardy observed that cold-induced hand pain involves reduced arterial pulses followed by vasodilation and erythema, indicating a local vascular effect [20]. Similarly, in cold stimulus headaches, cerebral blood flow changes occur, with reduced mean blood flow velocities in the middle cerebral arteries noted in patients who develop headaches, as shown by transcranial Doppler ultrasonography [21]. The diagnosis of hypnic headache requires the exclusion of secondary causes, making cerebral neuroimaging essential, as several symptomatic cases, such as hemangioblastoma of the cerebellum, nonfunctioning pituitary macroadenoma, growth hormone-secreting pituitary tumor, posterior fossa meningioma, and brainstem lesions, have been documented [22–26]. In conclusion, for these rare primary headaches, neuroimaging as a routine examination is essential to exclude secondary causes; however, there is currently a lack of recognized imaging biomarkers (Table 9.1).

Table 9.1 Neuroimaging studies of NDPH: significant findings

Authors, years	Subjects	Type of measurements	Main findings
Steffen Naegel et al. [2]	23 NDPH 23 HCs	Gray matter changes	No gray matter changes
Yanliang Mei et al. [3]	21 NDPH 25 HCs	Microstructural abnormalities	Widespread abnormalities in the white matter of the brain in NDPH
Wei Wang et al. [4]	29 NDPH 31 HCs	Functional connectivity	Patients with NDPH showed aberrant FC in multiple brain regions involved in perception and regulation of emotion and pain
Wei Wang et al. [5]	29 NDPH 37 HCs	Functional connectivity of brainstem nuclei	Patients with NDPH have abnormal FC of brainstem nuclei involved in the perception and regulation of pain and emotions
Xueyan Zhang et al. [6]	30 NDPH 30 HCs	ReHo, ALFF, and functional connectivity	Both increased ReHo and ALFF values of the left middle occipital gyrus (MOG_L) were found in the NDPH
Dong Qiu et al. [7]	28 NDPH 37 HCs	Brain structural changes and neural activity patterns	Patients with NDPH showed a significant decrease in cortical thickness of the left rostral cortex in the middle frontal gyrus, decreased cortical surface area of the left fusiform gyrus, decreased gray matter volume of the left superior frontal gyrus and the left middle frontal gyrus, and increased gray matter volume of the left calcarine
Xue Zhang et al. [8]	27 NDPH 33 HCs	Glymphatic function	No glymphatic dysfunction
Xiaoyan Bai et al. [9]	15 NDPH 15 HCs	Cerebral perfusion variances	NDPH were found to have decreased CBF and aCBV values in multiple regions in the right hemisphere
Tong Chen et al. [10]	21 NDPH 22 HCs	GABA and Glx levels in both periaqueductal gray and dentate nucleus	No significant differences
Dong Qiu et al. [11]	35 NDPH 40 HCs	Cortical functional network topological characteristics	The lateral occipital cortex and superior frontal gyrus FC were increased in NDPH groups

Note: *NDPH* new daily persistent headache, *HC* health control

References

1. Headache Classification Committee of the International Headache Society (IHS) The International Classification of Headache Disorders, 3rd edition (2018) Cephalalgia 38:1–211.
2. Naegel S, Zeller J, Hougard A, et al. No structural brain alterations in new daily persistent headache – a cross sectional VBM/SBM study. Cephalalgia. 2022;42:335–44.
3. Mei Y, Wang W, Qiu D, et al. Micro-structural white matter abnormalities in new daily persistent headache: a DTI study using TBSS analysis. J Headache Pain. 2023;24:80.

4. Wang W, Yuan Z, Zhang X, et al. Mapping the aberrant brain functional connectivity in new daily persistent headache: a resting-state functional magnetic resonance imaging study. J Headache Pain. 2023;24:46.
5. Wang W, Qiu D, Mei Y, et al. Altered functional connectivity of brainstem nuclei in new daily persistent headache: evidence from resting-state functional magnetic resonance imaging. CNS Neurosci Ther. 2024;30:e14686.
6. Zhang X, Wang W, Bai X, et al. Alterations in regional homogeneity and multiple frequency amplitudes of low-frequency fluctuation in patients with new daily persistent headache: a resting-state functional magnetic resonance imaging study. J Headache Pain. 2023;24:14.
7. Qiu D, Wang W, Mei Y, et al. Brain structure and cortical activity changes of new daily persistent headache: multimodal evidence from MEG/sMRI. J Headache Pain. 2023;24:45.
8. Zhang X, Wang W, Zhang X, et al. Normal glymphatic system function in patients with new daily persistent headache using diffusion tensor image analysis along the perivascular space. Headache. 2023;63:663–71.
9. Bai X, Wang W, Zhang X, et al. Cerebral perfusion variance in new daily persistent headache and chronic migraine: an arterial spin-labeled MR imaging study[J]. J Headache Pain. 2022;23:156.
10. Chen T, Bai X, Wang W, et al. Gamma-aminobutyric acid and glutamate/glutamine levels in the dentate nucleus and periaqueductal gray in new daily persistent headache: a magnetic resonance spectroscopy study. J Headache Pain. 2024;25:142.
11. Qiu D, Ge Z, Mei Y, et al. Mapping brain functional networks topological characteristics in new daily persistent headache: a magnetoencephalography study. J Headache Pain. 2023;24:161.
12. Thunstedt DC, Schmutzer M, Fabritius MP, et al. Headache characteristics and postoperative course in Chiari I malformation. Cephalalgia. 2022;42:879–87.
13. Donnet A, Valade D, Houdart E, et al. Primary cough headache, primary exertional headache, and primary headache associated with sexual activity: a clinical and radiological study. Neuroradiology. 2013;55:297–305.
14. Levin M. Classification and diagnosis of primary headache disorders. Semin Neurol. 2022;42:406–17.
15. Edward JA, Cornwell WK. 3rd. Impact of exercise on cerebrovascular physiology and risk of stroke. Stroke. 2022;53:2404–10.
16. Ling YH, Chen SP. Narrative review: headaches after reversible cerebral vasoconstriction syndrome. Curr Pain Headache Rep. 2020;24:74.
17. Boitet R, de Gaalon S, Duflos C, et al. Long-term outcomes after reversible cerebral vasoconstriction syndrome. Stroke. 2020;51:670–3.
18. Maynard P, Pace A. Primary headache associated with sexual activity: a review of the literature. Curr Pain Headache Rep. 2024;28:627–32.
19. Ducros A, Bousser MG. Thunderclap headache. BMJ. 2013;346:e8557.
20. Wolf S, Hardy JD. Studies on pain. Observations on pain due to local cooling and on factors involved in the "cold pressor" effect. J Clin Invest. 1941;20:521–33.
21. Chebini A, Dilli E. Cold stimulus headache. Curr Neurol Neurosci Rep. 2019;19:46.
22. Mullally WJ, Hall KE. Hypnic headache secondary to haemangioblastoma of the cerebellum. Cephalalgia. 2010;30:887–9.
23. Garza I, Oas KH. Symptomatic hypnic headache secondary to a nonfunctioning pituitary macroadenoma. Headache. 2009;49:470–2.
24. Valentinis L, Tuniz F, Mucchiut M, et al. Hypnic headache secondary to a growth hormone-secreting pituitary tumour. Cephalalgia. 2009;29:82–4.
25. Peatfield RC, Mendoza ND. Posterior fossa meningioma presenting as hypnic headache. Headache. 2003;43:1007–8.
26. Moon HS, Chung CS, Hong SB, et al. A case of symptomatic hypnic headache syndrome. Cephalalgia. 2006;26:81–3.

Chapter 10
Neuroimaging Studies of Painful Lesions of the Cranial Nerves

Robert Semnic, Stefan Stojanoski, and Miloš Vuković

10.1 Classification of Trigeminal Neuralgia

TN is a chronic pain disorder with one of the most severe pains one can suffer. The incidence of TN is 4–20/100,00, and women are affected more often than men [1, 2]. TN can be triggered by s, peaking, eating, or touching the skin. Typically, no neurologic deficits are clinically evident.

The latest classification of the International Headache Society [3] distinguishes between classical (CTN), secondary (STN), and idiopathic TN (ITN). NVC is the main cause of CTN.

STN is less common in cases involving pathology in different anatomical compartments, such as the cisternal space and Meckel's cave (e.g., trigeminal schwannoma (Fig. 10.1a, b), meningioma (Fig. 10.2a, b), epidermoid, and carcinomatosis). It can also occur at the skull base due to various tumors or in the extracranial space due to perineural spread of head and neck neoplasms (Fig. 10.1c). In multiple sclerosis (MS) patients, plaque can affect the root entry zone (REZ) and cisternal segment in 3–23% of patients [4] (Fig. 10.2c), but NVC can still be present. Broggi and colleagues evaluated patients with MS who underwent MVD for intractable TN, and 74% had MS lesions in the brainstem, with 46% also having severe NVC at surgery [5].

R. Semnic (✉)
Center for Imaging and Functional Medicine, Uppsala University Hospital, Uppsala, Sweden

Department of Diagnostic and Interventional Radiology, Dubrava University Hospital, Zagreb, Croatia
e-mail: robert.semnic@akademiska.se

S. Stojanoski · M. Vuković
Department of Radiology, Oncology Institute of Vojvodina, Sremska Kamenica, Serbia

Faculty of Medicine, University of Novi Sad, Novi Sad, Serbia
e-mail: stefan.stojanoski@mf.uns.ac.rs; milos.vukovic@mf.uns.ac.rs

I. Petrušić, Y. Wang (eds.), *Neuroimaging of Headache Disorders*, Headache,
https://doi.org/10.1007/978-3-031-85402-6_10

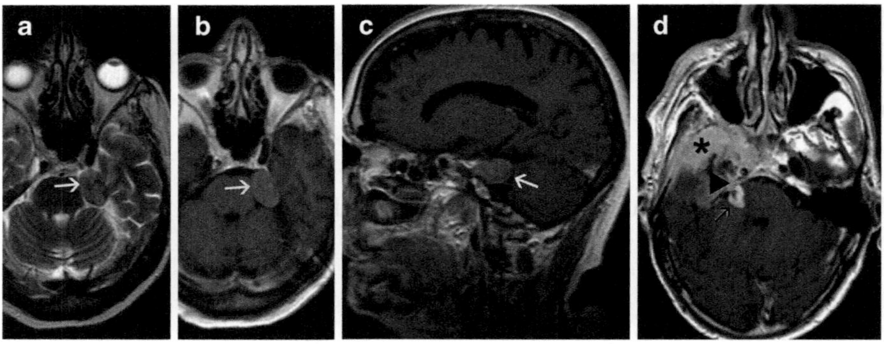

Fig. 10.1 Transverse T2-weighted image (**a**), transverse (**b**), and sagittal (**c**) contrast-enhanced images show a trigeminal schwannoma on the left side with mild and homogeneous contrast enhancement (→). Contrast-enhanced T1-weighted transverse image in another patient (**c**) depicts the perineural spread of squamous cell carcinoma of the upper lip, involving the right masticatory space (*), pterygopalatine fossa, and cavernous sinus (**c**). The maxillary nerve is involved at the foramen ovale (▶), along with the cisternal part of the right trigeminal nerve (↗)

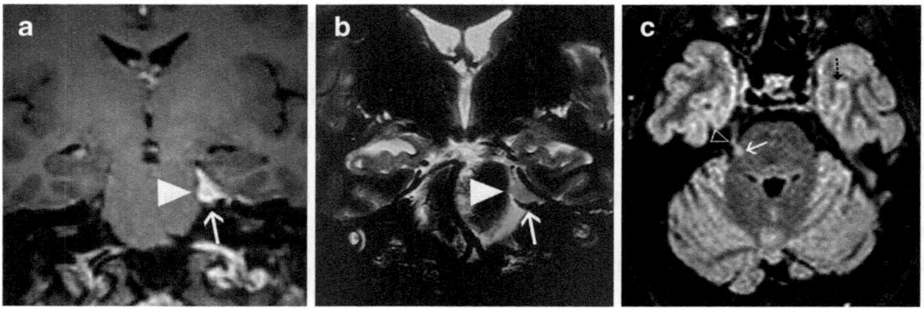

Fig. 10.2 Contrast-enhanced T1-weighted transverse image (**a**) and coronal T2-weighted image (**b**) in patient with tentorial meningioma on the left side (**a**, **b**, ▷). The trigeminal nerve is compressed, deformed, and dislocated downward (**a**, **b**, ↑). FLAIR transverse image at the level of pons (**c**). MS lesions are visible at the REZ of the right trigeminal nerve (←) and within a cisternal segment of the nerve (▷). Additionally, MS plaque is present in the periventricular white matter of the left temporal horn (⇣)

In ITN, a small number of patients remain with undetermined etiology where neither MRI nor electrophysiological tests show abnormalities.

10.2 Histological Landmarks of the Brainstem and Trigeminal Nerve

The root entry zone (REZ) represents the exact junction between the n.V and the brainstem, and the transition zone (TZ) represents the myelin transition area from central myelin (oligodendrocytes) to peripheral myelin (Schwann cells). The term

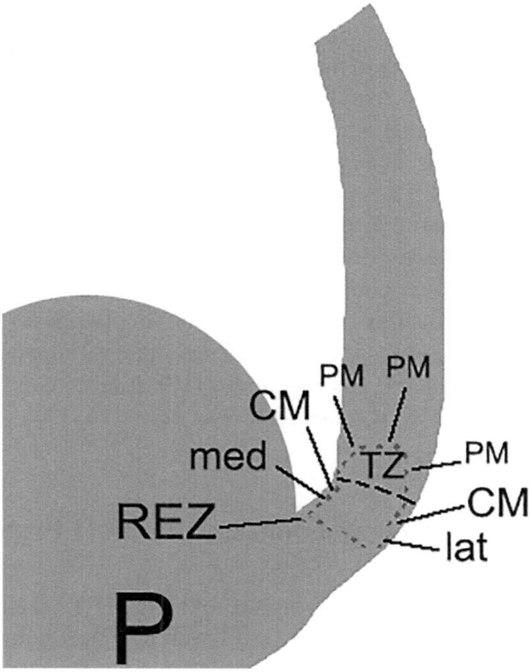

Fig. 10.3 A schematic representation of a horizontal section through the pons at the level of the trigeminal nerve. Central myelin (CM) is visible on both the lateral (CM lat) and medial (CM med) sides of the nerve at the transition zone (TZ). The TZ forms an arch (dashed line), with the line at its base connecting the junction points of central myelin (CM) and peripheral myelin (PM) on the medial and corresponding lateral aspects of the n.V. The root entry zone (REZ) is located at the junction between the nerve and the pons (P)

"REZ" includes TZ, the central myelin root portion, and the adjacent brainstem surface (Fig. 10.3). TZ is an anatomic area with increased mechanical vulnerability [7] and appears to be more relevant in patients with TN. TZ is not always located in the same position as REZ; therefore, those two landmarks should not be used interchangeably.

Peker studied 100 nerves from 50 cadavers and demonstrated that central myelin extends up to 4.9 mm from the REZ and TZ is 2.5 mm away from the brainstem [8]. NVC at the root entry and TZ (<3 mm from the brainstem) is more likely to be symptomatic than contact with a more distal cisternal segment [7].

Peripheral myelin is more resistant to compression and damage, which explains why NVC at the distal part of the nerve can occur in individuals without any TN history [9].

10.3 Pathogenesis of Classical TN

Cisternal segment neurovascular conflict is the most common cause of TN accounting for 80–90% of cases [10]. Elongation of cerebral arteries with aging [10] and repetitive vascular microtrauma cause focal axonal injury, central oligodendroglial demyelination, axonal loss, and dysmyelination [11, 12], which enables the sensory ephaptic afterdischarge between axons. Arteries cause symptomatic NVC more than veins due to the higher pressure and pulsatility [13].

In 88% of patients, the elongated superior cerebellar artery (SCA) descends to the trigeminal nerve and causes compression, while in 25% of patients, the compression is caused by the anterior inferior cerebellar artery (AICA) coming from below [12]. Less often, NVC is caused by the basilar and vertebral arteries (VA) [14]. Arterial NVC was visualized more proximally to the brainstem than venous compressions [15]. Purely venous causes of neurovascular compression are significantly less common (8–10%), with the transverse pontine vein and superior petrosal vein accounting for a majority of venous causes [16]. In contrast to arterial compression, venous neurovascular conflict is more commonly within the mid-cisternal segment and porus trigeminus [17]. Additionally, the presence of both arterial and venous NVC is found in 38% of cases [16, 17].

10.4 Recommendations for MRI Protocol

The combination of high-resolution 3D T2-weighted imaging with 3D time-of-flight angiography and 3D T1-weighted gadolinium-enhanced sequences is considered to be the optimal approach for the detection of NVC (Table 10.1) [15, 16]. Those sequences are used for surgical planning and may predict treatment response. They also increase the sensitivity and improve the specificity, allowing the detection of purely venous compression or veins associated with arterial conflicts, as well as the differentiation of their exact anatomical origin [18–20].

According to several studies, sensitivity and specificity for detecting NVC on MRI were 97% and 50% [20], 87% and 50% [22], and 97% and 100% [23], respectively.

Table 10.1 Recommended MRI protocol in patients with TN

Name of the MR sequence	Type of sequence; *characteristics*	Goals in the visualization of NVC	Sequence disadvantage
CISS[a] FIESTA[b] SSFP [c] BFFE[d] SPACE[e] DRIVE[f] BTFE[g]	3D heavily T2-weighted sequences *volumetric acquisition with multiplanar reformats; thin slices (0.6 mm)*	High anatomical details of the cisternal portion of the nerve and contrast between CSF and neurovascular structures in the CPA cistern	Poor contrast between vessel and nerve
Contrast-enhanced CISS		Enhancement of the artery/vein with better visualization of higher-grade NVC compared to non-enhanced CISS [21]	
Contrast-enhanced T1-weighted sequences	3D T1 sequences with i.v. gadolinium contrast *volumetric acquisition with multiplanar reformats; thin slices*	Visualization of contrast-enhanced veins and arteries in contrast to the trigeminal nerve	
3D TOF MR angiography	Flow-related enhancement of spins entering into an imaging slice in arteries *multiplanar reformats*	An artery with fast blood flow as a structure of high signal intensity and a nerve as a structure of intermediate signal intensity	Poor contrast between vessel and nerve; slow blood flow vessels are not displayed

CPA cerebellopontine angle cistern
Acronyms of MRI sequences: [a]Constructive interference in steady state
[b]Fast imaging employing steady-state acquisition
[c]steady-state free precession
[d]3D balanced fast field echo
[e]Sampling perfection with application-optimized contrasts using different flip-angle evolutions (general electric's name of their "SPACE" sequence is CUBE (not an acronym) and Philips' name of their "SPACE" sequence is VISTA (volume isotropic turbo spin echo acquisition)
[f]Driven equilibrium radiofrequency reset pulse
[g]Balanced turbo field echo

10.5 Localization of NVC and Clinical Implications

NVC was more prevalent on the symptomatic (89%) compared to the asymptomatic side (78%), and the presence of NVC was significantly associated with the pain side. NVC involving an artery was more prevalent on the symptomatic side (74% versus 56%). NVC on the affected n.V was more severe than on the contralateral or unaffected n.V [25]. NVC was more severe in patients who underwent surgery for TN compared to those who were treated with medication [26].

Trigeminal sensory root has somatotopic organization at the REZ with ophthalmic nerve fibers predominantly located superior within the nerve, V2 fibers run medially, and V3 fibers located more caudolaterally (Fig. 10.4) [27].

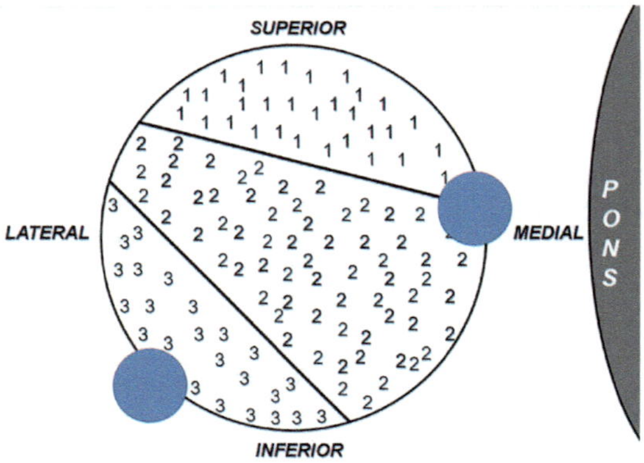

Fig. 10.4 Schematic of the coronal cross section through the trigeminal nerve at the REZ with fibers of the second branch (V2-mandibular nerve) widely distributed medially, third branch (V3-maxillary nerve) distributed laterally, and first branch (V1-ophthalmic nerve) located on the superior part. Small gray-colored circles represent arteries at the most common sites of NVC, either superomedially or laterally

Yoshino and colleagues reported a similar distribution correlating preoperative MRI with the distribution of symptoms in TN patients. Moreover, 89% of patients with symptoms related to the V2 division had NVC at the medial site of the REZ, and 76% of patients with neuralgic symptoms related to the mandibular division (V3) had NVC at the lateral site of the REZ [28]. Thus, lateral and inferior NVC corresponded to symptoms predominantly in the V3 distribution. Compression along the superior and medial surface of the trigeminal nerve responded with symptoms in the V1 and V2 distribution [28].

SCA usually compress the nerve superomedially [12]. Leal and colleagues reported that 82% of the cases with higher grades of NVC (grades 2 and 3) were located at the REZ and 17.3% at the distal part of the nerve [15]. Furthermore, 25% of grade 1 NVC were located at REZ and 75% at the distal part of the nerve.

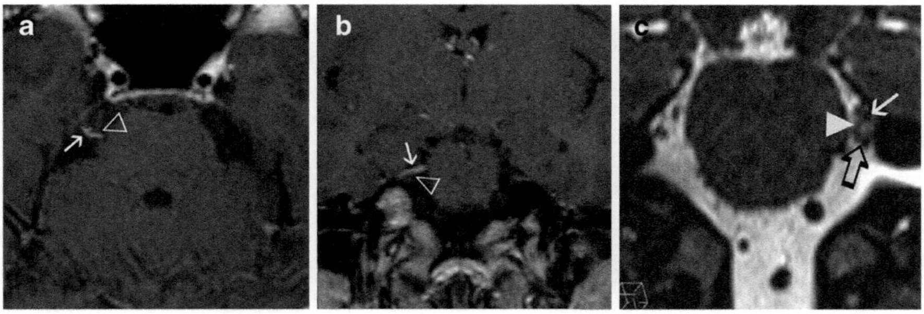

Fig. 10.5 Contrast-enhanced T1-weighted image in transverse (**a**) and coronal plane (**b**). NVC between transverse pontine vein (→) at the mid-cisternal part of the n.V (◁). SPACE sequence in coronal plane (**c**). Multiple NVC artery (←) on top of n.V (▷) and vein (⇒) under the nerve

In the same study, 85% of arterial NVC were located at REZ and 14% at the distal part of the nerve. On the other hand, in NVC caused by veins, only 30% were found at REZ and others at the mid-cisternal or juxtapetrous segment (Fig. 10.5a–c) [15].

10.6 Grading of Vascular Compression on MRI

Lial proposed a 4-point scale as follows: grade 0, neurovascular relation without contact; 1, contact when vessel touches the nerve without distortion; 2, displacement or distortion of the root but without indentation; and 3, indentation of the root [24]. Contact is present when the vessel touches the nerve and no cerebrospinal fluid is visible between the nerve and the vessel. Indentation exists if the NVC results in concavity of the nerve. On the other hand, Maarberg and colleagues considered nerve atrophy as the highest grade (Figs. 10.6, 10.7, 10.8 and 10.9) [25].

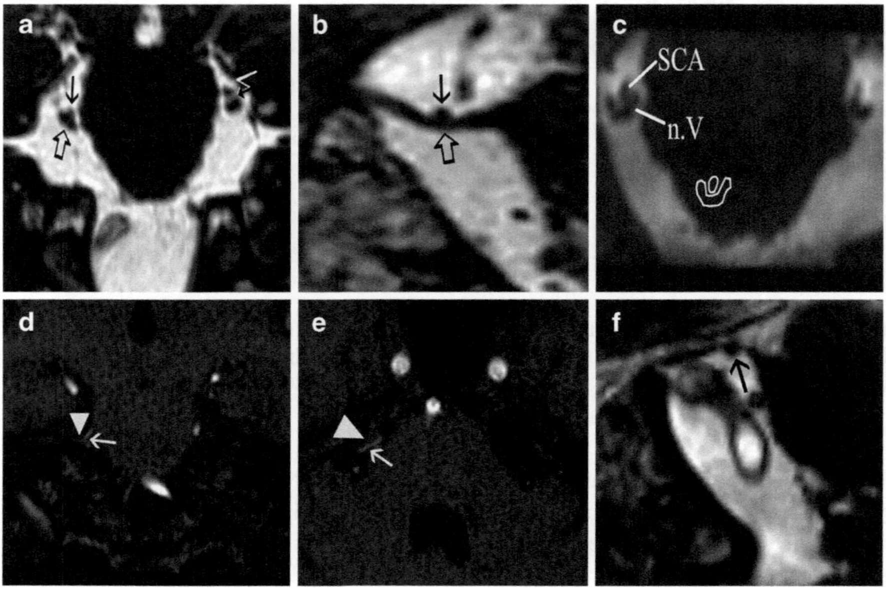

Fig. 10.6 DRIVE sequence in the coronal plane (**a**) with mild inferior displacement of right n.V (⇒) by SCA (↓). Signal of CSF is present between the left n.V and SCA (↯). DRIVE sequence in the sagittal plane (**b**) in the same patient. CISS sequence in coronal plane (**c**). SCA makes an indentation/concavity in n.V with schematic representation. Source images of 3D TOF cerebral MR angiography in coronal (**d**) and transverse plane (**e**). Right SCA (←) as a high signal intensity vessel due to high flow signal dislocates n.V (▷) presented as a structure with intermediate signal intensity. DRIVE sequence in sagittal plane (**f**). AICA coming from below and dislocating n.V upward

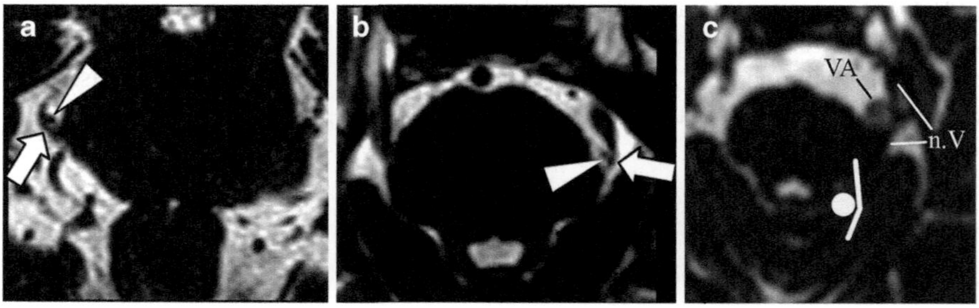

Fig. 10.7 DRIVE sequence in the coronal plane (**a**) with inferior displacement of n.V (⇒) by SCA (▽), 3 mm from REZ. DRIVE sequence in the transverse plane (**b**) with lateral displacement of n.V (⇒) by SCA (▽). DRIVE sequence in the transverse plane (**c**). Elongated VA dislocates n.V (⇒) at REZ with indentation. (Schematic representation of NVC is available)

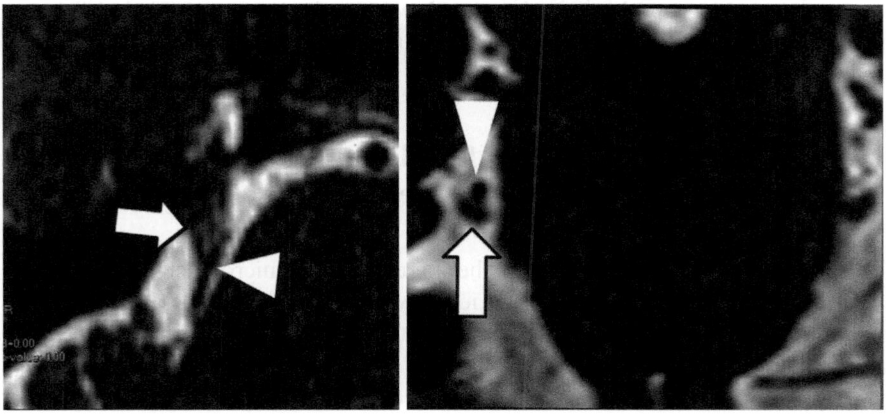

Fig. 10.8 DRIVE sequence in the transverse (**a**) and coronal plane (**b**). Neurovascular contact between the right n.V) (⇒) and the superior cerebellar artery (SCA) (◁), with no visible cerebrospinal fluid (CSF) signal between the nerve and artery

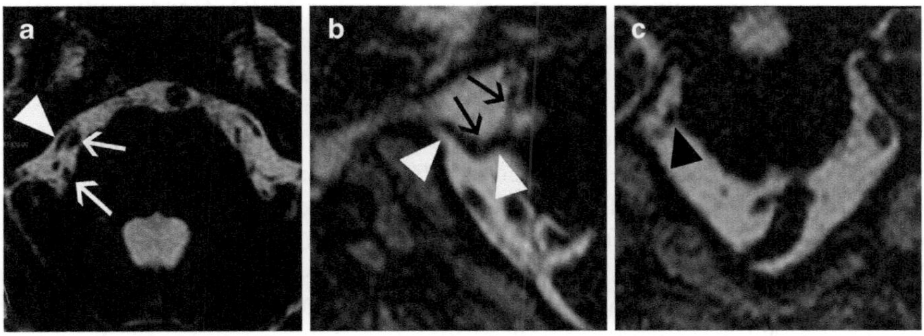

Fig. 10.9 CISS sequence in the transverse (**a**), sagittal (**b**), and coronal plane (**c**). High-graded NVC due to tortuous right SCA (**a**, **b**, → →) with the loop at the REZ as well at the mid-cisternal segment of the right n.V (▷). Atrophy of the nerve (**a** ▷, **b** ▲). Note the normal volume of the left n.V

10.7 Atrophy of the Affected Trigeminal Nerve

TN is associated with atrophy of the affected n.V [29–31] secondary to axonal loss and demyelination. Trigeminal NVC on MRI is likely to be symptomatic when it is accompanied by nerve atrophy (Fig. 10.9a, c) [30]. Nerve diameter and cross-sectional area were 20–28% smaller on the symptomatic side compared with the asymptomatic side [29]. The loss of volume on the affected side compared with that on the non-affected side (15.5%) in patients with TN was greater than the difference between the right and left sides in the control group (2.3%). There was a positive correlation between the degree of n.V indentation and nerve atrophy [32]. The loss of trigeminal nerve tissue is believed to be the result of chronic physical stress caused by vascular compression. This is supported by the fact that up to 42% of symptomatic nerves have gross atrophy [33]. Greater nerve atrophy was associated with more severe n.V indentation and better long-term outcomes following MVD [32].

10.8 MRI: Decision-making for Microvascular Decompression and Outcome

The primary goal in determining whether to recommend microvascular decompression (MVD) to patients with TN is to identify those who are likely to benefit from this treatment since alternative treatments such as percutaneous or radiosurgical alternatives are available.

Higher grades (grades 2 or 3) of NVC were specific to the symptomatic side, which implies that NVC is sufficient but not necessary to trigger TN. Patients with low-grade or without NVC were less likely to be free from pain after MVD compared with patients with high-grade NVC [21].

In these patients, other etiology can be considered, and a rhizotomy of the trigeminal ganglion could be an optional procedure for MVD. Good results after MVD in high-grade cases were around 80% after 15 years [34]. Atrophy of the trigeminal nerve is often associated with significant neurovascular conflicts, and patients with this condition tend to have good surgical outcomes [31].

Brînzeu and colleagues compared the degree of conflict on MRI and findings at surgery, and grade was underestimated in 45% of all conflicts, exactly estimated in one-third, and overestimated in 22%. The majority of overestimations were found in patients with grade 1 conflict or no conflict, while 90% of underestimations were in high-grade conflicts (grades 2 or 3). When MRI shows a grade 1 NVC, it can be challenging to determine whether to proceed with MVD. In such cases, it is important to consider the patient's overall health, clinical presentation, and alternative treatment options [20].

Sheehan and colleagues noted improved outcomes after Gamma Knife therapy when higher radiation doses were prescribed to the point of vessel impingement [35].

Surgical outcomes were better in cases in which vascular compression was detected on preoperative MRI/ MRA and when the compression occurred at the REZ region intraoperatively [36].

10.9 MRI Findings in Trigeminal Neuralgia Without NVC

NVC might not be found during surgical explorations, with broad incidence from 4 to 89% [37].

Imaging studies reported the following anatomical differences in patients with TN on the affected side compared to the unaffected side:

1. Smaller and sharper petrous ridge (Fig. 10.10b, c) [38].
2. Smaller cross-sectional area of the cerebellopontine angle cistern (Fig. 10.11a, b) [39].

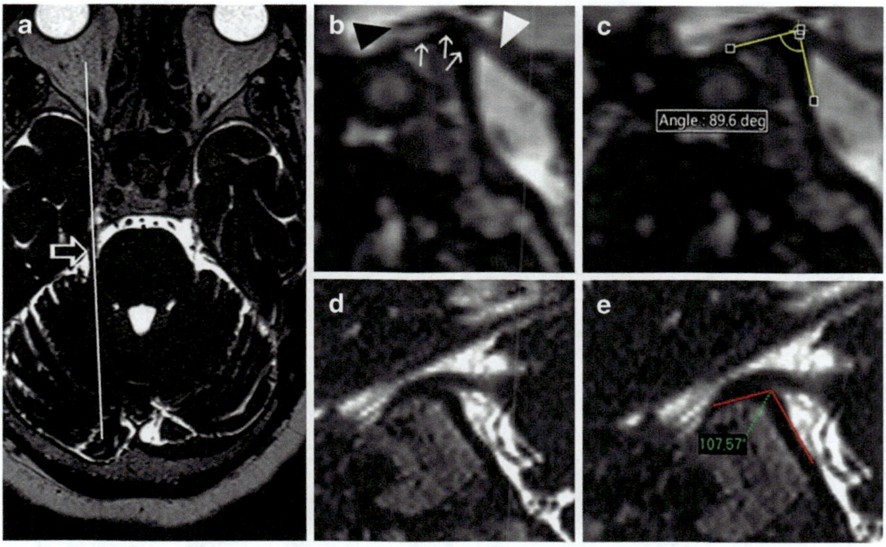

Fig. 10.10 The CISS sequence in the transverse plane (**a**) is centered on the cisternal segment of n.V (**a**, ⇒), and then an oblique sagittal view was obtained by placing slices along the course of the cisternal segment (**a**-draw line). The angle of the petrous ridge (**b** ↑↑↑) is measured following the upper ridge of the petrous bone in the patient (**b**, **c**) and a control subject (**d**, **e**). The angle of the petrous ridge is sharper in the patient with TN. Note the cisternal segment of the n.V (**b**, ▽) and part of the n.V at the Meckel's cave (**b**, ▶)

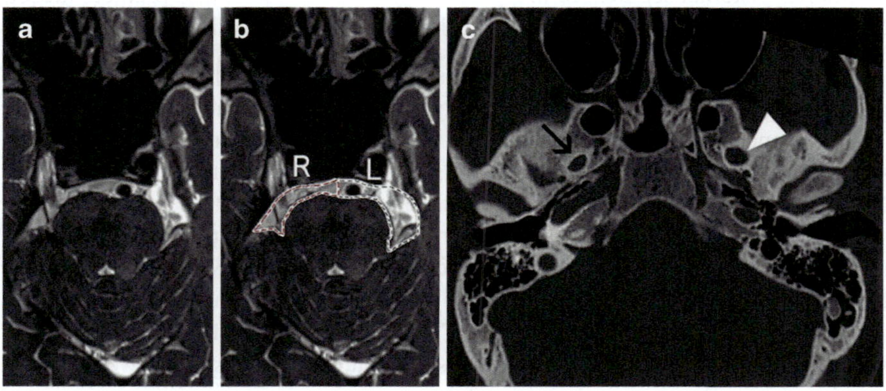

Fig. 10.11 DRIVE sequence in the transverse plane (**a**) and outlined cross-sectional area of the right (R) and left (L) CPA cistern on the same slice (**b**). The right CPA cistern (red dashed line) has a smaller cross-sectional area compared to the contralateral side. CT scan of the skull base with smaller foramen ovale on the right side (↘) in a patient with right-sided TN. Note the size of the normal-sized left foramen ovale (◁)

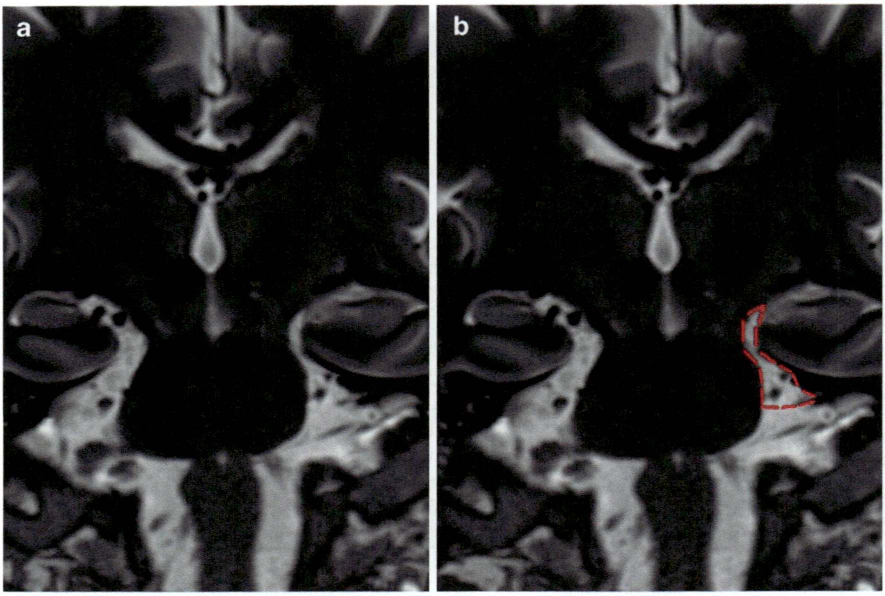

Fig. 10.12 SSFP sequence in the coronal plane (**a**) and outlined cross-sectional area of the left pontomesencephalic cistern (red dashed line) on the same slice (**b**). The cross-sectional area of the cistern on the affected side is smaller compared to the right side

3. Atrophy of the n.V (Fig. 10.9a, b) [40].
4. Shorter cisternal segment of n.V [40].
5. Smaller volume of the pontomesencephalic cistern (Fig. 10.12a, b [41].

It is assumed that smaller basal cisterns (Figs. 10.11a, b and 10.12) and sharper petrous ridge (Fig. 10.10) can lead to a closer nerve–vessel relationship.

Natsis and colleagues found a smaller width of the foramen ovale on the right side in the cadaveric study, and male skulls had a larger foramen than females [42]. Neto and colleagues reported that TN occurs more often in females and on the right side, where the foramen ovale is narrower [43]. High-resolution CT has reported a narrower foramen ovale on the affected side in patients with TN (Fig. 10.11c) [44]. It had been presumed that mechanical irritation of the trigeminal nerve may occur along its peripheral branches; therefore, CT has been suggested in patients without visible NVC on MRI [44]. Transcutaneous procedures or radiosurgery would probably be a better therapeutic choice for these cases.

All abovementioned radiological findings can be used as additional imaging markers supporting the clinically based diagnosis of TN.

10.10 Diffusion Tensor Imaging in Patients with TN

The degree of directionality of diffusion can be measured with fractional anisotropy (FA), which is a marker of microstructural integrity. DTI enables examining trigeminal nerve microstructure in vivo where lower FA in the affected REZ might reflect an alternating process of loss of myelin and remyelination—“remodeling” of the myelin sheaths. The same results were obtained for arterial and venous NVC, which support the hypothesis that both arteries and veins can cause TN and can be eligible candidates for MVD. Altered FA is also present in patients without visible NVC on MRI which may support the decision to perform MVD in those patients with the typical clinical presentation of a neurovascular compression-related TN [45]. The correlation between FA reduction and pain on the Visual Analog Scale suggests FA as a potential objective MRI biomarker to confirm TN diagnosis and monitor clinical severity [46]. In addition, pathological low FA showed reversibility after effective MVD [47].

Comparing brain FA between TN and healthy control groups showed lower FA in white matter tracts connecting regions engaged in the experience of pain, attention, and compensatory pain-avoiding motor behaviors such as corpus callosum, the cingulum, the posterior corona radiata, and the superior longitudinal fasciculus. The DTI changes in analyzed white matter fibers may result from decreased fiber organization [48].

10.11 Voxel-based Morphometry of Brain Cortex in Patients with TN

It is becoming increasingly understood that TN pathophysiology is associated with both trigeminal nerve and brain abnormalities. Voxel-based morphometry (VBM) is a whole-brain technique capable of revealing subtle, specific changes in gray matter (GM) by applying voxelwise statistics. Cortical thickness and volume of subcortical GM structures were measured using VBM from T1-weighted MRI scans in patients with right-sided TN. Increased GM volume has been found in the thalamus, amygdala, periaqueductal gray, and basal ganglia compared to healthy controls. The TN patients also had thicker cortex in the contralateral primary somatosensory cortex and frontal pole and thinner cortex in the pregenual cingulum, the insula, and the orbitofrontal cortex, areas exposed to “increased nociceptive input to the brain, and impaired descending modulation system that does not adequately inhibit pain, and increased motor output to control facial movements to limit pain attacks” (cited from DeSouza and colleagues) [49].

Obermann and colleagues found similar results in brain regions responsible for the perception and processing of pain throughout the trigeminal nociceptive system reflecting a cortical adaptation to chronic pain [50].

DeSouza and colleagues found that after successful MVD intervention, reversal of the decreased GM thickness occurred in the ipsilateral anterior insula, most probably due to decreased nociceptive input from the trigeminal afferents to the central nervous system. The same authors reported GM volume decrease within the anterior cingulate cortex, parahippocampus, and temporal lobe correlated with increasing disease duration [47].

10.12 Functional MRI in Patients with TN

Functional MRI helps understand the changes in brain activity associated with light tactile stimulation of the cutaneous trigger zone in patients with TN where induced pain is associated with pathologic activation of the whole trigeminal nociceptive system and structures involved in pain modulation, suggesting a state of maintained sensitization. After effective treatment, activation induced by stimulation of the trigger zone was confined to primary and secondary somatosensory cortices, suggesting that sensitization of the trigeminal nociceptive system in patients with TN depends on microstructural abnormalities in the nerve itself [51].

10.13 Radiomics in Patients with TN

Radiomics is a medical research field that extracts a large number of features from routine MRI images using data characterization algorithms and converts these features into data that can enhance the understanding of pathophysiology of particular diseases and support clinical decision algorithms. Complex radiomics pipeline in the research area of patients with TN includes the following: collecting data from MRI of the trigeminal nerve, segmentation of the trigeminal nerves with a deep learning algorithm, feature extraction (image texture, shape, and intensity), and finally predictive modeling. Radiomics features can identify patterns and correlations that are hidden from human readers.

Although Maarbjerg and colleagues [25] had shown that severe NVC was more common on the symptomatic side, they also found that NVC was common on both sides of symptomatic and asymptomatic sides of healthy people and most patients, which implies subjectivity of diagnosis in structural MRI, based on the opinions of the neuroradiologist. Therefore, developing a model based on feature information (radiomics) is a promising option.

Radiomics features calculated from MRIs of n.V correlate with pain status. In other words, pathological changes in involved trigeminal nerves may be extracted using radiomics analysis [52].

In a study involving a radiomics model applied to 350 patients with TN and 100 control participants, the model demonstrated excellent diagnostic capability in predicting TN [53].

Danyluk and colleagues compared MRI texture features derived from brain regions such as the anterior cingulate, insula, thalamus, and brainstem between TN patients and healthy subjects and reported differences between the two groups, and these results can enable automatic detection and classification of TN using imaging features from routine anatomical MRI [54].

10.14 Neuroimaging Studies of Other Painful Lesions of the Cranial Nerves

10.14.1 Glossopharyngeal Nerve Neuralgia

Glossopharyngeal nerve neuralgia (GPN) is characterized by a sudden, unilateral, stabbing pain in areas innervated by glossopharyngeal nerve (n. IX) and related branches. This pain often affects the ear, base of the tongue, tonsillar area, and jaw and may radiate to the eye, nose, chin, or shoulder, sometimes with vagal symptoms like cough or bradycardia. Common triggers include swallowing, talking, or coughing. It can be classified into pharyngeal, otalgic, and vagal types, with vago-glossopharyngeal neuralgia including additional symptoms like asystole or syncope [3].

GPN is rare, affecting about 0.8 per 100,000 people annually. GPN is categorized as classical (due to neurovascular compression), secondary (due to another condition), or idiopathic (with no clear cause). Structural compression includes tumors located at the base of the skull or cerebellopontine angle and those in proximity to cranial nerves such as meningiomas, epidermoid tumors, or schwannomas. Vascular compression can be present due to arteriovenous malformations, persistent hypoglossal artery, and vertebral artery dissections that can compress the glossopharyngeal nerve. Infectious and inflammatory conditions are rare causes of GPN (complications after surgery, infections, and inflammatory diseases).

High-resolution 3D T2-weighted sequences in combination with time-of-flight (TOF) MR angiography (MRA) are crucial for assessing n.IX and nearby blood vessels; postcontrast T1-weighted sequence is necessary to exclude other pathologies and preoperative planning [10]. For patients unable to undergo MRI, CT cisternography and CT angiography are useful alternatives. Accurate differentiation from similar conditions, such as TN or nervus intermedius neuralgia, is essential due to symptom overlap and differing treatments [55].

For n.IX, the TZ is located about 1.5 mm from the brainstem, where NVC is most commonly observed (95%). The posterior inferior cerebellar artery (PICA) is the most frequent cause of NVC in GPN (68%) (Fig. 10.13), followed by the VA (2%), venous structures (6%), or multiple vessels (23%) [7].

DTI in GPN showed FA, which indicates demyelination or myelin reorganization [10]. Studies have shown significantly lower ADC values on the affected side, which normalize after MVD [56].

Initial treatment for classical GPN usually involves medical therapy. If this fails, MVD is highly effective, particularly when preoperative nerve root atrophy is present. When NVC is not found on MRI, surgical rhizotomy may be considered. Vein compression often predicts poorer outcomes [57].

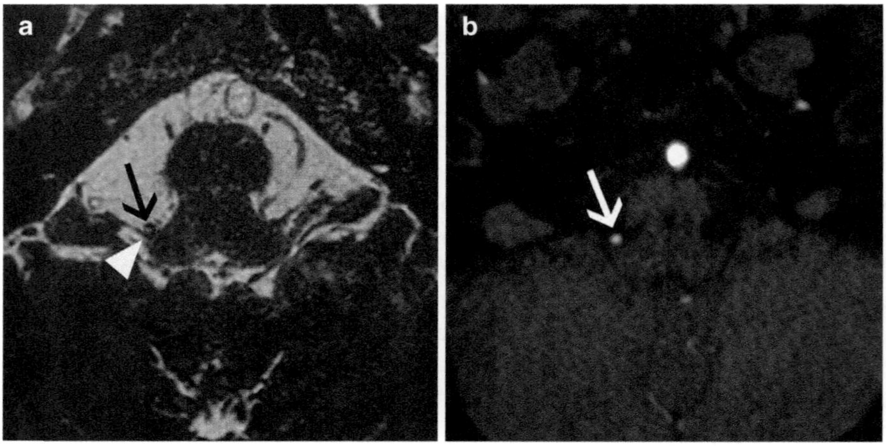

Fig. 10.13 FIESTA sequence in the transverse plane at the level of n.IX-XI (**a**) and 3D TOF MR angiography at the same level (**b**). NVC between right PICA (↓) at REZ of n.IX (**a**, ▷)

10.14.2 Pain Attributed to Nervus Intermedius

Two main painful disorders affecting the intermedius nerve are nervus intermedius neuralgia (previously known as geniculate neuralgia) and painful nervus intermedius neuropathy. The main difference between these conditions is the duration and characteristics of pain; neuralgia is characterized by recurrent, sudden attacks of unilateral pain, whereas neuropathy typically involves continuous or nearly continuous pain.

10.14.2.1 Nervus Intermedius Neuralgia

Nervus intermedius neuralgia is a rare disorder characterized by brief paroxysms of pain felt deeply in the auditory canal, in the region of the mastoid process, and sometimes can radiate to the angle of the mandible. Pain is provoked by stimulation of a trigger area in the posterior wall of the auditory canal and/or periauricular area. Occasionally, disorders such as lacrimation, salivation, and taste can accompany the pain.

Nervus intermedius neuralgia is further divided into classical, secondary, and idiopathic. The classical form develops without apparent cause other than NVC; secondary is caused by an underlying disease (e.g., multiple sclerosis or tumor); meanwhile, in the idiopathic form, there is no evidence of NVC or underlying disease. Given that sensory innervation of the ear canal is complemented with branches of the n.V, IX, and X cranial nerves, it can be challenging to rule out TN and GPN from the differential diagnosis [58].

Nervus intermedius is not always seen in imaging studies due to its small diameter, although detection improves by using higher field strengths and dedicated

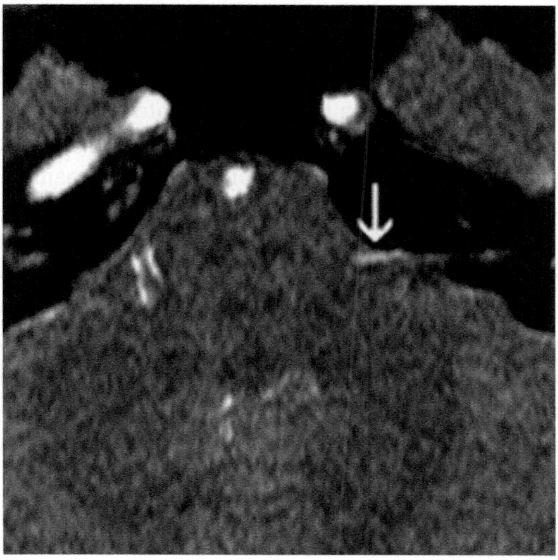

Fig. 10.14 TOF MR angiography. Left AICA (↓) compresses n.VII at REZ in a patient with nervus intermedius neuralgia

protocols. MR protocol includes high-resolution T2-weighted sequences with thin slices and 3D TOF MR angiography to detect potential NVC as well as postcontrast T1-weighted sequence to exclude the presence of other disorders (e.g., tumors) [10]. NVC typically occurs near the REZ and is caused by AICA (Fig. 10.14), rarely VA or PICA. Onoda suggests using 3D MR cisternography/MR angiography fusion to obtain a 3D view of the facial–vestibulocochlear nerve complex, n.V, and n.IX for the presurgical planning [59].

10.14.2.2 Nervus Intermedius Neuropathy

Painful nervus intermedius neuropathy (PNIN) is a rare disorder characterized by continuous pain in the auditory canal, auricle, or in the region of the mastoid process. Paroxysmal pain can sometimes be present, but it is not the predominant type, as in nervus intermedius neuralgia. Subgroups of painful nervus intermedius neuropathy, according to the International Headache Society [3], include painful nervus intermedius neuropathy attributed to herpes zoster, post-herpetic neuralgia of nervus intermedius, painful nervus intermedius neuropathy attributed to other disorders, and idiopathic painful nervus intermedius neuropathy.

PNIN attributed to herpes zoster, often associated with facial paresis, is clinically recognized as Ramsay Hunt syndrome. The hallmark of Ramsay Hunt syndrome is the unilateral, continuous, or near-continuous pain in the auditory canal, auricle, and/or mastoid process region. This pain may be persistent or occasionally interrupted by brief paroxysms. The discomfort is deeply localized within the auditory canal and is directly attributable to a herpes zoster infection of the nervus intermedius, after reactivation of the virus in the geniculate ganglion. Clinical confirmation in acute stages involves the detection of vesicles on the tympanic membrane, auditory canal, auricle, and/or skin over the mastoid process, sometimes on the anterior third of the tongue or hard palate. Pain may precede herpetic eruptions. Since viral spread may extend to other cranial nerves, including n. VIII, IX, X, and XI, additional symptoms may be noted such as tinnitus, hearing loss, vertigo, nausea, hoarseness, and dysphagia.

The natural progression of painful nervus intermedius neuropathy attributed to herpes zoster is not well documented, but the pain can persist beyond 3 months. In such chronic cases, the condition should be reclassified as post-herpetic neuralgia of the nervus intermedius [60].

On volumetric T1-weighted postcontrast and FLAIR images, typical findings include thickening, increased FLAIR signal, and enhancement of the affected facial nerve (Fig. 10.15), as well as dural enhancement in the internal auditory canal and petrous ridge. Dural enhancement and enhancement of the vestibulocochlear nerve and inner ear structures are findings that can distinguish Ramsay Hunt syndrome from Bell's palsy. Since viral spread can occur, contrast enhancement of the other cranial nerves can be found [61].

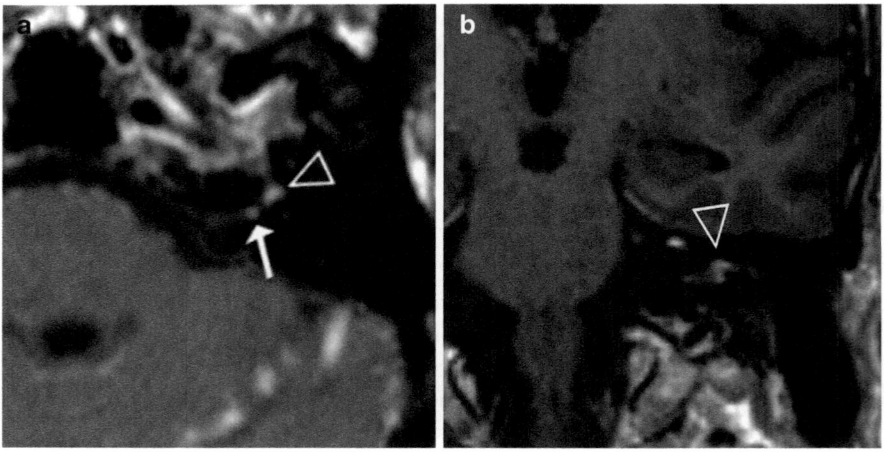

Fig. 10.15 Contrast-enhanced T1-weighted image in transverse (**a**) and coronal plane (**b**). Patient with *varicella-zoster* infection of the left earlobe (with vesicles), pain, and Bell's palsy. Contrast enhancement of the facial nerve in the fundus of the inner auditory meatus (↑) as well as in the geniculate ganglion (◁)

10.14.3 Occipital Neuralgia

Occipital neuralgia is a disorder characterized by unilateral or bilateral paroxysmal stabbing pain in the posterior scalp, in the innervation zones of greater, lesser, and/or third occipital nerves. It is commonly associated with tenderness over the involved nerves and is sometimes accompanied by diminished sensation or dysesthesia in the affected area. Occipital neuralgia can be caused by compression of the occipital nerve by PICA; dural arteriovenous fistula or cervical spine cavernoma; schwannoma in the craniocervical junction; occipital nerve schwannoma, due to C1–C2 arthrosis; or neoplastic lesions in the C1 and C2 region [62].

For the direct visualization of the occipital nerves, the imaging modality of choice is magnetic resonance neurography. The use of 3D PSIF and contrast-enhanced black-blood 3D STIR TSE sequences can detect thickening and signal alterations of the nerves. Van der Cruysse suggests the use of contrast-enhanced black-blood 3D STIR sequence to suppress the signal of fat around cranial and occipital nerves [63] to visualize pathological thickening and signal alteration.

10.14.4 Neck–Tongue Syndrome

Neck–tongue syndrome (NTS) is a rare headache disorder characterized by sudden unilateral pain in the neck or occipital region. This pain is often accompanied by a temporary sensory disturbance in the ipsilateral tongue, triggered by abrupt neck movements. The anatomical structures implicated in NTS include the C1–C2 facet joints, the C2 and C3 nerve roots, and the inferior oblique muscle in the atlanto-axial area [64]. Complicated NTS arises from degenerative joint disease, rheumatoid arthritis, inflammatory conditions, or anatomical variations. Uncomplicated NTS, on the other hand, can be idiopathic, hereditary, or associated with trauma.

MRI and CT scans can aid in diagnosis by revealing disc herniations, osteophytes, joint degenerative changes, or other pathological findings that may lead to nerve root compression [65].

10.14.5 Headache Attributed to Ischemic Ocular Motor Nerve Palsy

Ischemic ocular motor nerve palsy is a condition marked by the impaired function of one or more of the cranial nerves responsible for eye movement (n. III, IV, and VI), due to inadequate blood supply. This condition commonly affects patients with high vascular risk factors such as diabetes mellitus, hypertension, hyperlipidemia, and atherosclerosis.

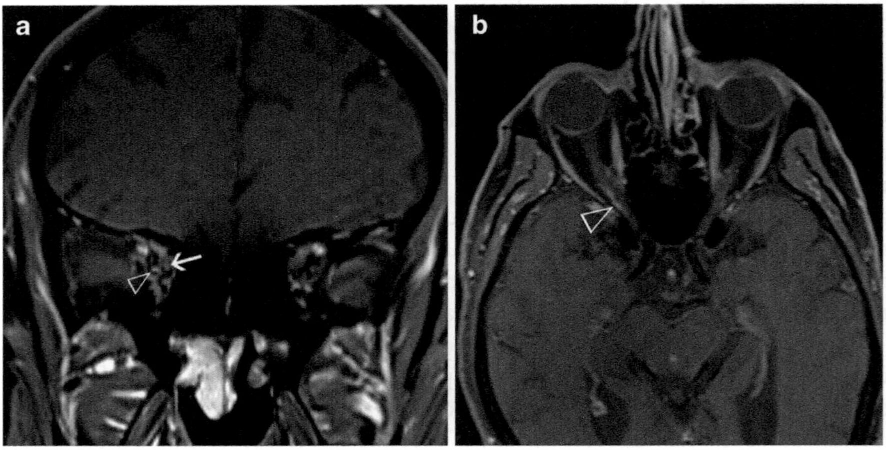

Fig. 10.16 Coronal (**a**) and transverse (**b**) contrast-enhanced T1-weighted sequence with fat saturation. Patient with sudden right-sided palsy of the n.III. Ischemic lesions of the nerve presented as thickening and enhancement of the nerve in the right orbital apex (**a**, **b**, ▷), lateral to the optic nerve (**a** ←)

Clinically, the presentation typically includes the sudden onset of diplopia, ptosis, and restricted eye movement in specific directions, depending on the cranial nerve involved. For instance, if the oculomotor nerve is affected, it can result in ptosis, a dilated pupil, and impaired eye movement upward, downward, and medially. In cases where the abducens nerve is involved, there is an inability to move the eye laterally. Trochlear nerve palsy, on the other hand, is characterized by diplopia when looking downward. Additionally, patients often experience unilateral frontal and/or periorbital pain [66].

High-resolution T2-weighted sequences and high-resolution T1-weighted sequences with fat suppression and thin slices can evaluate the cavernous and orbital segments of n. III, IV, and VI. Ischemic lesions of cranial nerves typically present as thickening of the nerve with contrast enhancement, most commonly seen in the cavernous segment and extending to the orbital apex (Fig. 10.16). The cisternal segments are rarely involved [67]. Roques suggested that the contrast-enhanced CISS sequence can aid in detecting ischemic lesions in the cavernous segment of the oculomotor nerve [68]. Aneurysm, neoplasm, infection, and inflammation should be ruled out on MRI.

10.14.6 Tolosa–Hunt Syndrome

Tolosa–Hunt syndrome (THS) is a rare idiopathic disorder characterized by painful ophthalmoplegia caused by nonspecific granulomatous inflammation of the cavernous sinus, superior orbital fissure, or orbital apex. It is primarily diagnosed through

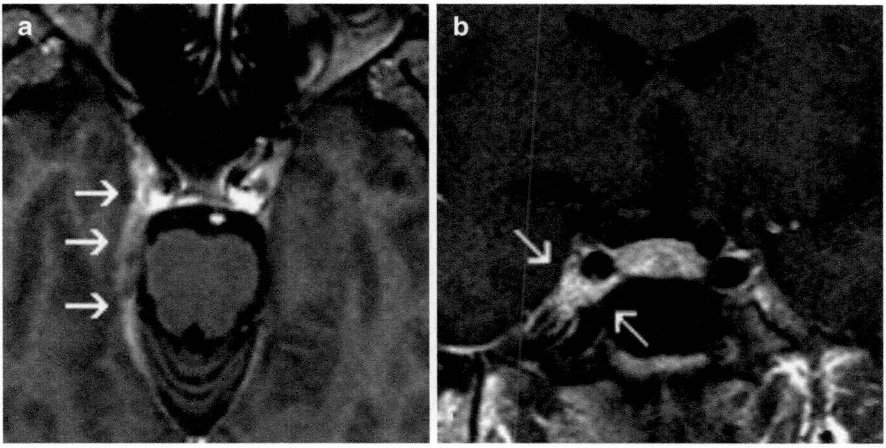

Fig. 10.17 Transverse (**a**) and coronal (**b**) contrast-enhanced T1-weighted sequence in a patient with Tolosa-Hunt syndrome. Contrast-enhanced soft tissue in the region of the right cavernous sinus (**a**, **b** →)

exclusion. The incidence of THS is approximately 1 case per million people per year, with an average age of presentation around 40 years [69].

MRI changes before and after steroid therapy can confirm the diagnosis of THS, although the resolution of radiological changes may take several months [70]. Findings suggestive of THS include enlargement of the cavernous sinus with T1-weighted hypointense and T2-weighted hypointense or isointense lesions, accompanied by significant contrast enhancement (Fig. 10.17). However, despite MRI's high sensitivity in detecting lesions, it lacks specificity, as similar presentations can be observed in conditions such as sarcoidosis, IgG4-related disease, meningioma, and lymphoma [68].

10.15 Conclusion

Classical TN is typically caused by NVC, and identifying the offending vessel, the precise location of compression, and grading of NVC represents key information for clinicians and surgery planning. Emerging MRI techniques such as DTI and voxel-based morphometry are showing promise in elucidating pathological changes within the trigeminal nerve (n.V) itself and in understanding how the brains of TN patients adapt to chronic pain.

Standardized MRI protocols and multi-institutional studies are essential to enhance diagnostic reliability and improve clinical outcomes in patients with TN and other cranial nerve-related pain disorders.

References

1. Maarbjerg S, Gozalov A, Olesen J, et al. Trigeminal neuralgia: a prospective systematic study of clinical characteristics in 158 patients. Headache. 2014;54:1574–82.
2. Manzoni GC, Torelli P. Epidemiology of typical and atypical craniofacial neuralgias. Neurol Sci. 2005;26 Suppl 2:s65–7.
3. Headache Classification Committee of the International Headache Society (IHS) The International Classification of Headache Disorders, 3rd edition (2018) Cephalalgia 38:1–211.
4. Nakashima I, Fujihara K, Kimpara T, et al. Linear pontine trigeminal root lesions in multiple sclerosis: clinical and magnetic resonance imaging studies in 5 cases. Arch Neurol. 2011;58:101–4.
5. Broggi G, Ferroli P, Franzini A, et al. Operative findings and outcomes of microvascular decompression for trigeminal neuralgia in 35 patients affected by multiple sclerosis. Neurosurgery. 2004;55:830–8.
6. Manzoni GC, Torelli P. Epidemiology of typical and atypical craniofacial neuralgias. Neurol Sci. 2005;26:s65–7.
7. Haller S, Etienne L, Kövari E, et al. Imaging of neurovascular compression syndromes: trigeminal neuralgia, hemifacial spasm, vestibular paroxysmia, and glossopharyngeal neuralgia. AJNR Am J Neuroradiol. 2016;37:1384–92.
8. Peker S. Microanatomy of the central myelin-peripheral myelin transition zone of the trigeminal nerve. Neurosurgery. 2006;59:354–9.
9. Nurmikko TJ, Eldridge PR. Trigeminal neuralgia-pathophysiology, diagnosis and current treatment. Br J Anaesth. 2001;87:117–32.
10. Donahue JH, Ornan DA, Mukherjee S. Imaging of vascular compression syndromes. Radiol Clin North Am. 2017;55:123–38.
11. Jannetta PJ. Neurovascular compression in cranial nerve and systemic disease. Ann Surg. 1980;192:518–25.
12. Sindou M, Howeidy T, Acevedo G. Anatomical observations during microvascular decompression for idiopathic trigeminal neuralgia (with correlations between topography of pain and site of the neurovascular conflict): prospective study in a series of 579 patients. Acta Neurochir. 2002;144:1–12.
13. Devor M, Amir R, Rappaport ZH. Pathophysiology of trigeminal neuralgia: the ignition hypothesis. Clin J Pain. 2002;18:4–13.
14. Borges A, Casselman J. Imaging the trigeminal nerve. Eur J Radiol. 2010;74:323–40.
15. Leal PR, Hermier M, Souza MA, et al. Visualization of vascular compression of the trigeminal nerve with high-resolution 3T MRI: a prospective study comparing preoperative imaging analysis to surgical findings in 40 consecutive patients who underwent microvascular decompression for trigeminal neuralgia. Neurosurgery. 2011;69:15–25.
16. Hong W, Zheng X, Wu Z, et al. Clinical features and surgical treatment of trigeminal neuralgia caused solely by venous compression. Acta Neurochir. 2011;153:1037–42.
17. Sade B, Lee JH. Microvascular decompression for trigeminal neuralgia. Neurosurg Clin N Am. 2014;25:743–9.
18. Hitchon PW, Zanaty M, Moritani T, et al. Microvascular decompression and MRI findings in trigeminal neuralgia and hemifacial spasm. A single center experience. Clin Neurol Neurosurg. 2015;139:216–20.
19. Zhou Q, Liu ZL, Qu CC, et al. Preoperative demonstration of neurovascular relationship in trigeminal neuralgia by using 3D FIESTA sequence. Magn Reson Imaging. 2012;30:666–71.
20. Brînzeu A, Drogba L, Sindou M. Reliability of MRI for predicting characteristics of neurovascular conflicts in trigeminal neuralgia: implications for surgical decision making. J Neurosurg. 2018;130:611–21.
21. Blitz AM, Northcutt B, Shin J, et al. Contrast-enhanced CISS imaging for evaluation of neurovascular compression in trigeminal neuralgia: improved correlation with symptoms and prediction of surgical outcomes. AJNR Am J Neuroradiol. 2018;39:1724–32.

22. Hitchona PW, Bathlab G, Moritanib T, et al. Predictability of vascular conflict by MRI in trigeminal neuralgia. Clin Neurol Neurosurg. 2019;182:171–6.
23. Sindou M. Trigeminal neuralgia: a plea for microvascular decompression as the first surgical option. Anatomy should prevail. Acta Neurochir (Wien). 2010;152(2):361–4.
24. Leal PRL, Roch JA, Hermier M, et al. Structural abnormalities of the trigeminal root revealed by diffusion tensor imaging in patients with trigeminal neuralgia caused by neurovascular compression: a prospective, double-blind, controlled study. Pain. 2011;152:2357–64.
25. Maarbjerg S, Wolfram F, Gozalov A, et al. Significance of neurovascular contact in classical trigeminal neuralgia. Brain. 2015;138:311–9.
26. Satoh T, Omi M, Nabeshima N, et al. Severity analysis of neurovascular contact in patients with trigeminal neuralgia: assessment with the inner view of the 3D MR cisternogram and angiogram fusion imaging. AJNR Am J Neuroradiol. 2009;30:603–7.
27. Pelletier VA, Poulos DA, Lende RA. Functional localization in the trigeminal root. J Neurosurg. 1974;40:504–13.
28. Yoshino N, Akimoto H, Yamada I, et al. Trigeminal neuralgia: evaluation of neuralgic manifestation and site of neurovascular compression with 3D CISS MR imaging and MR angiography. Radiology. 2003;228:539–45.
29. Erbay SH, Bhadelia RA, O'Callaghan M, et al. Nerve atrophy in severe trigeminal neuralgia: noninvasive confirmation at MR imaging-initial experience. Radiology. 2006;238:689–92.
30. Antoninia G, Di Pasqualea A, Cruccub G, et al. Magnetic resonance imaging contribution for diagnosing symptomatic neurovascular contact in classical trigeminal neuralgia: a blinded case-control study and meta-analysis. Pain. 2014;155:1464–71.
31. Leal PR, Barbier C, Hermier M, et al. Atrophic changes in the trigeminal nerves of patients with trigeminal neuralgia due to neurovascular compression and their association with the severity of compression and clinical outcomes. J Neurosurg. 2014;120:1484–95.
32. Cheng J, Meng J, Liu W, et al. Nerve atrophy in trigeminal neuralgia due to neurovascular compression and its association with surgical outcomes after microvascular decompression. Acta Neurochir. 2017;159:1699–705.
33. Devor M, Govrin-Lippmann R, Rappaport ZH. Mechanism of trigeminal neuralgia: an ultrastructural analysis of trigeminal root specimens obtained during microvascular decompression surgery. J Neurosurg. 2002;96:532–43.
34. Sindou M, Leston J, Decullier E, Chapuis F. Microvascular decompression for primary trigeminal neuralgia: long-term effectiveness and prognostic factors in a series of 362 consecutive patients with clear-cut neurovascular conflicts who underwent pure decompression. J Neurosurg. 2007;107:1144–53.
35. Sheehan JP, Ray DK, Monteith S, et al. Gamma Knife radiosurgery for trigeminal neuralgia: the impact of magnetic resonance imaging-detected vascular impingement of the affected nerve. J Neurosurg. 2010;113:53–8.
36. Tucer B, Ekici MA, Demirel S, et al. Microvascular decompression for primary trigeminal neuralgia: short-term follow-up results and prognostic factors. J Korean Neurosurg Soc. 2012;52:42–7.
37. Patel NK, Aquilinia K, Clarke Y, et al. How accurate is magnetic resonance angiography in predicting neurovascular compression in patients with trigeminal neuralgia? A prospective, single blinded comparative study. Br J Neurosurg. 2003;17:60–4.
38. Zhong H, Zhang W, Sun S, Bie Y. MRI findings in trigeminal neuralgia without neurovascular compression: implications of petrous ridge and trigeminal nerve angles. Korean J Radiol. 2022;23:821–7.
39. Gunesli A, Tufan K. Significance of the Cerebellopontine cistern cross-sectional area and trigeminal nerve anatomy in trigeminal neuralgia: an anatomical study using magnetic resonance imaging. Turk Neurosurg. 2020;30:271–6.
40. Park SH, Hwang SK, Lee SH, et al. Nerve atrophy and a small cerebellopontine angle cistern in patients with trigeminal neuralgia. J Neurosurg. 2009;110:633–7.

41. Rasche D, Kress B, Stippich C, et al. Volumetric measurement of the pontomesencephalic cistern in patients with trigeminal neuralgia and healthy controls. Neurosurgery. 2006;59:614–20.
42. Natsis K, Repousi E, Sofidis G, et al. The osseous structures in the infratemporal fossa: foramen ovale, bony spurs, ossified ligaments and their contribution to the trigeminal neuralgia. Acta Neurochir. 2015;157:101–3.
43. Neto HS, Camilli JA, Marques MJ. Trigeminal neuralgia is caused by maxillary and mandibular nerve entrapment: greater incidence of right sided facial symptoms is due to the foramen rotundum and foramen ovale being narrower on the right side of the cranium. Med Hypotheses. 2005;65:1179–82.
44. Liu P, Zhong W, Liao C, Liu M, Zhang W. Narrow foramen Ovale and Rotundum: a role in the etiology of Trigeminal Neuralgia. J Craniofac Surg. 2016;27:2168–70.
45. Lutz J, Thon N, Stahl R, et al. Microstructural alterations in trigeminal neuralgia determined by diffusion tensor imaging are independent of symptom duration, severity, and type of neurovascular conflict. J Neurosurg. 2016;124:823–30.
46. Liu Y, Li J, Butzkueven H, Duan Y, et al. Microstructural abnormalities in the trigeminal nerves of patients with trigeminal neuralgia revealed by multiple diffusion metrics. Eur J Radiol. 2013;82:783–6.
47. DeSouza DD, Davis KD, Hodaie M. Reversal of insular and microstructural nerve abnormalities following effective surgical treatment for trigeminal neuralgia. Pain. 2015;156:1112–23.
48. DeSouza DD, Hodaie M, Davis KD. Abnormal trigeminal nerve microstructure and brain white matter in idiopathic trigeminal neuralgia. Pain. 2014;155:37–44.
49. Desouza DD, Moayedi M, Chen DQ, et al. Sensorimotor and pain modulation brain abnormalities in trigeminal neuralgia: a paroxysmal, sensory-triggered neuropathic pain. PLoS One. 2013;8:e66340.
50. Obermann M, Rodriguez-Raecke R. Gray matter volume reduction reflects chronic pain in trigeminal neuralgia. NeuroImage. 2013;74:352–8.
51. Moisset X, Villain N, Ducreux D, et al. Functional brain imaging of trigeminal neuralgia. Eur J Pain. 2011;15:124–31.
52. Mulford KL, Moen SL, Grande AW, et al. Identifying symptomatic trigeminal nerves from MRI in a cohort of trigeminal neuralgia patients using radiomics. Neuroradiology. 2022;64:603–9.
53. Wang F, Ma A, Wu Z, et al. Development and validation of radiomics models for the prediction of diagnosis of classic trigeminal neuralgia. Front Neurosci. 2023;17:1188590.
54. Danyluk H, Ishaque A, Ta D, et al. MRI texture analysis reveals brain abnormalities in medically refractory trigeminal neuralgia. Front Neurol. 2021;12:626504.
55. Khan M, Nishi SE, Hassan SN, et al. Trigeminal neuralgia, glossopharyngeal neuralgia, and myofascial pain dysfunction syndrome: an update. Pain Res Manag. 2017;2017:7438326.
56. Szmyd B, Sołek J, Błaszczyk M, Jankowski J, et al. The underlying pathogenesis of neurovascular compression syndromes: a systematic review. Front Mol Neurosci. 2022;15:923089.
57. Kuncz A, Yoros E, Barzó P, et al. Comparison of clinical symptoms and magnetic resonance angiographic (MRA) results in patients with trigeminal neuralgia and persistent idiopathic facial pain. Medium-term outcome after microvascular decompression of cases with positive MRA findings. Cephalalgia. 2006;26:266–76.
58. Inoue T, Shima A, Hirai H, et al. Nervus Intermedius Neuralgia treated with microvascular decompression: a case report and review of the literature. NMC Case Rep J. 2017;4:75–8.
59. Onoda K, Kawaguchi A, Takaya Y, et al. A case of Nervus Intermedius Neuralgia. World Neurosurg. 2020;137:89–92.
60. Choi JW, Nahm H, Shin JE, et al. Atypical clinical manifestations of herpes zoster oticus: diagnostic usefulness of magnetic resonance imaging. J Neurovirol. 2019;25:874–82.
61. Kuya J, Kuya K, Shinohara Y, et al. Usefulness of high-resolution 3D multi-sequences for peripheral facial palsy: differentiation between bell's palsy and Ramsay hunt syndrome. Otol Neurotol. 2017;38:1523–7.
62. Hwang L, Dessouky R, Xi Y, et al. MR neurography of greater occipital nerve neuropathy: initial experience in patients with migraine. AJNR Am J Neuroradiol. 2017;38:2203–9.

63. Van der Cruyssen F, Croonenborghs TM, Renton T, et al. Magnetic resonance neurography of the head and neck: state of the art, anatomy, pathology and future perspectives. Br J Radiol. 2021;94:20200798.
64. Kim H, Lee S, Cho N, Song S. A systematic review of case reports on the neck-tongue syndrome. Medicina (Kaunas). 2021;57:1097.
65. Gelfand AA, Johnson H, Lenaerts ME, et al. Neck-tongue syndrome: a systematic review. Cephalalgia. 2018;38:374–82.
66. Kim JH, Kim M, Bae YJ. Magnetic resonance imaging in diplopia: neural pathway, imaging, and clinical correlation. Korean J Radiol. 2022;23:649–63.
67. Choi KD, Choi SY, Kim JS, et al. Acquired ocular motor nerve palsy in neurology clinics: a prospective multicenter study. J Clin Neurol. 2019;15:221–7.
68. Roques M, Biotti D, Darcourt J, et al. Microvascular ischemic isolated oculomotor nerve palsy revealed by contrast-enhanced 3D-CISS imaging. J Neuroradiol. 2021;48:466–7.
69. Ramirez JA, Ramirez Marquez E, Torres G, et al. Tolosa hunt syndrome: MRI findings. Cureus. 2023;15:e46635.
70. Nóbrega PR, Rodrigues PGB, de Sousa PI, et al. Steroid responsive cavernous sinus syndrome due to Rosai-Dorfman disease: beyond Tolosa-Hunt syndrome – a case report. BMC Neurol. 2021;21:264.

Chapter 11
Neuroimaging Studies of Headache Disorders in Pediatric and Adolescent Populations

Laura Papetti and Massimiliano Valeriani

11.1 Pediatric and Adolescent Headaches

Headache is the most common neurological disorder in pediatric patients and the primary reason for visits to pediatric neurology clinics. According to many epidemiological studies, headaches, particularly migraines, are usually first seen in childhood, with an increase in prevalence around the age of 8–10 years [1]. About 30–60% of children will experience at least one headache episode in their lifetime by the age of 6 [2]. Headaches during childhood could impact both family life and the patient's performance in both school and recreational activities. Early and accurate diagnosis and appropriate treatment are necessary to reduce disability associated with childhood headaches. The diagnosis of headache type is based on specific clinical and historical criteria, as defined by the "International Classification of Headache Disorders—ICHD 3." The criteria used for adult headaches may not always accurately reflect primary or secondary headaches in children.

Migraine is the most common cephalalgic disorder in children, with a prevalence ranging from 5% among children 5–10 years old to approximately 15% among teens [3]. However, the duration and side criteria for diagnosis of migraine can be difficult to apply in children, as attacks often last less than 2 h or are bilateral. The description of pain characteristics can be confusing, especially for younger patients

L. Papetti
Pediatric Headache Center, Developmental Neurology Unit,
Bambino Gesù Children' s Hospital, IRCCS, Rome, Italy

M. Valeriani (✉)
Systems Medicine Department, Tor Vergata University of Rome, Rome, Italy

Translational Pain Neuroscience and Precision Medicine, CNAP, Dept. of Health Science and Technology, School of Medicine, Aalborg University, Aalborg, Denmark
e-mail: massimiliano.valeriani@opbg.net

I. Petrušić, Y. Wang (eds.), *Neuroimaging of Headache Disorders*, Headache,
https://doi.org/10.1007/978-3-031-85402-6_11

who may struggle with articulating their symptoms. Medical history and general and neurological exams are intended to identify potential risk factors ("red flags") for secondary headaches.

11.1.1 Indication for Neuroimaging in Children and Adolescents

Risk stratification based on clinical history and physical examination is necessary before performing an imaging study for a child with headache. In the majority of cases, headaches are primary and can be classified as migraines or tension-type headaches. Most children who seek emergency care for headaches do not have a dangerous underlying cause for their symptoms. Secondary headaches that are life-threatening are limited to 6% of cases [4]. Patients with red flags in the clinical history and physical examination should be selected for brain neuroimaging (Table 11.1). The relevance of certain red flags, like night awakenings, occipital localization, and age, has been questioned recently.

Mas et al. and Bear et al. demonstrated that in the absence of atypical history or abnormalities on clinical examination, nocturnal awakenings/headache upon waking and occipital headaches in children are not more likely to be associated with intracranial pathology than headaches in other locations or children with normal sleep patterns [5, 6]. Additionally, a retrospective multicenter study re-evaluated the critical concept of age, showing that headaches in preschool-aged children (<6 years), though typically challenging diagnosis, are not in themselves sufficient to suggest a secondary cause [7].

The choice of radiological investigation, whether computed tomography (CT) or brain magnetic resonance imaging (MRI), is guided by the type of clinical suspicion as well as the setting in which the patient is located (emergency, outpatient, regular hospitalization). The short execution time of CT scan makes it a more important tool in emergency departments. Nonetheless, its primary function is to detect major vascular events or compressive lesions. Low-dose radiation CT protocols have been used in pediatric centers to mitigate the long-standing problem of ionizing radiation, which reduces the risk of malignancy later in life. MRI is the

Table 11.1 Red flags and questionable red flags

Red flags	Questionable red flags
Acute onset	Nocturnal awakenings
Changes in headache pattern	Headache upon waking
Abnormalities on neurological examination	Occipital side
Fundus oculi alterations (papilledema)	< 6 years
Comorbidities (neoplasms, CHD, CV shunts)	

CHD congenital heart disease; *CV* shunts cerebral ventricular shunts preferred neuroimaging method for children and adolescents due to the lack of radiation exposure. MRI has been found to be more sensitive in detecting white matter alterations, vascular malformations, and lesions in the posterior cranial fossa compared to CT. The use of brain MRI in emergency settings for pediatric patients is significantly restricted due to the relatively long execution times and the requirement for procedural sedation.

About 20–30% of patients with primary headaches who undergo neuroimaging exhibit incidental findings of brain abnormalities [8]. These findings are usually not significant and cannot be assumed to be the cause of the patient's headache. The most frequent findings include pineal cysts, focal areas of gliosis, arachnoid cysts, dilatation of the Virchow–Robin spaces, and mild herniation of the cerebellar tonsils [9]. Although the relationship between these findings and the headache disorder cannot be established in many cases, they can cause concern for families and lead to further examinations, increasing both costs and resource utilization. Neuroimaging in pediatric patients should only be recommended by specialists experienced in pediatric headaches.

11.2 Neuroimaging in Pediatric and Adolescent Primary Headache

11.2.1 Migraine and Tension-Type Headache

In children and adolescents, the most common primary headaches are migraines and tension-type headaches [2]. According to the ICHD-3, diagnosis is based on clinical and historical criteria. Differentiating the type of headache that affects the child can be a challenge. Pediatric migraines can have subtle and less clearly defined characteristics than adults, particularly in younger children. Additionally, migraine attacks in children often last less than 2 h. Distinguishing between migraine and tension-type headache in childhood can be challenging, as some symptoms overlap. In fact, tension-type headache can evolve into migraine and vice versa. According to the continuum model, tension-type headache and migraine are part of the same physiological spectrum. From this perspective, MRI findings are also similar in the two conditions, particularly with regard to small white matter hyperintensities [10].

The findings of brain MRI in pediatric migraine are typically normal, as migraine is a functional neurological disorder that does not have structural abnormalities. In certain situations, MRI may be utilized to rule out other causes of headache or if there are any alarming symptoms [11].

Some nonspecific findings can occasionally be observed, which may include white matter (WM) lesions (WMLs). WMLs are small hyperintense lesions that appear on T2-weighted FLAIR sequences during MRI. They are usually considered benign and do not correlate with the severity of symptoms [12].

Incidental WMLs were found in about 4–5% of pediatric patients imaged for headache, and all of the patients had primary headaches [13, 14]. Regarding the type of primary headache, WMLs are found in about 10% of pediatric patients with migraine [15]. The lower frequency of lesions in the pediatric population compared to adults could be explained by the reduced duration of the disease and by the lower incidence of migraine with aura in the populations studied [15].

It is thought that demyelination and axonal injury are the causes of these white matter hyperintensities. WMLs in children with primary headache are not indications for extensive cerebral imaging or blood tests for underlying systemic autoimmune illnesses [13].

Alterations in the white substance have been reported in pediatric migraine, even outside of the WMLs. Diffusion tensor imaging (DTI) studies have demonstrated widespread abnormalities of diffusivity indexes occurring in the WM of pediatric patients with migraine. Such abnormalities were characterized by decreased mean (MD), axial (AD), and radial (RD) diffusivity along WM tracts located in the brainstem, thalamus, and fronto-temporo-occipital lobes, bilaterally. Patients also experienced increased fractional anisotropy (FA) of the optical radiation. There was no connection between abnormalities in the WM tract and the duration and frequency of the disease [15, 16].

Numerous studies have explored migraine features derived from advanced MRI, which has expanded the scientific literature on migraine in recent years [17]. A better understanding of the pathological mechanisms of migraine can be achieved through morphological, functional, and perfusion studies of migraine patients using brain MRI. Furthermore, they are providing insight into the changes that occur in a brain that is subjected to migraine attacks, which will aid in the management of migraine patients. The majority of these studies are focused on adult populations, with only a few addressing pediatric patients.

Advanced MRI studies have shown that gray matter abnormalities are present in children with migraine, similar to those observed in adult patients. The use of advanced MRI techniques in the pediatric migraine population allows us to study these alterations at an early stage of the disease. Significant cortical changes in regions within the pain matrix may be observed in pediatric patients affected by migraine [16, 18–20].

Various structural brain changes have been revealed by studying cortical thickness (CoT) in pediatric patients with migraine [16, 18, 20]. CoT undergoes dynamic changes throughout life as a result of normal development and diseases [21]. Studies on pediatric migraine show a reduction in CoT in regions associated with pain processing, such as the insula, cingulate cortex, and prefrontal cortex. The involvement of these areas in nociceptive processing and emotional regulation of pain suggests a possible structural basis for migraine pathophysiology in children. Other regions, such as parts of the somatosensory cortex, may exhibit increased CoT. It is possible that these changes are compensatory in response to recurrent migraine attacks or altered sensory processing [16, 18–20]. Reduced CoT in specific regions has also been linked to cognitive impairments, such as difficulties with attention, memory, and executive functioning, which are sometimes observed in pediatric migraine sufferers [18]. Increased CoT in the pars opercularis of the inferior frontal gyrus was observed in patients who had nausea and/or vomiting during headache attacks [18].

Gray matter changes also appear to be related to age and sex. CoT abnormalities are more pronounced in older adolescents (>12 years) when compared to those younger than 12 years. This finding may reflect a structural–functional imbalance in the "developmental" brain, potentially leading to altered pain perception and processing between children and adolescents. Adolescents exhibited these anomalies in regions associated with executive function and nociceptive networks compared to younger patients [18].

Gyrification has been observed to vary based on gender in pediatric age. Female patients showed a decreased local gyrification index (LGI) in the right superior, middle, and transverse temporal gyri, right postcentral gyrus, and supramarginal gyrus compared to male patients. An increased volume of these gyri may explain patient deficits in auditory stimuli processing, characterized by hypersensitivity to sound during migraine attacks, the onset of migraine attacks with auditory triggers, and the atypical sensory perception during the interictal phase [18]. Compared to healthy controls, patients demonstrated lower LGI in both the left superior parietal lobule and the left inferior parietal lobule, especially in the supramarginal gyrus [18]. The finding of an altered LGI in these areas could explain the executive function deficits found in migraine patients during both ictal and interictal phases [22]. An abnormal LGI in the superior and inferior parietal lobules may alter patients' pain sensory discrimination abilities and the complex modulatory mechanism taking part in pain processing [18].

Further modification of the pain circuit in migraine patients has been detected by functional magnetic resonance imaging studies. Distinct differences in resting-state functional connectivity across different brain regions of children and adolescents with migraine are observed in these techniques. Adolescents have been observed to have stronger resting-state functional connectivity in the cerebellar network than young adults, and young adults have stronger connectivity in the executive and sensorimotor networks [23]. The descriptions indicate changes in both intra- and internetwork connectivity in brain regions involved in multisensory processing and cognitive control of pain [24]. Connectivity within the visual and salience networks in children with migraine can be affected by age-related interaction effects. Compared to controls, prepubertal children with migraines had weaker connectivity in the lateral occipital cortex, but this connectivity increased in these children during early puberty. The evidence suggests that differences in visual network connectivity in migraine begin at an early age, with a significant increase as children enter puberty. Within the frontoparietal network, children with migraine in early puberty demonstrated stronger connectivity in the inferior frontal gyrus, whereas those in mid-late puberty showed weaker connectivity in this region compared to controls. These findings reveal that there is a significant increase in connectivity in early puberty, followed by a decline in mid-late puberty [25].

Cognitive behavioral therapy (CBT) has demonstrated the ability to modify brain connectivity in adolescents suffering from migraine. After an 8-week CBT intervention, which led to reduced headache frequency, neuroimaging studies revealed enhanced functional connectivity in key regions involved in nociceptive processing, cognitive function, and emotional regulation, particularly within the amygdala. These findings suggest that CBT can effectively modulate pain-related neural circuits, highlighting its potential in the prevention and management of migraines through targeted neuropsychological interventions [26].

The use of resting-state MRI to measure functional connectivity has yielded valuable insights into how pain circuits are affected in young migraine patients, highlighting age-related differences. Patient-specific characteristics of headache perception are explained by these variations, which are influenced by factors such as sex, age, and individual differences. In pediatric patients, there is still no understanding of how pain therapy, especially when it comes to medication overuse headaches and chronic migraine, might affect the pain matrix [25].

Cortical structural differences in pediatric migraine patients have been observed by some authors in relation to the presence of aura [27, 28]. The volume of the left fusiform gyrus is selectively increased in patients who have migraine with aura. In contrast, this structure had a decreased volume in migraine without aura. The fusiform gyrus has a functional role in high-order visual processing, which includes color and form perception and stereopsis [28]. Compared with healthy control subjects and patients without aura, patients with aura had bilateral thickening of regions in the inferior parietal lobule, as well as thinning of the right central sulcus and insula, while patients without aura had an increased cortical thickness of the left middle temporal gyrus [27]. The inferior parietal lobule is primarily responsible for controlling executive functions and attentional processing from a top–down perspective [29]. The anterior region of the insula is thought to be a pivotal point in a brain network that subordinates cognition–emotion integration [30].

Perfusion studies are part of other brain neuroimaging studies in pediatric patients who have migraine with aura.

Transient hypoperfusion has been observed on the side opposite to the aura using MR perfusion imaging techniques, such as dynamic susceptibility contrast (DSC) and arterial spin labeling (ASL). Venous dilation can be detected in hemiplegic migraines, especially when using susceptibility-weighted imaging (SWI) opposite the hemiparesis [31, 32]. Cerebral blood flow is reduced in brain regions related to aura symptoms when MRI is conducted within 14 hours of onset, and it increases if the MRI is performed 17 h or more after the onset [33].

In conclusion, children and adolescents with migraines are found to have white and gray matter abnormalities in brain areas related to nociceptive pathways [16, 18]. The conclusion was reached that migraine is not just a temporary problem, but it can have long-term effects on the development and structure of the brain. In order to fully understand how these changes change over time and their significance in the clinical course of pediatric migraine, more research is required.

11.2.2 Trigeminal Autonomic Cephalalgias

Neuroimaging data on pediatric-onset TACs is scarce. Diagnostic uncertainty and concerns about a secondary cause for the disorder often result in the use of neuroimaging. However, the few studies available in the literature show that in patients with non-alternating, localized headache, with or without TAC-specific features and in the absence of neurological signs, brain imaging was either normal or revealed non-significant abnormalities. The idea that neuroimaging should not be routinely evaluated in the diagnostic workup for TACs is supported by this. Nonetheless, given the rarity of the disorder, it is essential that patients are referred to specialized pediatric headache centers to properly assess the etiology and determine if neuroimaging, such as MRI, is warranted [34].

11.3 Neuroimaging in Pediatric and Adolescent Secondary Headaches

According to the ICHD 3, secondary headaches in pediatric age can also result from head and/or neck trauma, cranial or cervical vascular disorder, nonvascular intracranial disorder, substance use, infection, a disorder of homeostasis, facial or cervical structure, or psychiatric disorder. In this section, we will talk about the most frequent forms of secondary headache in children and adolescents,

11.3.1 Headache Attributed to Infections

Infections are frequently the cause of headaches in children, and they are not restricted to cerebral infections like meningitis or encephalitis. Headaches can be caused by significant cytokine responses triggered by systemic viral or bacterial infections. If a child has fever and headache, neuroimaging may be recommended if there are signs that suggest a possible brain infection. These symptoms include acute neurological deficits, neck stiffness, vomiting, seizures, or altered consciousness.

CT scans are especially helpful in emergency situations to identify lesions that cause intracranial hypertension, like brain abscesses. In instances of suspected meningitis, a lumbar puncture should not be postponed for imaging, as early diagnosis and treatment are crucial [35]. MRI with contrast enhancement on postcontrast sequences is a common result of meningeal inflammation in bacterial meningitis. Postcontrast enhancement can also involve cranial nerves in more severe cases. Both vasogenic and cytotoxic cerebral edema occur due to disruption of the blood–brain barrier and appear as hyperintense signals on T2-weighted and FLAIR sequences, as well as on DWI [36]. Hypointense lesions with peripheral ring enhancement on postcontrast imaging may indicate the formation of intracerebral abscesses in advanced or complicated infections. Subdural empyema, characterized by the accumulation of pus in the subdural or epidural spaces, can appear as hyperintense areas on T2-weighted images, with peripheral enhancement, and as extra-axial fluid collections showing restricted diffusion on DWI [35].

Certain neuroimaging findings may be more susceptible to certain infections. Herpes simplex virus (HSV) type 1 has a particular affinity for the temporal lobes and can cause subtle changes in the cortico-subcortical signal (Fig. 11.1). In contrast, HSV type 2 mainly affects infants, particularly newborns, with a more widespread pattern of involvement and necrotizing lesions. Varicella–zoster virus can cause acute encephalitis, but it can also cause vasculopathy, leading to arterial ischemic strokes years later. Deep brain structures are frequently affected by Epstein–Barr and cytomegalovirus, leading to swelling of the deep gray nuclei [37]. Brainstem involvement can complicate encephalitis caused by enterovirus and parvovirus, which is often paucisymptomatic, and can lead to severe or fatal outcomes [38].

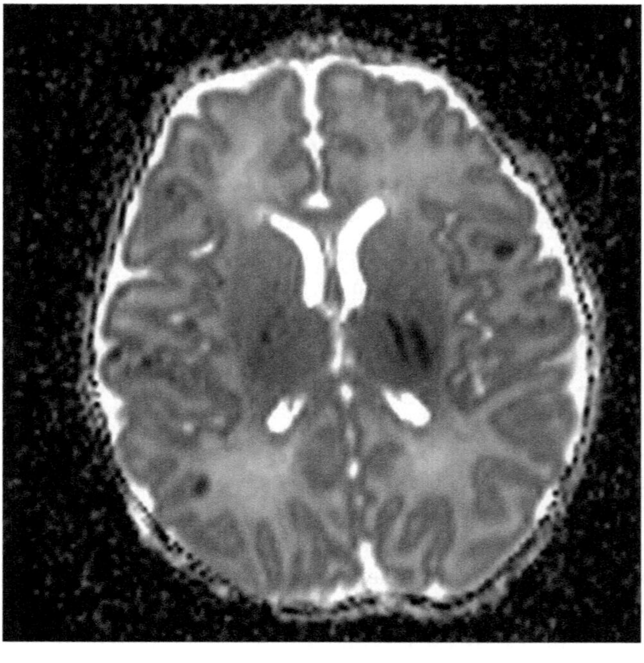

Fig. 11.1 Axial apparent diffusion coefficient (ADC) sequence. Brain MRI of an 18-day-old baby girl affected by HSV1 encephalitis

11.3.2 Headache Attributed to Intracranial Hypertension Secondary to Hydrocephalus

The accumulation of CSF within the cerebral ventricles in hydrocephalus can result in increased intracranial pressure. Hydrocephalus can result from either increased production of cerebrospinal fluid (CSF) or an obstruction in its drainage. Congenital conditions like aqueductal stenosis or Chiari malformation are the most common causes in pediatric patients. Acquired forms may arise from infectious processes (such as meningitis) or space-occupying masses, such as cerebral hemorrhages or brain tumors [39–41].

To diagnose and evaluate hydrocephalus in pediatric patients, MRI is essential, as it allows observation of structural changes in the cerebral ventricles and their effects on the surrounding brain tissue. MRI images must be evaluated accurately for treatment planning and monitoring the progression of the condition. For patients with elevated intracranial pressure and suspicion of intracranial neoplasm, pre-contrast and postcontrast MRI is the preferred method. Excessive CSF accumulation results in the dilated appearance of the cerebral ventricles, especially the lateral ventricles, third ventricle (triventricular hydrocephalus), and fourth ventricle (quadriventricular hydrocephalus). Atrophy or thinning of the surrounding cortical tissue can result from elevated pressure within the ventricles. The cerebral sulci may appear flattened or reduced because of the ventricles expanding and pressing on the cortical structures. The position and shape of the cerebellum and brainstem may be altered by hydrocephalus, which can compress adjacent brain structures like the basal nuclei. Chronic or severe hydrocephalus can lead to an expansion of the sella turcica, which can be seen as an increased volume in the cavity that houses the pituitary gland [41].

11.3.3 Headache Attributed to Chiari Malformation

Chiari malformations are frequently found during imaging performed for other reasons than headache. Additionally, given the high prevalence of primary headaches in pediatric patients, it is not uncommon to detect cerebellar tonsillar herniation in patients with primary headache, where such findings have limited clinical significance and are not considered causative of the headache [40]. The type and severity of the malformation can affect the distinctive characteristics of headache associated with Chiari malformations. The pain is usually located at the back of the neck and is characterized by a dull, pulsating, or pressing pain, with a sensation of pressure or tightness around the head. Physical activity, coughing, sneezing, or straining can exacerbate headaches. For patients who are suspected of having Chiari malformation, it is recommended to have MRI of the brain and cervical spine (Fig. 11.2). Abnormalities in CSF flow, especially at the craniocervical junction, can be detected by MRI. Neuroimaging is crucial for an accurate diagnosis and for planning

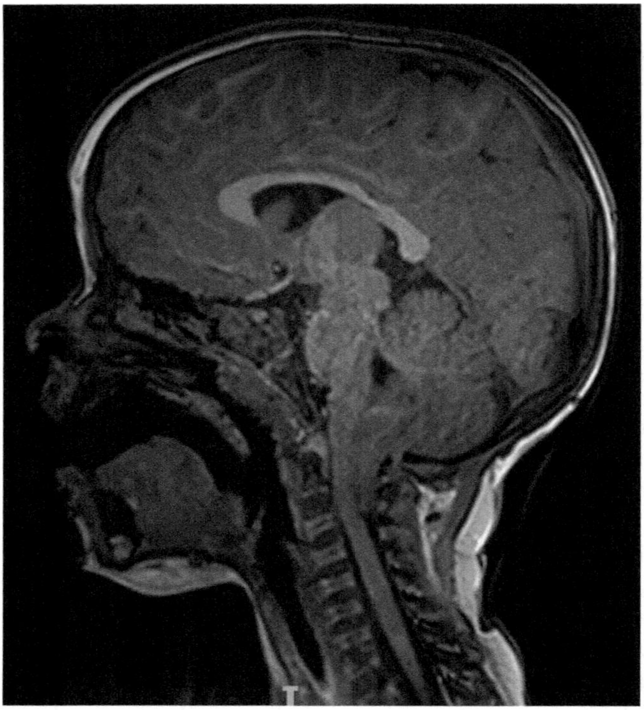

Fig. 11.2 Sagittal T1-MPRAGE sequence. MRI of a 2-year-old girl with Chiari type 1 malformation

appropriate treatment, which may range from conservative management to surgical intervention aimed at relieving spinal cord compression and restoring CSF flow [41].

11.3.4 Headache Attributed to Alterations of Cerebrospinal Fluid Pressure

Idiopathic intracranial hypertension (IIH) in pediatric patients is a condition characterized by increased CSF pressure without an obvious cause and without ventricular enlargement on neuroimaging. The most common symptom is headache, which is often described as diffuse and severe. Optic nerve compression is a common cause of visual disturbances, such as blurred vision and/or diplopia and papilledema. Females and overweight or obese children and adolescents are more susceptible to IIH. The presence of papilledema and elevated CSF pressure is necessary for a definitive diagnosis of IIH in both adults and children. Patients with elevated opening pressure and abducens nerve palsy or characteristic imaging findings may still be diagnosed with IIH despite not having papilledema [42].

On MRI, IIH may show indirect signs of increased intracranial pressure: distension of the optic nerve sheaths, optic disc swelling, flattening of the posterior aspect of the globe, retinal and choroidal folds, optic nerve tortuosity, flattening of the pituitary gland (also called "empty sella"), and minimal tonsillar herniation (usually less than 5 mm) (Fig. 11.3). Narrowing of the transverse sinus is a frequent finding linked to IH. Although some authors suggest that this stenosis could be a primary cause of IIH, there remains ongoing debate as to whether transverse sinus stenosis is a primary or secondary phenomenon [43].

Headaches caused by intracranial hypotension occur when CSF pressure within the skull drops below normal levels. A leak of CSF, which can be spontaneous or caused by trauma, surgery, or medical procedures like lumbar punctures, is the usual cause of intracranial hypotension. The headache is usually worse when standing or sitting up, but improves when lying down (orthostatic headache). Symptoms of intracranial hypotension include neck stiffness, nausea, dizziness, tinnitus, and visual disturbances [44]. Brain MRI should show some key findings, including brain sagging and dilated dural venous sinuses. A diffuse, linear dural enhancement can frequently be observed when contrast is used, which indicates irritation of the dura due to CSF volume depletion. Subdural fluid collections can take the form of subdural hygromas or subdural hematomas, which can be bilateral. Due to venous engorgement, the pituitary gland may appear swollen or enlarged, but it usually resolves once the CSF pressure is normalized [45].

A spinal MRI can help identify the location and cause of the leak. Spinal MRI is capable of detecting a CSF leak at the location of a dural tear or weakness. The spine may have fluid accumulation, and the MRI can reveal areas where CSF is leaking from the dural space. Sometimes the epidural space may show signs of abnormal fluid collection, which suggests a CSF leak. The T2-weighted images can make this fluid look hyperintense (Fig. 11.4). The dura can be enhanced during spinal MRIs with gadolinium contrast due to irritation caused by CSF loss. This can aid in confirming the diagnosis of CSF leak [45]. Detecting spinal CSF leaks could require magnetic resonance myelography (MRM). MRM can aid in localizing the site of the leak by highlighting areas where CSF is leaking from the spinal dura.

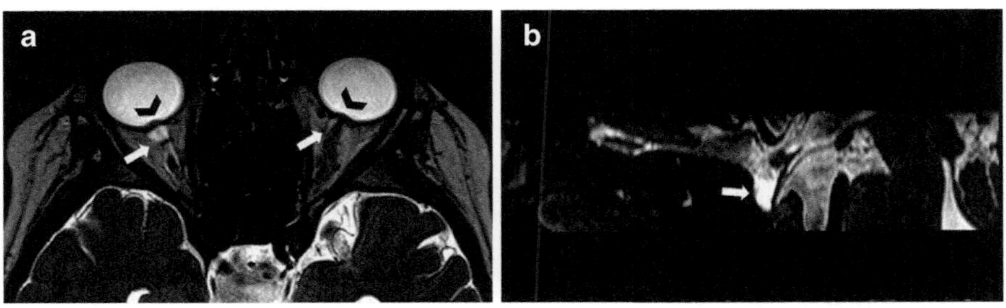

Fig. 11.3 Axial T2-weighted and sagittal T1-MPRAGE sequences. MRI of a 12-year-old boy affected by idiopathic intracranial hypertension. Bilateral prominent subarachnoid space around the optic nerves, intraocular protrusion of the optic nerves, flattening of the posterior globes, tortuous optic nerves (**a**), and partially empty sella (**b**)

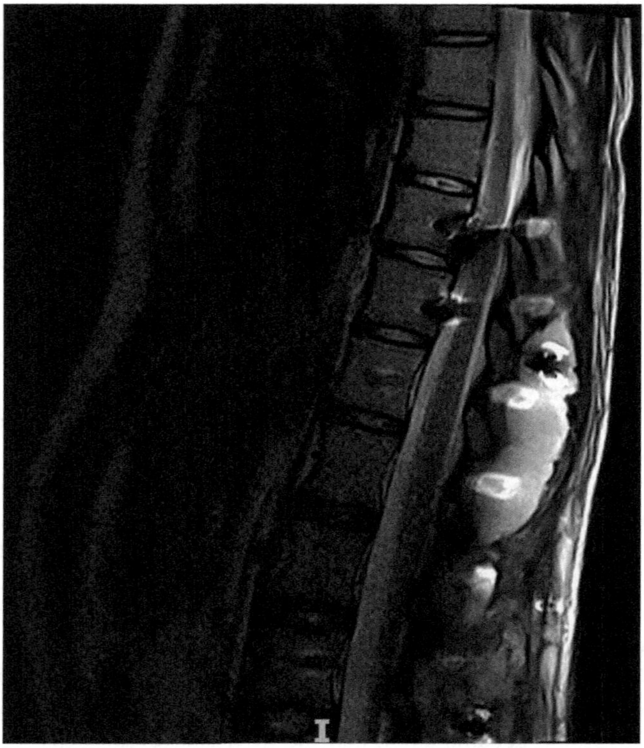

Fig. 11.4 Sagittal T2 turbo spin-echo (TSE) sequence. Dorsal spine MRI of a 17-year-old girl suffering from CSF hypotension. Imaging shows the results of surgery for scoliosis and the presence of a dorsal CSF collection

Computed tomography myelography (CTM) can be used if MRM is inconclusive. To identify any leaks along the spinal dura, CTM imaging is used after injecting contrast dye into the spinal canal. It is particularly useful for pinpointing precise leak sites, particularly when planning surgical repair [45, 46].

References

1. Stewart WF, Lipton RB, Celentano DD, Reed ML. Prevalence of migraine headache in the United States. Relation to age, income, race, and other sociodemographic factors. JAMA. 1992;267:64–9.
2. Szperka C. Headaches in children and adolescents. Continuum (Minneap Minn). 2021;27:703–31.
3. Nieswand V, Richter M, Gossrau G. Epidemiology of headache in children and adolescents – another type of Pandemia. Curr Pain Headache Rep. 2020;24:1–10.
4. Conicella E, Raucci U, Vanacore N, Vigevano F, Reale A, Pirozzi N, Valeriani M. The child with headache in a pediatric emergency department. Headache. 2008;48:1005–11.

5. Ahmed MAS, Ramseyer-Bache E, Taylor K. Yield of brain imaging among neurologically normal children with headache on wakening or headache waking the patient from sleep. Eur J Paediatr Neurol. 2018;22:797–802.
6. Bear JJ, Gelfand AA, Goadsby PJ, Bass N. Occipital headaches and neuroimaging in children. Neurology. 2017;89:469–74.
7. Raucci U, Parisi P, Ferro V, Margani E, Vanacore N, Raieli V, et al. Children under 6 years with acute headache in Pediatric emergency departments. A 2-year retrospective exploratory multicenter Italian study. Cephalalgia. 2023;43:03331024231164361.
8. Webb ME, Amoozegar F, Harris AD. Magnetic resonance imaging in pediatric migraine. Can J Neurol Sci. 2019;46:653–65.
9. Lewis DW, Ashwal S, Dahl G, Dorbad D, Hirtz D, Prensky A, Jarjour I. Practice parameter: evaluation of children and adolescents with recurrent headaches: report of the quality standards Subcommittee of the American Academy of neurology and the practice Committee of the Child Neurology Society. Neurology. 2002;59:490–8.
10. Toker RT, Mutlucan IO, Tanrıverdi C, Demir AB. MRI findings in children with migraine or tension-type headache. BMC Pediatr. 2023;23:435.
11. Camargo A, Kanekar S. Neuroimaging in pediatric headache. Neurol Clin. 2022;40:679–98.
12. Schwedt TJ, Guo Y, Rothner AD. Benign imaging abnormalities in children and adolescents with headache: CME. Headache. 2006;46:387–98.
13. Yılmaz Ü, Çeleğen M, Yılmaz TS, Gürçınar M, Ünalp A. Childhood headaches and brain magnetic resonance imaging findings. Eur J Paediatr Neurol. 2014;18:163–70.
14. Bayram E, Topcu Y, Karaoglu P, et al. Incidental white matter lesions in children presenting with headache. Headache. 2013;53:970e6.
15. Eidlitz-Markus T, Zeharia A, Haimi-Cohen Y, Konen O. MRI white matter lesions in pediatric migraine. Cephalalgia. 2013;33:906–13.
16. Messina R, Rocca MA, Colombo B, Pagani E, Falini A, Comi G, Filippi M. White matter microstructure abnormalities in pediatric migraine patients. Cephalalgia. 2015;35:1278–86.
17. Ellingson BM, Hesterman C, Johnston M, Dudeck NR, Charles AC, Villablanca JP. Advanced imaging in the evaluation of migraine headaches. NeuroImaging Clin. 2019;29:301–24.
18. Guarnera A, Bottino F, Napolitano A, Sforza G, Cappa M, Chioma L, et al. Early alterations of cortical thickness and gyrification in migraine without aura: a retrospective MRI study in pediatric patients. J Headache Pain. 2021;22:79.
19. Rocca MA, Messina R, Colombo B, et al. Structural brain MRI abnormalities in pediatric patients with migraine. J Neurol. 2014;261:350–7.
20. Frye RE, Liederman J, Malmberg B, et al. Surface area accounts for the relation of gray matter volume to reading-related skills and history of dyslexia. Cereb Cortex. 2010;20:2625–35.
21. Aldemir A, Yucel K, Güven H, et al. Structural neuroimaging findings in migraine patients with restless legs syndrome. Neuroradiology. 2020;62:1301–13.
22. Shallice T, Burgess PW. Deficits in strategy application following frontal lobe damage in man. Brain. 1991;114:727–41.
23. Colon E, Ludwick A, Wilcox SL, Youssef AM, Danehy A, Fair DA, et al. Migraine in the young brain: adolescents vs. young adults. Front Hum Neurosci. 2019;13:87.
24. Messina R, Rocca MA, Colombo B, Valsasina P, Meani A, Falini A, Filippi M. Dysregulation of multisensory processing stands out from an early stage of migraine: a study in pediatric patients. J Neurol. 2020;267:760–9.
25. Bell T, Khaira A, Stokoe M, Webb M, Noel M, Amoozegar F, Harris AD. Age-related differences in resting state functional connectivity in pediatric migraine. J Headache Pain. 2021;22:1–12.
26. Nahman-Averbuch H, Schneider VJ, Chamberlin LA, Kroon Van Diest AM, Peugh JL, Lee GR, et al. Alterations in brain function after cognitive behavioral therapy for migraine in children and adolescents. Headache. 2020;60:1165–82.
27. Messina R, Rocca MA, Colombo B, et al. Cortical abnormalities in patients with migraine: a surface-based analysis. Radiology. 2013;268:170–80.

28. Rocca MA, Messina R, Colombo B, Falini A, Comi G, Filippi M. Structural brain MRI abnormalities in pediatric patients with migraine. J Neurol. 2014;261:350–7.
29. Weidner R, Krummenacher J, Reimann B, Müller HJ, Fink GR. Sources of top-down control in visual search. J Cogn Neurosci. 2009;21:2100–13.
30. Gu X, Liu X, Van Dam NT, Hof PR, Fan J. Cognition-emotion integration in the anterior insular cortex. Cereb Cortex. 2013;23:20–7.
31. Masuzaki M, Utsunomiya H, Yasumoto S, Mitsudome A. A case of hemiplegic migraine in childhood: transient unilateral hyperperfusion revealed by perfusion MR imaging and MR angiography. Am J Neuroradiol. 2001;22:1795–7.
32. Bosemani T, Burton VJ, Felling RJ, Leigh R, Oakley C, Poretti A, Huisman TA. Pediatric hemiplegic migraine: role of multiple MRI techniques in evaluation of reversible hypoperfusion. Cephalalgia. 2014;34:311–5.
33. Boulouis G, Shotar E, Dangouloff-Ros V, Grévent D, Calmon R, Brunelle F, et al. Magnetic resonance imaging arterial-spin-labelling perfusion alterations in childhood migraine with atypical aura: a case–control study. Dev Med Child Neurol. 2016;58:965–9.
34. Borrelli A, Valeriani M, Monte G, Ursitti F, Proietti Checchi M, Tarantino S, et al. Cluster headache: diagnosis, management, and treatment in pediatric headache. J Clin Med. 2024;13:1203.
35. Hayes LL, Palasis S, Bartel TB, Booth TN, Iyer RS, Jones JY, et al. ACR appropriateness criteria® Headache–Child. J Am Coll Radiol. 2018;15:S78–90.
36. Bykowski J, Kruk P, Gold JJ, Glaser CA, Sheriff H, Crawford JR. Acute pediatric encephalitis neuroimaging: single-institution series as part of the California encephalitis project. Pediatr Neurol. 2015;52:606–14.
37. Jayaraman K, Rangasami R, Chandrasekharan A. Magnetic resonance imaging findings in viral encephalitis: a pictorial essay. J Neurosci Rural Pract. 2018;9:556.
38. Messacar K, Spence-Davizon E, Osborne C, Press C, Schreiner TL, Martin J, et al. Clinical characteristics of enterovirus A71 neurological disease during an outbreak in children in Colorado, USA, in 2018: an observational cohort study. Lancet Infect Dis. 2020;20:230–9.
39. Kahle KT, Kulkarni AV, Limbrick DD, Warf BC. Hydrocephalus in children. Lancet. 2016;387:788–99.
40. Victorio MC, Khoury CK. Headache and Chiari I malformation in children and adolescents. Semin Pediatr Neurol. 2016;23:35–9.
41. Toldo I, Tangari M, Mardari R, Perissinotto E, Sartori S, Gatta M, et al. Headache in children with Chiari I malformation. Headache. 2014;54:899–908.
42. Friedman DI, Liu GT, Digre KB. Revised diagnostic criteria for the pseudotumor cerebri syndrome in adults and children. Neurology. 2013;81:1159–65.
43. Görkem SB, Doganay S, Canpolat M, et al. MR imaging findings in children with pseudotumor cerebri and comparison with healthy controls. Childs Nerv Syst. 2015;31:373–80.
44. Tay ASMS, Maya MM, Schievink WI. Spontaneous intracranial hypotension mimicking iatrogenic spinal cerebrospinal fluid leaks. Headache. 2024; https://doi.org/10.1111/head.14826.
45. Algin O, Taskapilioglu O, Zan E, Hakyemez B, Karaoglanoglu M. Detection of CSF leaks with magnetic resonance imaging in intracranial hypotension syndrome. J Neuroradiol. 2011;38:175–7.
46. Madhavan AA, Brinjikji W, Cutsforth-Gregory JK, Amrhein TJ, Kranz PG, Benson JC, et al. Myelographic techniques for the localization of CSF-venous fistulas: updates in 2024. Am J Neuroradiol. 2024;45:1403–12.

Chapter 12
Future Directions in Neuroimaging of Headache Disorders

Igor Petrušić

12.1 Future Directions in Neuroimaging of Headache Disorders in Clinical Practice

Imaging patients with headache poses significant challenges for clinicians, as they have to balance the need for accurate diagnosis against the potential for unnecessary procedures. Despite extensive guidelines and research underscoring the lack of cost-effectiveness for imaging patients who suffer from headache without red flags, neuroimaging continues to rise [1, 2]. This trend is driven by several factors, including the fear of overlooking a clinically significant lesion, ingrained habitual practices, patient demands, concerns about professional reputation, and regulatory penalties [2].

Since potential red flags significantly influence decision-making, improved evidence on which red flags should influence neuroimaging decisions is desperately needed. This information would allow future guidelines to be more precise in describing the specific clinical scenarios that should prompt neuroimaging [3]. One of the critical issues in this context is the so-called defensive medicine approach, where clinicians order imaging studies primarily to avoid legal repercussions rather than based on clinical necessity. This practice not only increases healthcare costs but also exposes patients to unnecessary procedures, which can lead to anxiety, incidental findings, and further unwarranted interventions [4]. The societal impact of this practice is significant, highlighting the need for a shift in how imaging decisions are made. Regulatory and legislative reforms are essential to fostering an environment where clinicians can follow evidence-based guidelines without the fear of professional sanctions. Such reforms could include the implementation of clearer

---

I. Petrušić (✉)
Laboratory for Advanced Analysis of Neuroimages, Faculty of Physical Chemistry, University of Belgrade, Belgrade, Serbia

I. Petrušić, Y. Wang (eds.), *Neuroimaging of Headache Disorders*, Headache, https://doi.org/10.1007/978-3-031-85402-6_12

legal protections for clinicians who adhere to established guidelines, as well as the promotion of educational initiatives that emphasize the importance of guideline-based care.

On the other hand, the value of negative imaging findings needs to be better appreciated within the healthcare community [2]. While often seen as noncontributory, these findings can play a crucial role in alleviating patient anxiety, confirming the absence of serious pathology, and guiding more appropriate and cost-effective management strategies. Furthermore, understanding the broader implications of negative results can help clinicians make more informed decisions about when imaging is truly warranted. Moreover, the integration of clinical decision support tools and artificial intelligence (AI) into routine practice offers a promising solution to these challenges [5]. These technologies can provide evidence-based recommendations tailored to individual patients, helping clinicians navigate the complexities of headache management with greater confidence. Moreover, the implementation of headache classification through artificial neural networks is a powerful tool that reduces the time to obtain accurate, reliable, and timely clinical diagnoses. By incorporating data from large patient cohorts and continuously updating algorithms with the latest research, these tools can improve diagnostic accuracy, reduce unnecessary imaging, and ultimately enhance patient outcomes [6]. Furthermore, the development of headache-specified magnetic resonance imaging (MRI) protocols, which include advanced imaging modalities, and the adoption of advanced machine learning techniques in imaging analysis could lead to more precise identification of subtle abnormalities that might be missed by traditional methods [7]. Furthermore developing a huge amount of MRI data adequately labeled with headache diagnosis and accompanied with specific metadata information, which is analyzed using AI, will allow better AI solutions for this purpose [8]. Besides, there are already machine learning techniques able to analyze imaging data from MRI and suggest migraine diagnosis or its classification [9–11]. In the next few years, such techniques will become more and more accurate and available so that migraine diagnosis will not be just clinical but even supported by neuroimaging data. This could help bridge the gap between the need for a thorough investigation and the avoidance of unnecessary imaging, ensuring that only those patients who truly require neuroimaging undergo the procedure and benefit from additional information necessary for receiving optimal treatment and prediction of disease outcome.

In summary, addressing the challenges of imaging in headache management requires a multifaceted approach that includes regulatory reform, education, a greater appreciation of the value of negative findings, and the integration of advanced decision-support technologies, as well as the implementation of advanced neuroimaging modalities in the imaging of headache. This allows a personalized imaging and a shorter path to adequate therapy and better evaluation of disease evolution and treatment outcome. By aligning clinical practice with evidence-based guidelines and leveraging the power of AI, the medical community can improve the quality and cost-efficiency of headache care, benefiting both patients and healthcare systems.

12.2 Future Directions in Neuroimaging of Headache Disorders in Research Practice

Primary headache disorders are highly prevalent and very disabling neurological disorders, yet comprehensive pathological substrate and pathomechanisms remain under investigation, and their diagnoses are solely based on clinical criteria. A shortcoming of these criteria is that they do not fully capture the heterogeneity of headache disorders and their subtypes, such as migraine spectrum of abundant manifestations, including the underlying genetic and neurobiological factors [12]. In the era of the advancement of neuroimaging modalities blended with new AI-driven technologies, the neurological and neuroimaging communities are called to focus on finding neuroimaging biomarkers for headache disorders and their subtypes to improve disease characterization and identify novel drug targets. Therefore, emerging neuroimaging techniques and future directions of headache research and treatment should consider radiomics AI-driven approach including multimodal neuroimaging, genetic and serum biomarkers, as well as deep phenotyping biomarkers to facilitate personalized medicine for headache treatment and revise the headache diagnostic criteria to reflect disease burden and prognosis [5]. Moreover, deep learning methods can automatically detect aberrations in the brain regions associated with different headache types, which uncovers the great potential of deep learning methods for the classification and automatic extraction of brain imaging-based biomarkers for headache disorders and their subtypes [10, 13]. In addition, longitudinal data will also give a better picture of disease progression [14]. Therefore, it is vastly important to use machine learning and big data approaches and encourage data-sharing initiatives among headache and neuroimaging researchers allowing publicly available neuroimaging datasets, which may help uncover hidden relationships in complex headache disorders and lead to precision medicine providing a more accurate diagnosis, appropriate treatment, and timely prevention strategies by considering patients' neuroimaging blueprint [15, 16]. However, this cannot be realized without integrating clinical and radiomics data in a data-sharing unified, secure, and decentralized framework that achieves large sample sizes and a great level of data harmonization. Furthermore, there is a great need for the formation of an expert consortium that will recommend best practices in research related to neuroimaging of headache disorders, focusing on reducing sources of heterogeneity in the broader field of functional MRI, including the variability in potential analysis methods for functional MRI datasets, and the heterogeneity in the selection of healthy controls and patients [17, 18]. All these approaches may lead to classification redefinitions of headache disorders (Fig. 12.1).

Numerous headache studies used advanced neuroimaging techniques to explore pathophysiology and differentiate primary headache disorders, as well as to predict disease evolution and response to therapy [9–11, 13, 19–27]. However, emerging neuroimaging modalities could provide new avenues in headache research (Fig. 12.2). For example, conventional functional MRI (fMRI) detects brain activity indirectly by measuring localized changes in regional blood flow, oxygenation, and

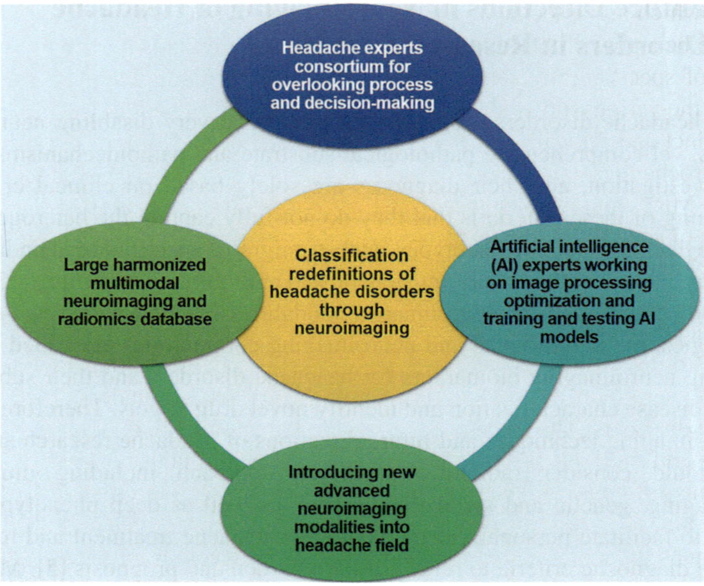

Fig. 12.1 Framework for achieving classification redefinitions of headache disorders through neuroimaging

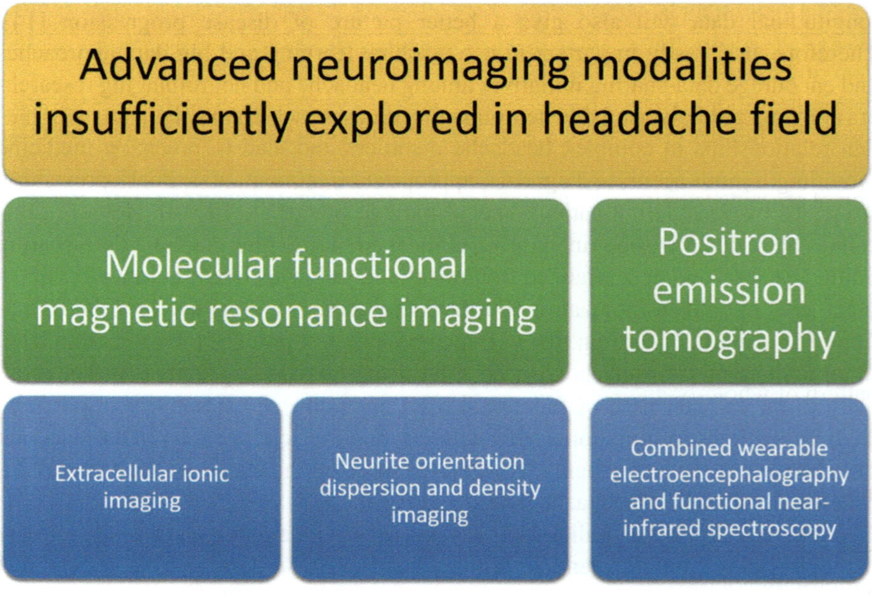

Fig. 12.2 Types of advanced neuroimaging modalities that are insufficiently explored in the headache field

volume, which are associated with neural activity. While hemodynamic fMRI has proven to be a powerful tool for analyzing brain function, it is inherently limited by its lack of specificity. In other words, the fMRI technique does not differentiate between the various molecules and cell types involved in neural processing, which play distinct and critical roles in brain function. Molecular fMRI, which can measure neurochemical signaling in the brain through the use of neurotransmitter-sensitive MRI contrast agents, addresses this limitation by permitting MRI-based detection of specific molecular processes in brain tissue [28–30]. Therefore, molecular fMRI expands the capabilities of traditional fMRI by targeting particular neurotransmitters, receptors, and other molecular markers crucial to neural communication and plasticity [31]. For example, molecular fMRI techniques can be designed to detect the presence and activity of specific neurotransmitters, such as dopamine, serotonin, or glutamate [32], which are vital to understanding various headache disorders. This capability allows investigators to map brain activity more precisely and investigate the underlying molecular mechanisms of brain dysfunction during different mental states or in response to stimuli throughout the ictal and interictal phases in different headache disorders. Moreover, molecular fMRI opens new avenues for studying the dynamic interplay between different cell types, such as neurons and glial cells, in real time [28]. Additionally, molecular fMRI could facilitate the monitoring of treatment effects at a molecular level, offering a powerful tool for evaluating the efficacy of pharmacological interventions [33]. Moreover, compared with positron emission tomography (PET) in combination with different specific radioligands, molecular fMRI affords poorer sensitivity but more versatile molecular detection mechanisms, higher spatial and temporal resolution, and logistical advantages because it does not rely on radioactive tracers [28]. In addition, researchers should exploit the next-generation MRI scanner designed for ultra-high-resolution human brain imaging at 7 Tesla with hardware advances that enable the assessment of cortical layer functional activity [34]. Although there is still a limitation of crossing the blood–brain barrier for newly developed contrast agents, focused transcranial ultrasound has emerged as a powerful technique for transient, spatially localized disruption of the blood–brain barrier, followed by an introduction of agents via the vasculature [35]. Additionally, combination approaches such as conventional or molecular fMRI and EEG, accompanied by increasingly sophisticated analytical techniques, can provide a unified perspective on the spatial and temporal pattern of whole-brain neural activity during ictal phases of different types of headache disorders.

Furthermore, extracellular calcium imaging optimized for MRI in humans could also provide new markers for the differentiation of headache disorders and their subtypes and help in understanding complex primary and secondary headache pathophysiologies, as well as in tracking therapy response. Since ionic fluctuations are closely coupled to neural activity and ions play a variety of neuromodulatory roles in the central nervous system [36], monitoring interstitial calcium concentrations in the brain can thus provide specific information about modulatory functions in headache patients who receive prophylactic treatment, potentially with greater spatiotemporal specificity than hemodynamic fMRI [29]. Although extracellular calcium imaging optimization for MRI in humans is still undergoing research, advances in molecular engineering, MRI physics, and contrast agent development could bring extracellular calcium imaging to clinical MRI within the next decade. It is also of interest to target MRI sensors toward neurochemicals that have not yet been addressed, such as neuropeptides or K+ ions [37].

Although several diffusion tensor imaging studies in the headache field showed compromised integrity of white matter microstructure and even disturbances in the glymphatic system in various headache disorders [38–44], findings lack validation and pathological specificity. A recently developed multicompartment diffusion imaging model (neurite orientation dispersion and density imaging—NODDI) may provide better insight into gray and white matter microstructure, addressing the current limitation of conventional diffusion tensor imaging [45, 46].

In addition, recent advances in PET hardware and tracer development have expanded the range of relevant biological targets in headache research, enabling focused assessment of neuroinflammation, synaptic function, and mitochondrial function [47]. For example, [18F]BCPP-EF, a PET tracer that binds to mitochondrial electron transport chain complex I, could have great potential to improve our understanding of mitochondrial dysfunction in migraine [48]. Among PET targets in headache research, the synaptic vesicle glycoprotein 2A (SV2A), a transmembrane protein of synaptic vesicles present in all synaptic terminals irrespective of neurotransmitter content, should also be listed because changes in PET measures of synaptic density are thought to reflect changes in the number of dendritic spines and thus a change in synapse health [49].

Another promising approach is to combine wearable brain electroencephalography and functional near-infrared spectroscopy for monitoring the ictal phase of various headache disorders, which could help in the early detection of headache attacks and provide new information regarding the different headache pathophysiologies [50]. Additionally, future studies that combine brain stimulation approaches with fMRI, EEG, and computational modeling will be useful in bridging the gap in understanding how different brain states influence the effectiveness of brain stimulation on neurophysiological processes and behavior in headache patients.

In any case, neuroimaging has the potential to be key in personalizing therapies, particularly neuromodulatory interventions. Finally, multidisciplinary teams that combine clinical and technological expertise are needed to apply these emerging neuroimaging technologies to answer headache-related questions and hopefully lead to translation to clinical care and improve patient lives and outcomes. In other words, the headache research field needs more engineers, and neuroscientists and clinicians have to make more effort to develop common ground with relevant stakeholders [5].

References

1. Do TP, Remmers A, Schytz HW, et al. Red and orange flags for secondary headaches in clinical practice. Neurology. 2019;92:134–44.
2. Jordan JE, Flanders AE. Headache and neuroimaging: why we continue to do it. AJNR Am J Neuroradiol. 2020;41:1149–55.
3. Reynolds EL, Burke JF, Evans L, et al. Headache neuroimaging: a survey of current practice, barriers, and facilitators to optimal use. Headache. 2022;62:36–56.
4. Fakes K. Patient experiences and anxiety related to medical imaging: challenges and potential solutions. J Med Radiat Sci. 2024;71:3–6.
5. Petrušić I, Ha W-S, Labastida-Ramirez A, et al. Influence of next-generation artificial intelligence on headache research, diagnosis and treatment: the junior editorial board members' vision—part 1. J Headache Pain. 2024;25:151.
6. Alowais SA, Alghamdi SS, Alsuhebany N, et al. Revolutionizing healthcare: the role of artificial intelligence in clinical practice. BMC Med Educ. 2023;23:689.
7. Mitrovic K, Savic AM, Radojicic A, et al. Machine learning approach for migraine aura complexity score prediction based on magnetic resonance imaging data. J Headache Pain. 2023;24:169.
8. Torrente A, Maccora S, Prinzi F, et al. The clinical relevance of artificial intelligence in migraine. Brain Sci. 2024;14:85.
9. Chong CD, Gaw N, Fu Y, et al. Migraine classification using magnetic resonance imaging resting-state functional connectivity data. Cephalalgia. 2017;37:828–44.
10. Siddiquee MMR, Shah J, Chong C, et al. Headache classification and automatic biomarker extraction from structural MRIs using deep learning. Brain Commun. 2022;5:fcac311.
11. Mitrovic K, Petrusic I, Radojicic A, et al. Migraine with aura detection and subtype classification using machine learning algorithms and morphometric magnetic resonance imaging data. Front Neurol. 2023;14:1106612.
12. Ashina M, Terwindt GM, Al-Karagholi MA-M, et al. Migraine: disease characterisation, biomarkers, and precision medicine. Lancet. 2021;397:1496–504.
13. Messina R, Sudre CH, Wei DY, et al. Biomarkers of migraine and cluster headache: differences and similarities. Ann Neurol. 2023;93:729–42.
14. Lin Y-K, Tsai C-L, Lin G-Y, et al. Pathophysiology of chronic migraine: insights from recent neuroimaging research. Curr Pain Headache Rep. 2022;26:843–54.
15. Davatzikos C. Machine learning in neuroimaging: Progress and challenges. NeuroImage. 2019;197:652–6.
16. Hranilovich JA, Legget KT, Dodd KC, et al. Functional magnetic resonance imaging of headache: issues, best-practices, and new directions, a narrative review. Headache. 2023;63:309–21.
17. Li X, Esper NB, Ai L, et al. Moving beyond processing- and analysis-related variation in restingstate functional brain imaging. Nat Hum Behav. 2024;8:2003–2017.
18. Coppola G, Renzo AD, Parisi V, et al. Comment on "lack of reproducibility of resting-state functional MRI findings in migraine with aura". Cephalalgia. 2024;44:3331024231225186.
19. Tu Y, Zeng F, Lan L, et al. An fMRI-based neural marker for migraine without aura. Neurology. 2020;94:e741–51.
20. Marino S, Jassar H, Kim DJ, et al. Classifying migraine using PET compressive big data analytics of brain's mu-opioid and D2/D3 dopamine neurotransmission. Front Pharmacol. 2023;14:1173596.
21. Hsiao F-J, Chen W-T, Pan L-LH, et al. Resting-state magnetoencephalographic oscillatory connectivity to identify patients with chronic migraine using machine learning. J Headache Pain. 2022;23:130.
22. Mu J, Chen T, Quan S, et al. Neuroimaging features of whole-brain functional connectivity predict attack frequency of migraine. Hum Brain Mapp. 2020;41:984–93.

23. Chong CD, Berisha V, Ross K, et al. Distinguishing persistent post-traumatic headache from migraine: classification based on clinical symptoms and brain structural MRI data. Cephalalgia. 2021;41:943–55.
24. Wei HL, Yang WJ, Zhou GP, et al. Altered static functional network connectivity predicts the efficacy of non-steroidal anti-inflammatory drugs in migraineurs without aura. Front Mol Neurosci. 2022;15:956797.
25. Wang Y, Wang Y, Bu L, et al. Functional connectivity features of resting-state functional magnetic resonance imaging may distinguish migraine from tension-type headache. Front Neurosci. 2022;16:851111.
26. Yang XJ, Liu L, Xu ZL, et al. Baseline brain Gray matter volume as a predictor of acupuncture outcome in treating migraine. Front Neurol. 2020;11:111.
27. Tso AR, Brudfors M, Danno D, et al. Machine phenotyping of cluster headache and its response to verapamil. Brain. 2021;144:655–64.
28. Wei H, Frey AM, Jasanoff A. Molecular fMRI of neurochemical signaling. J Neurosci Methods. 2021;364:109372.
29. Bartelle BB, Barandov A, Jasanoff A. Molecular fMRI. J Neurosci. 2016;36:4139–48.
30. Angelovski G, Toth E. Strategies for sensing neurotransmitters with responsive MRI contrast agents. Chem Soc Rev. 2017;46:324–36.
31. Koolschijn RS, Clarke WT, Ip IB, et al. Event-related functional magnetic resonance spectroscopy. NeuroImage. 2023;276:120194.
32. Brustad EM, Lelyveld VS, Snow CD, et al. Structure-guided directed evolution of highly selective p450-based magnetic resonance imaging sensors for dopamine and serotonin. J Mol Biol. 2012;422:245–62.
33. Ghosh S, Harvey P, Simon JC, et al. Probing the brain with molecular fMRI. Curr Opin Neurobiol. 2018;50:201–10.
34. Feinberg DA, Beckett A, Vu AT, et al. Next-generation MRI scanner designed for ultra-high-resolution human brain imaging at 7 Tesla. Nat Methods. 2023;20:2048–57.
35. Poon C, McMahon D, Hynynen K. Noninvasive and targeted delivery of therapeutics to the brain using focused ultrasound. Neuropharmacology. 2017;120:20–37.
36. Rasmussen R, O'Donnell J, Ding F, et al. Interstitial ions: a key regulator of state-dependent neural activity? Prog Neurobiol. 2020;193:101802.
37. Miller ADC, Ozbakir HF, Mukherjee A. Calcium-responsive contrast agents for functional magnetic resonance imaging. Chem Phys Rev. 2021;2:021301.
38. Petrušić I, Daković M, Kačar K, et al. Migraine with aura and white matter tract changes. Acta Neurol Belg. 2018;118:485–91.
39. Mei Y, Wang W, Qiu D, et al. Micro-structural white matter abnormalities in new daily persistent headache: a DTI study using TBSS analysis. J Headache Pain. 2023;24:80.
40. Wu C-H, Chang F-C, Wang Y-F, et al. Impaired glymphatic and meningeal lymphatic functions in patients with chronic migraine. Ann Neurol. 2024;95:583–95.
41. Király A, Szabó N, Párdutz Á, et al. Macro- and microstructural alterations of the subcortical structures in episodic cluster headache. Cephalalgia. 2018;38:662–73.
42. Chong CD, Peplinski J, Berisha V, et al. Differences in fibertract profiles between patients with migraine and those with persistent post-traumatic headache. Cephalalgia. 2019;39:1121–33.
43. Yang H-C, Nguyen T, Naugle KM et al. White matter microstructural changes in post-traumatic headache: a diffusion tensor imaging (DTI) study. medRxiv [Preprint]; 2024. https://doi.org/10.1101/2024.08.05.24310944
44. Vittorini MG, Sahin A, Trojan A, et al. The glymphatic system in migraine and other headaches. J Headache Pain. 2024;25:34.
45. Kraguljac NV, Guerreri M, Strickland MJ, et al. Neurite orientation dispersion and density imaging in psychiatric disorders: a systematic literature review and a technical note. Biol Psychiatry Glob Open Sci. 2023;3:10–21.
46. Li Z, Mei Y, Wang W, et al. White matter and cortical gray matter microstructural abnormalities in new daily persistent headache: a NODDI study. J Headache Pain. 2024;25:110.

47. Hadjikhani N, Albrecht DS, Mainero C, et al. Extra-axial inflammatory signal in parameninges in migraine with visual aura. Ann Neurol. 2020;87:939–49.
48. Kato Y, Yokokura M, Iwabuchi T, et al. Lower availability of mitochondrial complex I in anterior cingulate cortex in autism: a positron emission tomography study. Am J Psychiatry. 2023;180:277–84.
49. Rossi R, Arjmand S, Bærentzen SL, et al. Synaptic vesicle glycoprotein 2A: features and functions. Front Neurosci. 2022;16:864514.
50. Li B, Li M, Xia J, et al. Hybrid integrated wearable patch for brain EEG-fNIRS monitoring. Sensors (Basel). 2024;24:4847.

GPSR Compliance

The European Union's (EU) General Product Safety Regulation (GPSR) is a set of rules that requires consumer products to be safe and our obligations to ensure this.

If you have any concerns about our products, you can contact us on ProductSafety@springernature.com

In case Publisher is established outside the EU, the EU authorized representative is:

Springer Nature Customer Service Center GmbH
Europaplatz 3
69115 Heidelberg, Germany

Batch number: 10732044

Printed by Printforce, the Netherlands